Fundamentals of Sports Injury Management

SECOND EDITION

MARCIA K. ANDERSON, PhD, LATC
Professor and Director, Athletic Training Program
Department of Movement Arts, Health Promotion, Leisure Studies
Bridgewater State College
Bridgewater, Massachusetts

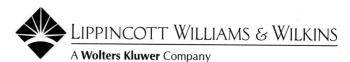

LIPPINCOTT WILLIAMS & WILKINS
A **Wolters Kluwer** Company

Philadelphia · Baltimore · New York · London
Buenos Aires · Hong Kong · Sydney · Tokyo

Editor: Pete Darcy
Managing Editor: Linda Napora
Marketing Manager: Christen DeMarco
Production Editor: Christina Remsberg
Compositor: In House Composition
Printer: Quebecor World

351 West Camden Street
Baltimore, Maryland 21201-2436 USA

530 Walnut Street
Philadelphia, PA 19106

Printed in the United States of America

First Edition, 1997

Library of Congress Cataloging-in-Publication Data

Anderson, Marcia K.

    Fundamentals of sports injury management/Marcia K. Anderson.–2nd ed.

    p.; cm.

    Includes bibliographical references and index.

    ISBN 0-7817-3272-7

    1. Sports injuries. I. Title

    [DNLM: 1. Athletic Injuries. 2. Sports Medicine. QT 261 A548f2002]

    RD97 .A527 2002

    617.1'027--dc21

                           2002072941

To purchase additional copies of this book, call our customer service department at **(800) 638-3030** or fax orders to **(301) 824-7390**. International customers should call **(301) 714-2324**.

Visit Lippincott Williams & Wilkins on the Internet: http://www.LWW.com. Lippincott Williams & Wilkins customer service representatives are available from 8:30 am to 6:00 pm, EST.

02 03 04 05
1 2 3 4 5 6 7 8 9 10

Fundamentals of
Sports Injury Management

SECOND EDITION

It was difficult to prepare the second edition of *Fundamentals in Sports Injury Management*. This text continues our commitment to provide a comprehensive, but challenging content in a "user-friendly" format that facilitates student learning and retention. In addition, the content addresses the professionals who provide immediate first aid care for physically active individuals across the lifespan. Following the publication of the second edition of *Sports Injury Management*, a more advanced text for the athletic training student, it was determined that the second edition of *Fundamentals* should be aimed at providing basic sports injury care guidelines for those individuals who may not have immediate access to a certified athletic trainer, but who are expected to provide initial care to an injured athlete. These individuals may include coaches, exercise science/health fitness professionals, physical education instructors, supervisors in recreational sports programs, and directors in YMCA or other community sports-related programs. *Fundamentals* can be used in an introductory athletic training class or sports first aid class. Because of the content, it is advisable that the student complete parallel coursework and receive current certification in cardiopulmonary resuscitation and airway management.

NEW FEATURES IN THIS EDITION

Fundamentals in Sports Injury Management has undergone extensive review from certified athletic trainers, leading to a more reader-friendly text that includes pertinent information that can be easily taught in a one-semester course. Expanded illustrations of anatomy, critical information boxes, tables, and field strategies highlight each chapter to enhance the learning process. Some of the many highlighted changes and additions are:

- Highlighted medical terms are defined within the text and in the glossary.
- Wherever possible, each condition has its own header and is defined or explained, signs and symptoms are identified, and general management protocols are provided. This helps clarify and highlight the importance of each condition.
- Chapter 1, *Introduction to Sports Injury Management*, introduces the student to the primary sports medicine team, its responsibilities, and the legal considerations in providing basic sports injury care to athletes.
- Chapter 2, *Emergency Procedures*, explains how to develop an emergency plan for a sports facility and discusses emergency conditions and their management. New to this edition is information on anaphylaxis and exercising in thunderstorms. Finally, the student is introduced to the HOPS format to assess sports-related injuries.
- Chapter 3, *The Sports Injury Process*, describes mechanisms of injury and details the three phases of the healing process.
- Chapter 4, *Wound Care*, introduces the student to the various types of body tissues that can be injured. Anatomical considerations are explained, injury classifications are provided where appropriate, and new information is presented on open and closed soft tissue wound care, including current universal precautions and infection control standards. General principles for moving an injured athlete are then explained followed by a discussion on using cold versus heat in the process of injury treatment.
- Chapters 5–12, expanded joint chapters, cover specific injuries or conditions organized by body regions. Organization of the chapters has been changed to reflect the flow through the body, beginning at the head and face; moving down the spine, thorax, and abdomen; then moving to the shoulder, elbow, wrist, and hand; and finally moving to the hip, knee, lower leg, ankle, and foot.
  - Each chapter opens with an expanded coverage of joint anatomy with detailed illustrations. Joint motions are demonstrated and the primary muscles responsible for the motions are listed. Injury prevention strategies including protective equipment are then discussed.
  - Chapters are organized to provide information on contusions, sprains, strains, overuse conditions, and fractures. Each condition is defined, signs and symptoms are identified, and management protocols are provided.
  - Assessment begins with a summary box detailing conditions or signs and symptoms that warrant immediate transportation to the nearest medical facility. Following the HOPS format, the student is then taken through a basic assessment to determine whether the injured individual should be referred to a physician for further care, or whether the individual can be treated on-site.
  - Some of the new sections discussed in the joint chapters include a comparison of the different classifications of cerebral concussions, standard criteria for return to competition after a head injury, posttraumatic headaches, postconcussion syndrome, injuries to the spinal cord and brachial plexus, cardiac tamponade, sudden death, bursitis

of the shoulder, thoracic outlet compression syndrome, slipped capital femoral epiphyseal fracture of the hip, testicular cancer, and knee dislocations.

- Chapter 13, *Respiratory Tract Conditions*, discusses common upper and lower respiratory conditions and their management, including bronchitis, bronchial asthma, and exercise-induced bronchospasm.
- Chapter 14, *Gastrointestinal Conditions*, includes information on gastroesophageal reflux, gastritis, gastroenteritis, indigestion, diarrhea, constipation, and irritable bowel syndrome.
- Chapter 15, *The Diabetic Athlete*, discusses the physiologic basis of diabetes, explains the two most common types of diabetes mellitus and complications that may arise from the disease, and provides exercise recommendations.

PEDAGOGICAL FEATURES

As an educator, I have highlighted and summarized information in the text by incorporating several pedagogical features to enhance the text's usefulness as a teaching tool. These features are designed to increase readability and retention of relevant and critical information. These in-text features include:

Learning Outcomes

Each chapter opens with a series of learning outcomes, the most important concepts in the chapter that the student should focus on during reading.

Medical Terminology

New and difficult medical terminology is bolded and defined in the text and can be found in the glossary.

Critical Information Boxes

A unique feature of this edition is the use of boxes interspersed throughout each chapter to list or summarize critical information that supplements the material in the text. In the joint chapters, for example, these boxes summarize signs and symptoms of specific conditions.

Tables

Several chapters have tables that expand upon pertinent information discussed in the text. This allows a large amount of knowledge to be organized in an easy-to-read summary of information.

Field Strategies

Another unique feature of this book is the use of Field Strategies to clinically apply cognitive knowledge. In the joint chapters, for example, the student can move step by step through a specific condition, learning how to provide immediate management for the injury.

Art and Photography Program

Art plays a major role in facilitating the learning process for visual learners. The editor and I worked hard to incorporate appropriate, detailed illustrations and photographs to supplement material presented in the text. The medical illustrator worked tirelessly to provide realistic and accurate figures that depict anatomical structures; innovative approaches illustrate injury mechanisms.

Summary

Each chapter has a summary of key concepts discussed in the text. The main points are noted here; the summary in no way denotes all of the critical information covered in the chapter.

References

Any valuable teaching tool must include a listing of cited references used to gather information for the text. I have tried to limit the references to a 5-year period, except where the reference is considered to be the original ground-breaking research. With an accurate bibliography, the instructor or student has resources to pursue topics for which additional information might be needed.

Glossary and Index

At the end of the book, the student will find an extensive glossary of terms from highlighted words in the individual chapters. Furthermore, the comprehensive index contains cross-referencing information to locate specific information within the text.

I hope the new format and level of the material is well received by my colleagues. It is difficult to please all educators who are looking for that one book that can meet all their needs. The goal of the second edition of *Fundamentals of Sports Injury Management* is to be that book. I look forward to your comments.

Marcia K. Anderson
Bridgewater, Massachusetts

I would like to thank several of my colleagues, many of whom assisted in the development of the text through their critical analysis and review of the initial drafts. These individuals include:

Susan J. Hall, Ph.D., University of Delaware, Wilmington, Delaware
Malissa Martin, Ed.D., Middle Tennessee State University, Murfreesboro, Tennessee
Other reviewers:
E. Mike Davis, AT, Humboldt State University, Arcata, California
Tim O'Brien, M.Ed., L/ATC, Mayville State University, Mayville, North Dakota
Lisa Stalens, MPH, ATC, LAT, University of Texas at Austin, Austin, Texas
Jane Steinberg, MA, ATC/L, Carson-Newman College, Jefferson City, Tennessee

I would also like to thank the talented, hard-working editors at Lippincott Williams & Wilkins: Pete Darcy, Linda Napora, and Nancy Peterson; and Lydia V. Kibiuk, medical illustrator. Their patience, attention to detail, and quest for excellence provided a strong foundation for *Fundamentals of Sports Injury Management—Second Edition.*

A special thanks to Victoria Bacon for her support and encouragement to stick to the project and meet the deadlines and to my new dog, Tory, who spent many hours laying quietly at my side while I worked on the computer to complete the text. And finally, a special thanks to my two colleagues in the athletic training program at Bridgewater State College, Professor Cheryl Hitchings and Dr. Kathleen Laquale. They have always been supportive of my writing and have reviewed numerous drafts of the chapters. A daunting task for anyone. Thank you to all!

Marcia K. Anderson

CONTENTS

Fundamentals of
Sports Injury Management

SECOND EDITION

Foundations of Sports Injury Management

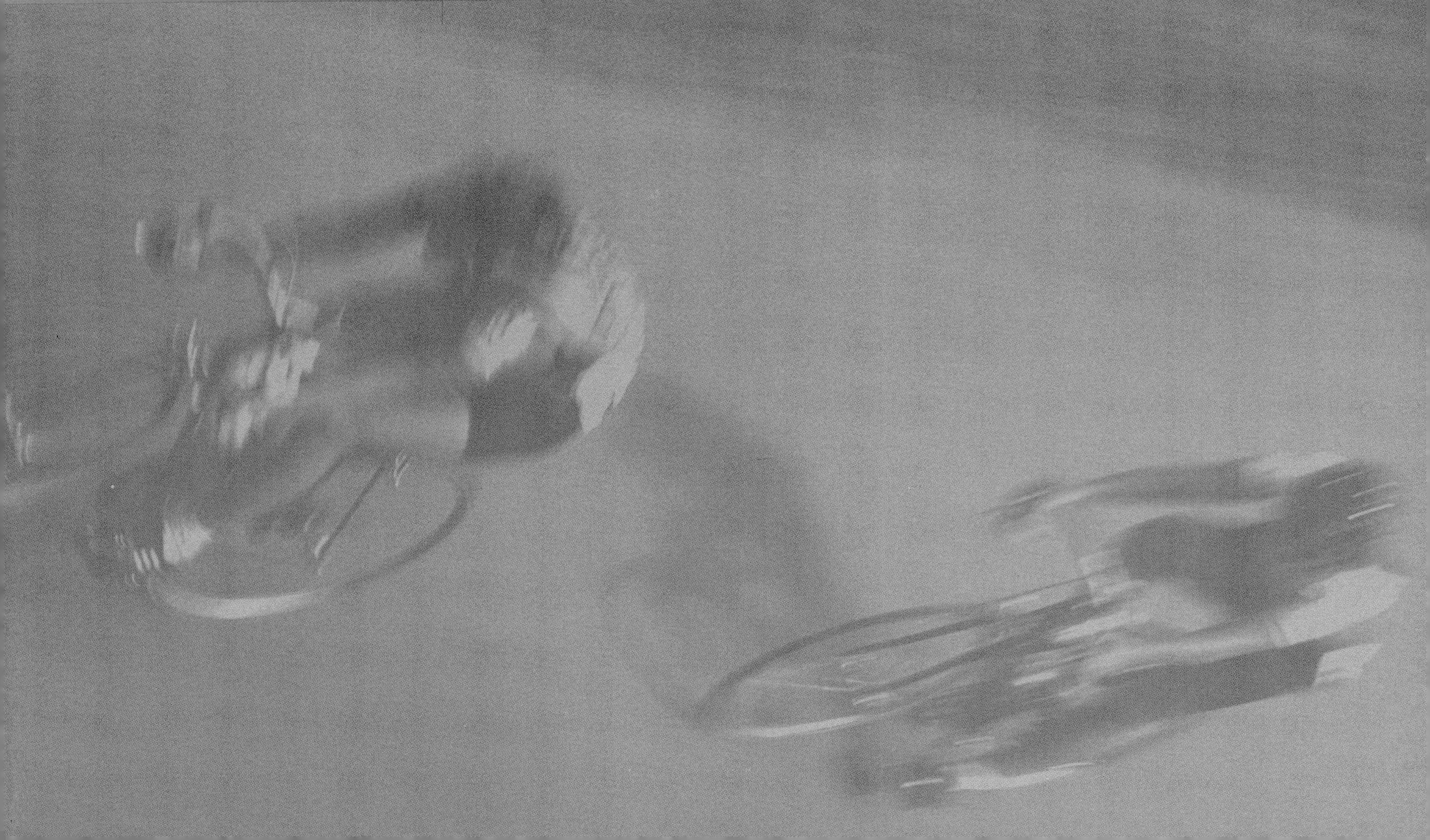

SECTION I

CHAPTER 1

Introduction to Sports Injury Management

KEY TERMS

Battery

Commission

Comparative negligence

Duty of care

Expressed warranty

Foreseeability of harm

Implied warranty

Informed consent

Omission

Sports medicine

Standard of care

Tort

OBJECTIVES

1. Define sports medicine.
2. Identify individuals who can provide immediate care to an injured athlete.
3. List responsibilities of a team physician and certified athletic trainer in caring for an injured athlete.
4. List responsibilities of a coach, recreational sport supervisor, or fitness coordinator in rendering emergency care to an injured athlete.
5. Explain standard of care and duty of care for individuals responsible for rendering on-site medical care to an athlete.
6. Identify the factors that must be proven to find an individual negligent.
7. Define and explain the legal liability of failure to warn, foreseeability of harm, informed consent, and product liability.
8. Explain the parameters of confidentiality of medical care.
9. Identify legal defenses, including assumption of risk, Good Samaritan laws, and comparative negligence.
10. Identify procedures that can reduce the risk of litigation in rendering medical care to an injured party.

Sport, with the inherent risks involved, leads to injury at one time or another for nearly all participants. In an organized sport setting such as interscholastic, intercollegiate, and professional level of play, team physicians and athletic trainers are responsible for the daily health and safety of sport participants. Furthermore, these individuals serve as a valuable resource to educate and counsel athletes to prevent chronic degenerative injuries and diseases through life-long, activity-related fitness and health education. Often, however, these individuals may not be readily accessible at all arenas and venues where sports injuries may occur. Therefore, other individuals, such as coaches, sport supervisors, fitness coordinators, and health employees may be called upon to render immediate sports injury care to an injured sport participant. Although the information provided in this book is intended for all of these individuals, for the sake of brevity, here they are referred to as coaches.

This chapter examines the parameters of providing immediate health care to an injured sport participant. Responsibilities of the team physician and certified athletic trainer are then briefly discussed. Most of the content focuses on the key responsibility of the supervising coach for immediate care of an injured athlete because this individual is often the first employee at the scene of a sport-related injury. Discussion then moves to legal considerations affecting coaches and fitness coordinators who are expected to render immediate sports injury care to an athlete who is using the sport facility or participating in programs sponsored by the facility.

THE PRIMARY SPORTS MEDICINE TEAM

Sports medicine is a broad and complex branch of health care, encompassing several disciplines. Essentially, it applies medical and scientific knowledge to prevent and care for injuries or illnesses related to sport, exercise, or recreational activity. In doing so, sports medicine enhances the health, fitness, and performance of the participant. Health care is safeguarded primarily by a group of individuals that make up the primary sports medicine team. This team includes the team physician, the primary care physician, the certified athletic trainer, and the coach. Although physicians and athletic trainers have a tremendous amount of expertise in injury care, coaches are often the only individuals on site during daily practices. They must therefore assume a larger responsibility for providing immediate first aid to an injured athlete until more advanced care arrives. Other professionals can also complement the primary sports medicine team and help provide a safe environment for all sport participants. These individuals include equipment managers, facility administrators, physical therapists, and other allied health care professionals.

Providing a safe, healthy, and accessible environment that is properly supervised can prevent many injuries. Because of the inherent risks in some sports and the forces involved in contact and collision activities, injuries still occur. Understanding the role and responsibilities of each member of the primary sports medicine team helps define the scope of care provided by each person within the team.

Team Physician

In organized sport, such as interscholastic, intercollegiate, or professional athletic programs, a team physician may be hired, or may volunteer his or her services, to direct the primary sports medicine team. This individual supervises the various aspects of health care and is the final authority on the mental and physical readiness of athletes in organized programs. This individual can be a valuable resource on current therapeutic techniques, facilitate referrals to other medical specialists, and provide educational counseling to sport participants, parents, athletic trainers, and coaches. In an athletic program, the team physician performs the following functions:

- Administers and reviews preseason physical examinations
- Diagnoses injuries
- Dispenses medications
- Directs rehabilitation programs
- Works with the athletic staff to develop an emergency plan
- Educates the staff on health care insurance coverage and legal liability
- Reviews all medical forms, policies, and procedures to ensure compliance with school and athletic association guidelines

In many high school and collegiate settings, financial constraints may prevent hiring a full-time team physician. Instead, several physicians rotate the responsibility of being present at competitions. Physicians may be paid a stipend, be contracted, or volunteer to cover games. Primary care physicians, orthopedists, and other specialists with an interest in sports injury care may serve as team physicians. The team physician should be present at competitions, particularly those that involve high-risk sports, such as football, hockey, or lacrosse. He or she can conduct emergency injury assessment and manage and treat any immediate injury or illness.

Primary Care Physician

In the absence of a team physician, the primary care physician or family physician assumes a pivotal role in providing health care to the sport participant. This individual can provide information on the growth and development of an adolescent and information on the athlete's immunization records and comprehensive medical history. In addition, the primary care physician may administer preparticipation examinations, provide initial clearance for sport participation, diagnose sports injuries, prescribe medication, and clear an individual for sport participation after an injury.[1]

Athletic Trainer

Athletic trainers are the critical link between the sport program and medical community, and they must be certified by the National Athletic Trainers' Association Board of Certification (NATABOC). Athletic trainers have a strong background in human anatomy and physiology, biomechanics, exercise physiology, nutrition, pharmacology, and general medical conditions and disabilities. Because of this broad background, athletic trainers are the facilitator and liaison between the physician and athlete, between the physician and coach, and among parents, administrators, and other allied health professionals. Their primary duties and responsibilities focus on twelve domains **(Box 1-1)**.[2]

Coach

The athletic coach is a critical component of the sports medicine team. These individuals know the physical and psychological demands of the sport. They may also be more familiar with any pre-existing conditions of the athletes, such as poor flexibility, tight heel cords, seasonal allergies, or exercise-induced bronchitis. In addition, coaches are often responsible for developing pre-season conditioning programs; supervising warm-up sessions prior to daily practices; instructing athletes on the proper progression of the various sport techniques; and supervising the daily use of protective equipment. No other individual has such a critical focus on the initial prevention of injury. Even if the institution has a certified athletic trainer on staff, it is impossible for the athletic trainer to be at all sporting events. Therefore, the coach must be able to recognize a potentially serious injury and be able to determine what immediate care must be provided. Responsibilities associated with injury prevention and immediate care include the following:

- Review preseason conditioning programs
- Assess the quality, effectiveness, and maintenance of protective equipment
- Assess the extent of injury
- Recognize the severity of injury
- Determine how best to intervene
- Initiate the emergency care plan

> ➤ ➤ Box 1-1

Domains of the Athletic Training Educational Competencies

- Risk management and injury prevention
- Therapeutic exercise
- Pathology of injuries and illness
- General medical conditions and disabilities
- Assessment and evaluation
- Nutritional aspects of injury and illness
- Acute care of injury and illness
- Psychosocial intervention and referral
- Pharmacology
- Health care administration
- Therapeutic modalities
- Professional development and responsibilities

- Contact emergency medical services (EMS), if needed
- Provide emergency first aid until advanced medical assistance arrives

Compared with an athletic trainer, most coaches will less likely be trained in advanced injury assessment and treatment protocols. Therefore, all coaches and fitness coordinators should complete a basic athletic training class and have current certification in standard first aid and cardiopulmonary resuscitation (CPR) as minimal protection against litigation. In addition, the entire athletic staff should meet regularly with community EMS workers to develop and practice emergency procedures, skills, and techniques. At least one staff person should have advanced training in emergency care.

LEGAL CONSIDERATIONS

Preventing injuries and reducing further injury or harm is a major responsibility for all sports injury care providers. Despite the best possible care, accidents do happen, some of which may result in legal action against the coach or athletic trainer. Legal action involving the practice of sports injury care is typically tried under tort law. A **tort** is a civil wrong done to an individual, whereby the injured party seeks a remedy for damages suffered. In lawsuits, actions are measured against a standard of care provided by individuals who have a direct duty to provide care.

Standard of Care

Standard of care is measured by what another minimally competent individual educated and practicing in that profession would have done in the same or similar circumstance to protect an individual from harm or further harm. One's expectations of standard of care differ depending on the profession. For example, an injured party would hold a physician to a higher standard of care for rendering medical services than would be expected of a coach.

Duty of Care

Duty of care is measured by what is learned, or should have been learned, in the professional preparation of an individual charged with providing health care. Individuals responsible for supervising athletes have a duty of care to teach proper and appropriate techniques for the age group, to supervise activity areas, to inspect and provide quality safety equipment, and to ensure a safe environment to everyone using the facility or participating in programs sponsored by the facility.

Clearance for Participation

The question may arise as to who is the final authority to clear an individual to participate after an injury. Because this decision legally falls outside the realm of most individuals, the final authority in measuring an individual's status for participation rests with the supervising team physician, regardless of the age of the participant. In the absence of a team physician, the final authority rests with the family physician. Parents of minors cannot assume the risk involved in sport for their child.

Negligence

Negligence can occur as a result of an action (**commission**) or lack of an action (**omission**) that a professional performs on an athlete who the professional had a legal duty of care to protect. Other terms often used in negligence cases are shown in **Box 1-2**.

Although a sport participant does assume some risk inherent in any sport, the individual does not assume the risk that professionals will breach their duty of care. To find an individual negligent, the injured person must prove that 1) there was a duty of care; 2) there was a breach of that duty; 3) there was harm (e.g., pain and suffering, permanent disability, or loss of wages); and 4) the resulting harm was directly caused by that breach of duty.[3] If a spectator notices a large hole in the field before a soccer game, and a player steps into the hole and breaks an ankle, the spectator is not liable because that individual has no duty of care to the player. A coach, however, does have a duty of care to the participants to check the field for hazards before competition. As such, the coach could be held liable for injury sustained by the

participant. Fortunately, the number of lawsuits brought against athletic trainers and coaches in the performance of their duties is rare.

Legal Liabilities

Athletic trainers and coaches can take several precautionary steps to limit the risk of litigation. These may involve:

- Informing the athlete about the inherent risks of sport participation
- Foreseeing the potential for injury and correcting the situation before harm occurs
- Obtaining informed consent from the athlete or their guardian prior to participation in the sport and prior to any treatment should an injury occur
- Using quality products and equipment that do not pose a threat to the athlete
- Maintaining strict confidentiality of all medical records

FAILURE TO WARN

Athletic trainers and coaches should inform potential sport participants and clients of the risks for injury during sport participation. Participants and parents of minor children should learn that risk for injury exists and must understand the nature of that risk for informed judgments on participation. Understanding and comprehending the nature of the risk is determined by the participant's age, experience, and knowledge of pertinent information about the risk. An advanced gymnast, for example, would know of, and appreciate, the risk of injury much more than a novice gymnast. Therefore, it is crucial to warn the novice of all inherent dangers in the activity and to continually reinforce that information throughout the entire sport season. Warnings may be communicated by having a preseason meeting with parents and participants, discussing them during prescreening when the client is first introduced into the fitness or health facility, posting visible warning signs around equipment, requiring protective equipment, and discouraging dangerous techniques. Other methods that can be used are listed in **Box 1-3**.

FORESEEABILITY OF HARM

To recognize the potential for injury first, then to remove that danger before an injury occurs, is another duty of care for coaches. **Foreseeability of harm** exists when danger is apparent, or should have been apparent, resulting in an unreasonably unsafe condition. This potential for injury can be identified during regular inspections of safety equipment, gymnasiums, weight training rooms, field areas, and swimming pools. For example, unpadded walls under the basketball hoops, glass or potholes on playing fields, slippery floors on a pool deck, exposed wiring, and weight training machines that do not operate properly all pose a threat to safety. Unsafe conditions

---

➤ ➤ **BOX 1-2**

Definition of Negligent Torts

Malfeasance (commission) occurs when an individual commits an act that is not his/her responsibility to perform. If a lower leg fracture is suspected due to the visible angulation of the involved bones, the coach could be liable if he or she decides to straighten out the leg and immobilize the limb in a splint

Misfeasance occurs when an individual commits an act that is his/her responsibility to perform, but uses the wrong procedure, or does the right procedure in an improper manner. If the coach asks two players to carry the injured athlete with the suspected lower leg fracture off the field in a seated position cradled in their crossed arms, the coach could be liable, since the leg was not properly immobilized prior to transport

Nonfeasance (omission) occurs when an individual fails to perform their legal duty of care. If the coach failed to provide any care to the injured athlete with the suspected lower leg fracture and went on with practice, he or she could be liable for delaying medical care

Malpractice occurs when an individual commits a negligent act while providing care

Gross negligence occurs when an individual has total disregard for the safety of others

➤ ➤ BOX 1-3

Strategies to Avoid Litigation

- Hire qualified coaches, athletic trainers, and fitness instructors, and establish strict rules for supervision and use of the facility
- Have an established preparticipation plan that includes the following:
  - Health and fitness examination
  - Emergency medical data information cards
  - Physician's clearance to participate
- Hold a preseason/preparticipation meeting to:
  - Inform participants and parents of the risks involved in sport participation
  - Obtain written informed consent to participate in the activity from the adult individual and from the parents of minor children
  - Obtain written informed consent from the adult participant and the parents of minor children to authorize standard medical and emergency medical care
- Have a well-established sports medicine team to:
  - Develop a total health care plan, including staff responsibilities during emergency situations
  - Obtain adequate secondary health insurance for participants and liability insurance for the staff
  - Establish a communication system at each field, pool, or gymnasium station
  - Maintain appropriate injury accident reports
  - Establish clearly defined standing orders for providing basic first aid care to athletes
  - Develop criteria to return an injured athlete to participation
  - Select and purchase quality safety equipment from a reputable dealer
  - Inspect safety equipment and supervise proper fitting, adjustment, and repair of equipment
  - Inspect equipment, facilities, and fields for hazards and prohibit their use if found to be dangerous
  - Establish policies for documentation, confidentiality, and storage of medical records
  - Keep accurate records of equipment purchases, reconditioning, and repairs
- Post warning signs in plain sight on and around equipment to inform of the risks involved in abuse of equipment, and to describe proper use of the equipment
- Post visible signs in the swimming pool area giving the depth of the pool and prohibiting diving in the shallow area
- Require participants to wear protective equipment regularly, including protective eyewear in appropriate racquet sports
- Provide continuing education for sport and fitness coordinators through in-service workshops and programs
- Act as a reasonably prudent professional in caring for all sport participants

should be identified, reported in writing to appropriate personnel, restricted from use, and repaired or replaced as soon as possible.

INFORMED CONSENT

Informed consent implies that an injured party has been reasonably informed of needed treatment for the services one performs, has been told of possible alternative treatments, and has been told of advantages and disadvantages of each course of action. To be valid, expressed consent can be obtained only from one who is competent to grant it; that is, an adult who is physically and mentally competent. In the case of children under 18, only the parent or guardian can grant consent on behalf of the minor. There are three exceptions to this rule. Implied consent exists when an unconscious individual is in a life-threatening situation. It is assumed that the individual would consent to appropriate lifesaving intervention. Secondly, consent is implied if emergency first aid begins and the injured party does not resist. Finally, for minors, exceptions exist in emergency situations when parents are unavailable.

Touching another person without his or her informed consent may constitute **battery**, which may be grounds for litigation. Although many courts require that intent to harm be present in an allegation of battery, written documentation of informed consent should be obtained from an individual or from parents of minors prior to treatment to avoid litigation. This consent can be obtained in writing prior to beginning sport participation. It also can be obtained during preparticipation meetings as part of the documentation depicting consent to participate in that activity.

REFUSING HELP

Although rare, an injured sport participant may refuse emergency first aid for several reasons: religious beliefs, cultural differences, avoidance of additional pain or discomfort, or the desire to be evaluated and treated by a more medically qualified individual. Regardless of the reason given to refuse help, the conscious and medically competent individual has the right to refuse treatment. An exemption to this standard may occur when failure to move the injured party could result in an increased risk for further injury to the injured party or to others in the vicinity of the accident. For example, during an organized bike race, if several bikers collide and fall down onto a busy road, it would be appropriate to move any injured individuals off the road so as not to endanger themselves or any approaching motorists. In this instance, the best option is to have another employee summon EMS while the immediate sports care provider tries to persuade the injured party to accept immediate care until the ambulance arrives. It is helpful to have a witness to the event—too often an injured individual initially refuses consent only to later deny having done so.

PRODUCT LIABILITY

Sport participants, parents, coaches, and athletic trainers place great faith in the quality and safety of equipment used in sport participation. Manufacturers have a duty of care to design, manufacture, and package equipment that will not cause injury to an individual when used as intended. This is called an **implied warranty**. An **expressed warranty** is a written guarantee that the product is safe for use. Strict liability makes the manufacturer liable for all defective or hazardous equipment that unduly threatens an individual's personal safety.[3,4]

Any alteration or modification to any protective equipment may negate the manufacturer's liability. Coaches should know the dangers involved in using sport equipment, and they have a duty to properly supervise its fitting and intended use. Furthermore, they should continually warn participants of the inherent dangers if the equipment is used incorrectly.

CONFIDENTIALITY

A major concern affecting all individuals providing health care to an athlete is an individual's right to privacy. If the athlete is older than 18 years of age, release of any medical information must be acknowledged in writing by the athlete. For individuals younger than 18 years of age, parents or legal guardians must provide consent for the dissemination of this information. This permission should identify what, if any, information should be shared with an individual other than the patient's physician. In many cases, schools and professional teams have a competitive athlete give consent that all medical information can be shared between the athletic trainers and the supervising physician.[5]

Coaches and fitness coordinators may become privy to information about the injured athlete that would be embarrassing to the individual, or to his or her family, if it were made public. Therefore, it is critical to share pertinent information about the athlete's condition with only those individuals who need to know. Some states, however, require that certain incidents, such as abuse, rape, and a stabbing or gunshot wound, be reported to the appropriate authorities.

Legal Defenses

If the threat of litigation exists, many athletic trainers and coaches rely on certain conditions to strengthen their case. These conditions include the athlete's assumption of risk in participating in sport, Good Samaritan laws, and comparative negligence.

ASSUMPTION OF RISK

Sport participants assume some risks inherent in their chosen sport. When they agree to participate in competitive activity, they should be informed of the risks of participa-tion, testing, and physical activity, and they should be advised that participation is voluntary. Many facilities require that each participant sign an express assumption of risk form. By signing the form, athletes acknowledge the material risks and anticipate and acknowledge that other injuries and even death is a possibility. The form also acknowledges that athletes have had an opportunity to ask questions and have them answered to their complete satisfaction. Finally, athletes affirm that they subjectively understand the risks of their participation in the activity and that they voluntarily choose to participate, assuming all risks of injury or even death due to their participation. These forms have helped the legal defense of individuals involved in providing health care to athletes. However, as mentioned earlier, athletes do not assume the risk that the professional will breach their duty of care.

GOOD SAMARITAN LAWS

Beginning in the early 1960s, several states enacted legislation to protect physicians or other recognized medical personnel from litigation that stemmed from emergency treatment provided to injured individuals at the scene of an accident. These laws, nicknamed "Good Samaritan Laws," were developed to encourage bystanders to assist others in need of emergency care by granting them immunity from potential litigation. Although the laws vary from state to state, immunity generally applies only when the emergency first aider 1) acts during an emergency; 2) acts in good faith to help the victim; 3) acts without expected compensation; and 4) is not guilty of any malicious misconduct or gross negligence toward the injury party (i.e., does not deviate from acceptable first aid protocol).[6]

Although Good Samaritan Laws were intended to protect physicians and medical personnel, several states have expanded the language to include laypersons serving as emergency first aid workers. However, these laws are easy to get around and will not protect rescuers from litigation regardless of their actions. It is therefore essential that sport and fitness coordinators be properly trained in emergency first aid and care of sports injuries if they are expected to supervise athletes and render immediate first aid.

COMPARATIVE NEGLIGENCE

When an athlete is injured and a lawsuit results, several individuals and their employers are named in the suit. These individuals can include physicians, surgeons, athletic trainers, coaches, and emergency personnel who provided medical services to the athlete. **Comparative negligence** refers to the relative degree of negligence on the part of the plaintiff and defendant, with damages awarded proportionate to each person's carelessness. For example, if the athlete was found to be 30% at fault for his or her own injury (contributory negligent) and the defendants were 70% at fault; on a $100,000 judgment, the defendants would be responsible for $70,000 in damages, and the athlete (plaintiff) would assume an equivalent of $30,000 in damages. The courts would also weigh the relative degree of negligence on the part of each defendant and then award payment of damages proportionate to each person's carelessness that led to the eventual injury.

Preventing Litigation

All individuals responsible for providing health care to athletes should be aware of their duty of care consistent with existing state laws. They should then complete that duty of care within established policies and standards of practice for their respective profession. Coaches and athletic trainers can take steps to reduce the risk of litigation. These precautions include regular inspection of athletic fields and facility design, doing safety checks of equipment and facilities, hiring qualified personnel, providing proper supervision and instruction, purchasing quality equipment, posting appropriate warning signs, having accurate medical records, and having a well-organized emergency care plan. Other steps are shown in **Box 1-3**.

Summary

1. Sports medicine is a branch of medicine that applies medical and scientific knowledge to improve sport performance.
2. The primary sports medicine team provides immediate on-site supervision to prevent injury and deliver immediate health care. This team includes the team physician, primary care physician in the absence of a team physician, athletic trainer, and coach.
3. In the absence of an athletic trainer, the coach should be able to:
   - Assess and recognize potentially severe injuries
   - Provide emergency first aid
   - Initiate appropriate referral for advanced medical care, if necessary
4. To find an individual liable, the injured person must prove that there was:
   - A duty of care
   - A breach of that duty
   - Harm directly caused by that breach of duty
5. Coaches and fitness coordinators have a duty of care to supervise and provide emergency sports injury care to all athletes using the sport facility and to those participating in programs sponsored by the facility. Supervisors are expected to teach proper and appropriate techniques for the age group, inspect and provide quality safety equipment, ensure a safe environment, and warn all participants of the risks for injury during sport participation so the participant can make an informed judgment about participation.
6. To recognize the potential for injury first, then to remove that danger before an injury occurs, is called foreseeability of harm.
7. Informed consent implies that an injured individual has been reasonably informed of needed treatment and consents to receiving that treatment.
8. Manufacturers have a duty of care to design, manufacture, and package equipment that will not cause injury to an individual when used as intended.
9. Sport and fitness coordinators cannot release any medical information about an injured individual without that person's written consent if the person is older than 18 years of age. Release of any medical information for individuals younger than 18 years of age must be granted by the child's parent or legal guardian.
10. Although Good Samaritan Laws were developed to encourage bystanders to assist others in need of emergency care by granting the bystanders immunity from potential litigation, these laws do not protect an employee of a sport or fitness facility who renders improper care to a client or sport participant. Sport and fitness coordinators should complete a basic athletic training class and be certified in standard first aid and cardiopulmonary resuscitation (CPR) as minimal protection against litigation.
11. Steps to reduce the risk of injury and subsequent litigation include:
    - Obtaining informed consent
    - Recognizing the potential for injury and correcting it
    - Warning participants of the risk of injury
    - Hiring qualified personnel
    - Providing proper supervision and instruction
    - Purchasing, fitting, and maintaining quality equipment
    - Posting appropriate warning signs
    - Maintaining accurate and complete health care records
    - Protecting confidentiality of medical history
    - Having a well-organized emergency care system

References

1. Mellion MB, and Walsh WM. The team physician. In *Sports medicine secrets*, edited by MB Mellion. Philadelphia: Hanley & Belfus, 1994.
2. NATA Board of Certification, Inc. Role Delineation Study, prepared by Columbia Assessment Services. Philadelphia: FA Davis, 1999.
3. Leverenz LJ, and Helms LB. 1990. Suing athletic trainers: part I, a review of the case law involving athletic trainers. Ath Train (JNATA) 25(3):212-216.
4. Leverenz LJ, and Helms LB. 1990. Suing athletic trainers: part II, implications for the NATA competencies. Ath Train (JNATA) 25(3):219-226.
5. Arendtp E. 1996. What every health care professional should know. NATA News Jan:20-21.
6. National Safety Council. First Aid and CPR. Sudbury, MA: Jones and Bartlett Publishers, 1997.

CHAPTER 2

Emergency Procedures

KEY TERMS:

Anaphylaxis

Apnea

Arrhythmia

Atherosclerosis

Cardiac asystole

Cold diuresis

Crepitus

Cyanosis

Diplopia

Diuretics

Hematoma

Homeostasis

Hyperhydrate

Hyperthermia

Hypertrophic
cardiomyopathy

Hypothalamus

Hypothermia

Myocardial infarction

Shock

Sign

Symptom

Syncope

Tachycardia

Thermoregulation

Triage

Unconsciousness

OBJECTIVES

1. Explain how to develop an emergency action plan.

2. Identify what role a coach should assume in rendering emergency sports injury care.

3. List the most common life-threatening conditions.

4. Differentiate between a partial and total airway obstruction.

5. Describe the various situations that can lead to sudden death from cardiac arrest.

6. Explain how a coach might assess an unconscious athlete to determine the severity of injury.

7. List the signs and symptoms of shock and explain how to manage the situation.

8. Describe how the human body gains and loses heat.

9. Explain methods used to prevent heat illness and cold-related injuries.

10. Identify the signs and symptoms of heat-related conditions and describe their management.

11. Differentiate between frostbite and systemic cooling, and describe the management of each.

12. Explain what steps to take if you are caught outdoors during lightning or a thunderstorm.

13. Describe the procedures for performing a secondary survey using the HOPS format.

14. List emergency conditions that warrant immediate action by emergency medical services (EMS).

This chapter first discusses how to develop an emergency action plan for a sport/fitness facility. The roles of facility personnel and local emergency medical services (EMS) workers who may care for an injured athlete are then explained. Next, conditions that may pose a threat to an athlete's life are introduced. Finally, a systematic assessment process is introduced to help the coach determine whether an emergency exists and EMS should be summoned.

THE EMERGENCY ACTION PLAN

Serious injuries can be frightening, particularly when breathing or circulation is impaired. As the first responder on the scene, the coach is expected to evaluate the situation, recognize life-threatening conditions, provide immediate care, and initiate any emergency procedures to ensure that the injured party is transported immediately to the nearest medical facility. An EMS system is a well-developed process that jointly activates the emergency health care services of the sport facility and community to provide immediate health care to an injured athlete.

Developing the Plan

The facility and staff charged with providing emergency sports injury care should meet annually with representatives from local EMS agencies to discuss, develop, and evaluate the emergency action plan. The questions listed in **Box 2-1** should be answered as the plan is developed. A written plan should be developed for each activity site, such as the gymnasium, pool area, weight training area, and outside fields. This is an excellent opportunity to review individual responsibilities and protocols for an emergency at the facility. The emergency response team should practice the emergency plan through regular educational workshops and training exercises. Everyone must work together during emergencies to ensure that medical attention is not delayed. For high schools and colleges, you may want to refer to the National Collegiate Athletic Association (NCAA) Emergency Action Plan template, which can be seen on their web site, http://www.ncaa.org.

Responsibilities of Medical Personnel

Members of the on-site emergency response team should be certified in first aid and cardiopulmonary resuscitation (CPR) and should know their responsibilities according to the emergency action plan. The on-site team should meet annually to review the location and proper use of medical supplies and equipment. This material must be easily accessible and operational. In a school setting, the athletic trainer is responsible for setting up the event area with appropriate equipment and supplies for the medical kit **(Box 2-2)** and emergency "crash" kit **(Box 2-3)**, as

> ➤ ➤ **BOX 2-1**

Questions to Answer in Establishing an Emergency Procedures Plan

- Who will render immediate care to the injured athlete?
- Does everyone know the location and have easy access to first aid supplies, splints, fire extinguishers, and a phone?
- Who will control the area and keep other participants away from the accident scene?
- What care will be provided by the on-site emergency response team?
- Who will call Emergency Medical Services (EMS), and what information will be given over the phone?
- Who will meet the ambulance and escort it through locked doors and gates?
- Who will contact the family of the injured athlete, and what information will be given over the phone?
- Who will supervise the other activity areas if a sport or fitness coordinator must leave his/her area to assist at the accident scene?
- What procedures will be implemented for the proper use and disposal of items and equipment exposed to blood or bodily fluids?

well as for providing a method of communication (e.g., two-way radio or cellular phone) to facilitate a call to summon EMS.

Should an accident occur, the most medically qualified on-site individual should assume the major responsibility of stabilizing and calming the injured party. In addition, he or she should:

- Assess any life-threatening condition
- Determine whether EMS should be summoned
- Direct other staff members to move spectators away from the accident scene
- Gather information about how the injury occurred
- Summon additional medical supplies or equipment if necessary
- Manage or stabilize the immediate injury if appropriate
- Supervise other staff members who may assist in the care of the injured party
- Treat the individual for shock until EMS arrives

EMS personnel include emergency medical technicians (EMTs) or paramedics trained in emergency care. Once on the scene, they assume the major responsibility of care. Their responsibilities may include:

- Controlling the scene and ensuring safety of the injured party
- Conducting a more detailed assessment of the injury
- Taking vital signs
- Providing additional care of the injury

Checklist for Athletic Training Medical Kit

- Adhesive bandages (assorted sizes)
- Adhesive Tape
  - 1/2 inch
  - 1 inch
  - 1 1/2 inch
  - 2 inch
- Airway (pocket mask and oropharyngeal)
- Alcohol (isopropyl)
- Antacid tablets or liquid
- Antifungal powder or spray
- Antiseptic/antibiotic ointment
- Antiseptic soap
- Aspirin tablets
- Blister tape
- (Dermiclear®)
- Butterfly bandage and Steri-strips
- Cloth ankle wraps
- Contact lens case and solution
- Cotton balls
- Cotton-tipped applicators
- Elastic wraps
  - 4 inch
  - 6 inch
- Double-length 6 inch
- Elastic tape (Elastikon® or Conform®)
  - 1 inch
  - 2 inch
  - 3 inch
- Emergency kit
  - Coins for pay phone
  - Emergency telephone numbers
  - Location of nearest trauma center
  - Health information cards
  - Injury reports
  - Insurance information
- Eyewash and eye cup
- Eyepatches (sterile)
- Felt (compression/horseshoe pads)
  - 1/4 inch
  - 1/2 inch
- Fingernail clipper

- Flexible collodion
- Foam padding
  - 1/8 inch
  - 1/4 inch
  - 1/2 inch
  - 1 inch
- Forceps (tweezers)
- Fungicide cream
- Gauze pads (sterile and nonsterile)
- Germicide solution
- Heel and lace pads
- Heel cups
- Hydrogen peroxide
- Latex gloves
- Mirror (hand-held)
- Moleskin
- Nasal pledget (plug)
- Nonadhering sterile pads
- Nonocclusive dressing
- Oral thermometer
- Penlight
- Paper, pen, or pencil
- Plastic bags for ice
- Ring cutter
- Scalpel and blades, disposable
- Scissors
- Bandage
- Heavy duty surgical taping
- Trainer's Angel®
- Second skin
- Skin lubricant (petroleum jelly)
- Sling or triangular bandages
- Stethoscope and blood pressure cuff
- Suntan lotion or sunblock
- Tape adherent
- Tape cutter
- Tape remover
- Tongue depressors
- Towlettes, moist
- Underwrap

- Lifting, securing, and immobilizing the injured party onto an appropriate stretcher
- Preparing and transporting the individual to the nearest medical facility for advanced care

EMERGENCY CONDITIONS

Injuries or conditions that impair, or have the potential to impair, vital function of the central nervous system and cardiorespiratory system are considered emergency conditions (Box 2-4). Many serious injuries are clearly evident and recognizable, such as lack of breathing or absence of a pulse. However, other serious injuries may not be as easy to determine.

To recognize an injury, subjective symptoms and objective signs are gathered. A **symptom** is information provided by the injured individual on his/her perception of the problem. These conditions or feelings include blurred vision, ringing in the ears, fatigue, dizziness, nausea, headache, pain, weakness, or an inability to move a body part. A **sign** is a measurable physical finding about the individual's condition that the emergency responder sees, feels, hears, or smells when assessing the individual. Interpreting the symptoms and signs is the foundation of recognizing and identifying the injury or condition. Management of these injuries is covered in the appropriate section. Because external hemorrhage and fractures are common wounds in sports participation, they are discussed in more detail in Chapter 4, "Wound Care."

OBSTRUCTED AIRWAY

The airway can become partially or totally blocked by a solid foreign object (mouth guard, bridgework, chewing gum, chaw of tobacco, or mud), fluids (blood clots from head injuries or vomitus), swelling in the throat caused by allergic reactions, or, more commonly, the back of the tongue (due to unconsciousness). An obstructed airway prevents adequate oxygen from being exchanged in the lungs and can lead to **cyanosis** and death.

Partial Airway Obstruction

When a person has a partial airway obstruction, there is still some air exchange in the lungs and the individual is able to cough. The individual typically grasps the throat in the universal distress signal for choking. If the individual is able to cough forcefully, do not interfere. Stand beside the person and encourage him or her to continue coughing in an attempt to dislodge the obstruction. An ineffective cough or a high-pitched noise during breathing indicates poor air exchange and should be treated as a total airway obstruction.

Total Airway Obstruction

In a total airway obstruction, no air is passing through the vocal cords, so the individual is unable to speak, breathe, or cough. In a conscious person, the universal distress signal is usually apparent. The Heimlich maneuver is used to dislodge the foreign object so breathing may resume. However, if the individual becomes unconscious, the coach must react quickly to clear the airway and stimulate the breathing process.

CARDIOPULMONARY EMERGENCIES

Cardiac arrest can result from strenuous physical activity in a dehydrated state, direct trauma, electrical shock, excessive alcohol or other chemical substance abuse, suffocation, drowning, or heart anomalies. Cardiac anomalies are the most direct cause of sudden death in athletes younger than 30 years; hypertrophic cardiomyopathy is the most common. In athletes older than 30 years, atherosclerotic coronary artery disease is the more likely cause of sudden death. Other reported cardiac-related causes include mitral valve prolapse, myocarditis, acquired valvular heart disease, coronary artery disease, and Marfan syndrome.

Hypertrophic cardiomyopathy (HCM), characterized by an abnormal thickening of the left ventricle wall, develops before age 20 and typically goes undetected during routine physical examination. Symptoms of cardiac dysfunction, which do not appear until early adulthood if at all, result in impaired ventricle filling. As a result, periods of **arrhythmia** (irregular heart beats) or blood flow obstruction can occur that may produce **syncope** (fainting and lightheadedness) during physical exertion. **Atherosclerosis** involves an excessive buildup of cholesterol within the coronary arteries, which narrows the diameter of the arteries and impedes blood flow. In turn, the amount of oxygen supplied to the heart is reduced. Because of the diminished oxygen, angina or chest pain during physical exertion is a common symptom. If excessive cholesterol buildup blocks a coronary artery, the person is at risk for a **myocardial infarction** (heart attack). If the blockage exists in a major coronary artery, death often occurs. Signs and symptoms that indicate a possible heart attack can be seen in **Box 2-5**.

UNCONSCIOUS ATHLETE

Head injuries are the leading cause of loss of consciousness in sport activity and are discussed in more detail in Chapter 5. Being fully alert and conscious implies that the individual is aware of the surroundings and can respond to questions. **Unconsciousness** identifies an individual who lacks conscious awareness and is unable to respond to superficial sensory stimuli, such as pinching in the armpit. Coma, the most depressed state of consciousness, occurs when the individual cannot be aroused even by stimuli as powerful as pin pricks.

One must assume that an unconscious athlete has a life-threatening condition that requires an immediate primary survey. Therefore, it is critical for all coaches to be certified in CPR because they are often the first people on the injury scene. The following guidelines help to assess an unconscious athlete:

1. Assume that a possible cervical spine injury is present until ruled out.
2. Activate the emergency action plan.
3. Place a hand on the athlete's head to prevent an unnecessary motion of the cervical spine during the assessment.
4. Note the athlete's body position, and determine level of consciousness and unresponsiveness. Assess the ABCs.
5. If the athlete is supine (face up) and breathing, nothing should be done until the athlete regains consciousness.
6. If the athlete is prone (face down) and breathing, nothing should be done until the athlete regains consciousness.
7. If the athlete is prone and not breathing, the athlete should be logrolled carefully into a supine position. Immediately assess the ABCs (airway, breathing, and circulation).

8. If a helmet is worn, do not remove the helmet until a full assessment is completed to determine the presence or absence of a cervical neck injury. Removal of a helmet without removal of the shoulder pads leads to hyperextension of the cervical spine. However, the face mask must be cut away and removed using a face-cutting tool, such as an Anvil Pruner or Trainer's Angel.
9. If CPR is necessary, the jersey and shoulder pad laces can be cut and the pectoral pads spread to access the sternum for hand placement.
10. Any necessary life support should be maintained and monitored until emergency personnel arrive.

HEMORRHAGE

Severe hemorrhage causes a decrease in blood volume and blood pressure. To compensate for this factor, the heart's pumping action must increase. Because there is less blood in the system, however, the strength of the pumping action is weakened, resulting in a characteristic rapid, weak pulse. Arterial bleeding from an oxygen-rich vessel is characterized by a spurting, bright red color. Major arteries, when completely severed, often constrict and seal themselves for a short period. If the artery is only punctured or partially severed, however, bleeding can be severe. Venous bleeding from an oxygen-depleted vessel is a dark, bluish-red, almost maroon color. The continuous steady loss of blood can be heavy. Most superficial veins collapse if they are cut, but bleeding from deep veins can be as profuse and difficult to control as arterial bleeding. Capillary bleeding is usually very slow and often described as oozing. The blood is red, but a duller shade than arterial blood. This type of bleeding clots easily.

External bleeding is best controlled with direct pressure and elevation. Using universal safety precautions (see Field Strategy 4-1), pressure is applied directly over the wound with a sterile gauze pad, compressing the region against the underlying bone. Elevation uses gravity to reduce blood pressure, and thus aids blood clotting. In more severe bleeding, indirect pressure points can also help control hemorrhage, but they should not be used if a fracture is suspected because of possible movement of the fractured bone ends.

Internal bleeding can result from blunt trauma or certain fractures (such as those of the pelvis, rib, or skull). Because internal hemorrhage is not visible, it can be overlooked, which can lead to shock. The history of injury (i.e., a fall, a deceleration injury, or severe blunt trauma), coupled with signs and symptoms of shock (**Box 2-6**), should indicate that possible internal bleeding exists.

FRACTURES

A fracture is a break in the continuity of a bone and is classified as open or closed, depending on whether the skin surface is penetrated. Because of infection, open fractures are more serious than closed fractures. Signs of fracture can be seen in **Box 4-4**, and their management is summarized in **Field Strategy 4-4.**

SHOCK

Shock can occur to some degree in any injury involving pain, bleeding, internal trauma, fracture, or spinal injury. This condition occurs when the heart is unable to exert adequate pressure to circulate enough oxygenated blood to the vital organs. Causes include a damaged heart that fails to pump properly, low blood volume from blood loss or dehydration, or dilated blood vessels, which leads to blood pooling in larger vessels away from vital areas. The heart pumps faster but, because of reduced volume, pulse rate is weakened and blood pressure drops (hypotension). This rapid, weak pulse is the most prominent sign of shock **(Box 2-6)**. As the individual's condition deteriorates, breathing becomes rapid and shallow. Vital body fluids pass through the weakened capillaries, leading to further circulatory distress. If not corrected, circulatory collapse can lead to unconsciousness and death.

If shock is suspected, activate the emergency action plan. The following guidelines may help manage this condition:

1. Secure and maintain an open airway.
2. Control any major bleeding, and splint any suspected fractures to slow bleeding and reduce pain.
3. If the athlete has a lower leg fracture, keep the leg level while splinting the fracture. Raise the leg only after it has been properly immobilized.
4. If you do not suspect a head or neck injury or a leg fracture, elevate the feet and legs 8 to 12 inches.
5. If there are breathing difficulties, the athlete might be more comfortable with the head and shoulders raised in a semi-reclining position.
6. If a head injury has been sustained, elevate the head and shoulders to reduce pressure on the brain.
7. In a suspected neck injury, keep the athlete lying flat.

8. Maintain body heat by keeping the athlete warm, but do not overheat. Remove any wet clothing if possible, and cover the athlete with a blanket. Keep the individual quiet and still. Avoid any rough or excessive handling.
9. Do not give the athlete anything by mouth in case surgery is indicated.
10. Monitor the vital signs every 2 to 5 minutes until emergency personnel arrive.

ANAPHYLAXIS

For most individuals, allergies cause simple rashes, itching, watery eyes, and some short-term discomfort. For a small group of people, however, a more powerful reaction to allergens, either eaten or injected, can lead to a life-threatening condition called anaphylaxis. **Anaphylaxis** is a shocklike, frequently fatal hypersensitive reaction to an allergen. Severe reactions may take place immediately, or they may be delayed 30 minutes or longer. Commonly known substances that cause anaphylaxis in hypersensitive individuals include:

- Medications (e.g., penicillin and related drugs, aspirin, sulfa drugs)
- Food and food additive (e.g., shellfish, nuts, berries, eggs, monosodium glutamate [MSG], nitrates, nitrites)
- Insect stings (e.g., honeybee, yellow jacket, wasp, hornet, fire ant)
- Inhaled substances (e.g., plant pollens, dust, chemical powders)
- Radiographic dyes

Signs and symptoms of anaphylactic shock occur within minutes of exposure to the involved substance, and they peak in 15 to 30 minutes, ending several hours later **(Box 2-7)**. The individual may have a history of such reactions, may wear a medical identification tag, and may have a self-administered epinephrine device (EpiPen®). Immediate treatment involves activating EMS and maintaining the cardiorespiratory functions of the individual. If a bee sting or insect bite is suspected, remove the stinger by scraping, not squeezing. Management of a bee sting and anaphylactic shock is covered in **Field Strategy 2-1**.

HEAT-RELATED CONDITIONS

The process by which the body maintains body temperature is called **thermoregulation**, which is primarily controlled by the **hypothalamus**, a region of the diencephalon forming the floor of the third ventricle of the brain. **Hyperthermia**, or elevated body temperature, occurs when internal heat production exceeds external heat loss. The hypothalamus gland maintains **homeostasis**, or a state of equilibrium within the body, by initiating cooling or heat retention mechanisms to achieve a relatively constant body core temperature between 36.1 and 37.8°C (97 to 100°F).

➤ ➤ **B o x 2 - 6**

Signs and Symptoms of Shock
- Rapid, weak pulse
- Cold, clammy moist skin; initially chalklike but later may appear cyanotic
- Shallow irregular breathing, but may also be labored, rapid, or gasping
- Profuse sweating and extreme thirst
- Nausea, vomiting, or both
- Dull, sunken eyes with dilated pupils
- Restlessness, anxiety, disorientation, or dizziness

➤ ➤ Box 2-7

Signs and Symptoms of Anaphylactic Shock

- Initially, a general feeling of warmth accompanied by intense itching, especially on the soles of the feet and palms of the hands
- Localized rash or swelling around the insect sting
- Dizziness, choking, wheezing, and shortness of breath
- Rapid and weak pulse
- Headache, nausea, and vomiting
- Dilated pupils
- Blueness around the lips and mouth
- Tightness and swelling in the throat and chest
- Swelling of the mucous membranes (tongue, mouth, nose), which can lead to respiratory distress and unconsciousness
- Seizures leading to sudden collapse and unconsciousness

Internal Heat Regulation

During exercise, the body gains heat from either external sources (environmental temperatures) or internal processes **(Fig. 2-1)**. Much of the internal heat is generated during muscular activity through energy metabolism. During exercise, the circulatory system must deliver oxygen to the working muscles and deliver heated blood from deep tissues (core) to the periphery (shell) for dissipation. The increased blood flow to the muscles and skin is made possible by increasing cardiac output and redistributing regional blood flow (i.e., blood flow to the visceral organs is reduced). As exercise begins, heart rate and cardiac output increase, while superficial venous and arterial blood vessels dilate to divert warm blood to the skin surface. Heat is dissipated when the warm blood flushes into skin capillaries. This is evident when the face becomes flushed and reddened on a hot day or after exercise. When the individual is in a resting state and the air temperature is below 30.6°C (87°F), about two thirds of the body's normal heat loss occurs as a result of conduction, convection, and radiation **(Box 2-8)**. As air temperature approaches skin temperature and exceeds 30.6°C, evaporation becomes the predominant means of heat dissipation.

Relative humidity is the most important factor in determining the effectiveness of evaporative heat loss. Relative humidity (the ratio of water in the ambient air to the total quantity of moisture that can be carried in air at a particular ambient temperature) is expressed in a percentage. For example, 65% relative humidity means that ambient air contains 65% of the air's moisture-carrying capability at the specific temperature. When humidity is high, the ambient vapor pressure approaches that of the

FIELD STATEGY 2.1   MANAGEMENT OF A BEE STING

- After sustaining a bee sting, immediately refrain from strenuous exercise.
- Remove the stinger with a fingernail; it should not be squeezed because this injects more venom.
- Apply ice to the site.
- Use systemic antihistamines to help with local reactions.
- Closely observe the individual for signs of anaphylactic shock, which include the following:
  - Apprehension
  - Paresthesia
  - Choking or signs of laryngeal edema
  - Wheezing, coughing, or difficulty breathing
  - Generalized urticaria or edema
  - Pupillary dilation
- If anaphylaxis occurs, perform the following steps:
  - Activate EMS.
  - Place the athlete supine with the feet elevated.
  - Apply a constriction band that occludes superficial venous and lymphatic return—but does not obstruct arterial flow—a few inches above the sting site.
  - Apply ice to further reduce venom absorption.
  - Check for a medical identification tag.
  - If the person has an EpiPen, inject the epinephrine into the thigh as instructed.
  - If a respiratory or cardiac arrest occurs, begin CPR.
  - Transport immediately to the nearest medical facility.
- Sensitive athletes who participate outdoors should use the following precautions:
  - Refrain from wearing bright, colorful, or floral clothing.
  - Refrain from using scented soaps, lotions, or aftershaves.

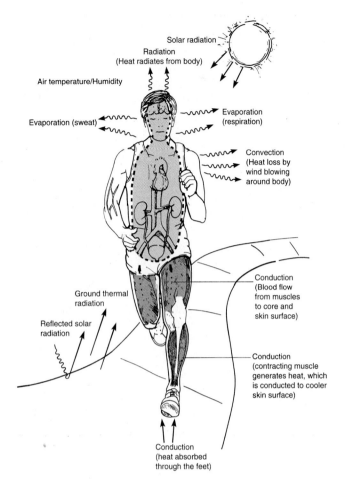

Solar radiation

Radiation
(Heat radiates from body)

Air temperature/Humidity

Evaporation (sweat)

Evaporation
(respiration)

Convection
(Heat loss by
wind blowing
around body)

Ground thermal
radiation

Conduction
(Blood flow
from muscles
to core and
skin surface)

Reflected solar
radiation

Conduction
(contracting muscle
generates heat, which
is conducted to cooler
skin surface)

Conduction
(heat absorbed
through the feet)

➤ FIGURE 2-1. Heat gain and heat loss. Heat produced within working muscles is transferred to the body's core and skin. During exercise, body heat is dissipated into the surrounding environment by radiation, conduction, convection, and evaporation.

moist skin, and evaporation is greatly reduced. Therefore, this avenue for heat loss is closed, even though large quantities of sweat bead on the skin and eventually roll off. This form of sweating represents a useless water loss that can lead to a dangerous state of dehydration, which increases the risk of heat illness. When temperature and relative humidity are combined, the values can be charted on the heat index to determine the risk of potential heat illness **(Fig. 2-2)**.

In addition to heat loss through sweating, a continuous evaporation of water occurs from the lungs, from the mucosa of the mouth, and through the skin. This averages about 350 ml of water as it seeps through the skin every day, and another 300 ml of water vaporized from mucous membranes in the respiratory passages and mouth. The latter is illustrated when you "see your breath" in very cold weather. Sport participants often lose 1.5 to 2.5 L per hour of water during exercise. This translates into a loss of 3 to 6 pounds of body weight per hour. During a 2 to 3 hour practice, an athlete could lose from 6 to 12 pounds of body weight. Although an individual may continually drink water throughout an exercise bout, less than 50% of the fluid lost is replenished.[1]

Therefore, an athlete should drink as much fluid as possible before exercise and before thirst is perceived during exercise. It is also critical to drink beyond the perception of satisfying one's thirst to **hyperhydrate** (overhydrate) the body to prevent voluntary dehydration.

Preventing Heat Emergencies

Several factors can affect one's tolerance to heat. Acclimatization and proper hydration are among the most critical in preventing heat illness.

ACCLIMATIZATION

Exercising moderately during repeated heat exposures can result in physiologic adaptation to a hot environment, which can improve performance and heat tolerance. In general, the major acclimatization occurs during the first week of heat exposure and is complete after 10 days. Only 2 to 4 hours of daily heat exposure are required. The first several sessions should be light and should last about 15 to 20 minutes. Thereafter, the duration and intensity of exercise sessions can progressively increase. Proper hydration is essential for an effective acclimatization process.

FLUID REHYDRATION

The primary objective of fluid replacement is to maintain plasma volume so that circulation and sweating occur at optimal levels. Dehydration progressively decreases plasma volume, peripheral blood flow, sweating, and stroke volume (quantity of blood ejected with each heart beat), and leads to a compensatory increase in heart rate, all of which can decrease physical performance and increase the risk of heat illness. Thirst is not an adequate indicator of water needs during exercise because an individual is already 1% dehydrated when thirst is perceived.[2] Cold liquids, especially water, empty from the stomach and small intestines significantly faster than warm fluids. The gastric emptying rate can be retarded when ingested fluids contain even the smallest traces of salt or simple sugars, whether glucose, fructose, or sucrose.

To prevent dehydration, fluids must be ingested and absorbed by the body **(Box 2-9)**. Running through sprinklers or pouring water over the head may feel cool and satisfying, but it does not prevent dehydration. A standard rule is to drink until thirst is quenched and then drink a few more ounces. An easy method to determine whether athletes are drinking enough fluids is to have them monitor the color and volume of their urine. An average adult's urine amounts to 1.2 quarts in a 24-hour period. Urination of a full bladder usually occurs four times each day. Within 60 minutes of exercise, passing a light-colored urine of normal to above-normal volume indicates adequate hydration. If the urine is dark yellow,

➤ ➤ BOX 2-8

Methods of Heat Exchange

- **Radiation**

  The loss of heat from a warmer object to a cooler object in the form of infrared waves (thermal energy) without physical contact. For example, when temperatures of surrounding objects in the environment, such as the sun or hot artificial turf, exceed skin temperature, radiant heat is absorbed by the body.

- **Conduction**

  The direct transfer of heat through a liquid, solid, or gas from a warm object to a cooler object. For example, a football player can absorb heat through the feet simply by standing on hot artificial turf.

- **Convection**

  Transfer of heat depends on conduction from the skin to the water or air next to it. The effectiveness of heat loss depends on how fast the air (or water) next to the body is exchanged once it becomes warmer. If air movement is slow, air molecules next to the skin are warmed and act as insulation. In contrast, if warmer air molecules are continually replaced by cooler air molecules, as occurs on a breezy day or in a room with a fan, heat loss increases as the air currents carry heat away. In water, the body loses heat more rapidly by convection while swimming than while lying motionless.

- **Evaporation**

  The most effective heat loss mechanism used to cool the body. Sweat evaporates when molecules in the water absorb heat from the environment and become energetic enough to escape as a gas. As core temperature rises during exercise or illness, peripheral blood vessels dilate and sweat glands are stimulated to produce noticeable sweat, which can amount to a loss of 1.5 to 2.5 L of body water in 1 hour. On a hot, dry day, sweating is responsible for more than 80% of heat loss. The total sweat vaporized from the skin depends on three factors:
  - The skin surface exposed to the environment
  - The temperature and relative humidity of the ambient air
  - The convective air currents around the body

---

is of a small volume, and has a strong odor, the athlete needs to continue drinking. However, ingesting vitamin supplements often results in a dark-yellow urine, so urine color, volume, and odor must all be considered when determining hydration status.[1,2]

ELECTROLYTE REPLACEMENT

The minerals sodium, chloride, magnesium, and potassium are called electrolytes because they are dissolved in the body as electrically charged particles called ions. Electrolytes regulate fluid balance, nerve conduction, and muscle contractions. Electrolyte solutions are unnecessary for individuals with normal diets. However, for athletes demanding peak performance in competitions greater than 1 hour or during intense intermittent exercise, carbohydrate drinks may benefit performance.[3] Commercial drinks may be used; however, they should be cooler than ambient temperature (between 15 to 22°C [59 to 72°F]) and should be flavored to enhance palatability. They should also range between 4 to 8% of multiple transportable carbohydrate and contain a small amount of sodium.[3,4] While maintaining hydration, the participant should avoid **diuretics** (substances that promote the excretion of urine) such as excessive amounts of protein, caffeinated drinks (soda, tea, coffee), chocolate, and alcoholic beverages.

➤ FIGURE 2-2. The heat stress index. If the relative humidity and ambient air temperature are known, the heat stress index can be consulted to determine the relative degree of heat stress. From McArdle WD, Katch FI, Katch VL. Exercise Physiology: Energy, Nutrition, and Human Performance. 5th ed. Philadelphia, Lippincott Williams & Wilkins, 2001:630.

CLOTHING

Light-colored, lightweight, porous clothing is preferred to dark, heavyweight, nonporous material. Cottons and linens readily absorb moisture. Evaporative heat loss occurs only when clothing is thoroughly wet and perspiration can evaporate. Changing into a dry shirt simply prolongs the time between sweating and cooling. Heavy sweat suits or rubberized plastic suits produce high relative humidity close to the skin and retard evaporation, severely increasing the risk of heat illness.

Even when football players are wearing only football helmets and loose-fitting, porous jerseys and shorts, 50% of their body surface can be sealed, limiting evaporative cooling. Increased metabolic rate needed to carry the weight of their equipment, as well as increased temperature on artificial surfaces, increase the risk of heat illness. To counter this, football players should initially practice in tee shirts, shorts, and low-cut socks. On hot, humid days, uniforms should not be worn; if possible, shoulder pads and helmets should be removed often to allow for radiation and evaporative cooling. Because much of the body's heat escapes through the head, helmets used in noncontact sports (like cycling or wrestling) should allow for adequate airflow and evaporation.

PRACTICE SCHEDULES

On hot, humid days, reschedule workouts, practices, and competitions to early morning or evening hours to avoid the worst heat of the day (11:00 AM to 3:00 PM). Allow for frequent water breaks (i.e., 10 minutes every half hour), shorten practices, and lessen the exercise intensity. Whenever possible, get the players out of the direct sunlight (shade trees and tents), and remove restrictive equipment (pads and helmets) frequently.

WEIGHT CHARTS

Measuring pre- and post-exercise weight can decrease the risk of heat illness. A rule of thumb is that for every pound of water lost, 24 oz (3 cups) of fluid should be ingested, meaning that 150% of the fluid loss during exercise is replenished.[5] In addition to fluids, carbohydrates should also be ingested within 30 minutes post-exercise, especially those with a high water content (like melons and tomatoes). Even under the best circumstances, 24 hours are needed to fully restore the fluids and muscle glycogen that are used during just 2 hours of strenuous exercise. Before the next exercise period, the athlete should ingest 3.5 to 4.5 g of carbohydrates per pound of body weight each day. Alcohol should be avoided. Lost fluid should be replaced and weight normalized before the next episode of exercise.

Heat Illnesses

If the signs and symptoms of heat stress (thirst, fatigue, lethargy, and visual disturbances) are not addressed, cardiovascular compensation begins to fail, and a series of progressive complications, termed heat illness, can result. The various forms of heat illness, in order of severity, include heat cramps, heat exhaustion, and heat stroke **(Table 2-1)**. Although symptoms often overlap between the conditions, failure to take immediate action can result in severe dehydration and possible death.

HEAT CRAMPS

Heat cramps are painful, involuntary muscle spasms, usually seen in the calf and abdominal muscles, caused by excessive water and electrolyte loss during and after intense exercise in the heat. Predisposing factors include lack of acclimatization, use of diuretics or laxatives, and sodium depletion in the normal diet. The condition can be prevented by ingesting copious amounts of water and increasing the daily intake of salt through a normal diet several days before the period of heat stress. Passive stretching of the involved muscles and ice massage over the affected area is helpful. The athlete should also ingest enough cool fluids that contain an electrolyte solution and drink beyond the point of satisfying his or her thirst. The individual should be watched carefully because this condition may precipitate heat exhaustion or heat stroke.

TABLE 2.1	MANAGEMENT OF HEAT-RELATED CONDITIONS	
Condition	**Signs/Symptoms**	**Treatment**
Heat cramps	Involuntary muscle spasms or cramps; normal pulse and respirations; profuse sweating and dizziness	Rest in cool place; massage cramp with ice and passive stretching; drink cool water with diluted electrolyte solution
Heat exhaustion	Thirst; headache; weakness; confusion; profuse sweating; skin is wet, cool, clammy, and may appear ashen; rapid, shallow breathing; weak pulse	Rest in cool place; remove equipment and clothing; execute rapid cooling of body; sponge or towel with cool water or use fan; discontinue activity until thoroughly recovered and cleared by a physician
Heat stroke	Sweating ceases; irritability progresses to confusion and hysteria; unsteady gait; pulse is rapid and strong; skin is hot, dry, red, or flushed; blood pressure falls; convulsions; seizures; coma	ACTIVATE EMS; rest in cool place; rapidly cool body with ice water immersion or place crushed ice packs on the neck, axilla, and groin; transport immediately to the nearest medical center

HEAT EXHAUSTION

Exercise-induced heat exhaustion is caused by ineffective circulatory adjustments compounded by a depletion of extracellular fluid, especially plasma volume, owing to excessive sweating. The condition usually occurs in unacclimatized individuals during the first few intense exercise sessions on a hot day. Those who wear protective equipment or heavy uniforms are also at greater risk because evaporation through the material may be retarded. Heat exhaustion is a "functional" illness and is not associated with organ damage. Blood pools in the dilated peripheral vessels, which dramatically reduces the central blood volume necessary to maintain cardiac output.

Thirst, headache, dizziness, mild anxiety, fatigue, a weak and rapid pulse (**tachycardia**), and low blood pressure in the upright position are common signs and symptoms. The individual may also appear ashen and gray and have an uncoordinated gait and a small urine output **(Fig. 2-3A)**. Sweating may be reduced if the person is dehydrated, but body temperature generally does not exceed 39.5°C (103°F). The individual should immediately be moved to a cool place, and all equipment and unnecessary clothing should be removed. **Table 2-1** explains the management of heat exhaustion.

HEAT STROKE

Heat stroke is the least common but most serious heat illness. In football, heat stroke is second only to head injuries as the most frequent cause of death. The condition is also seen in dehydrated distance runners and wrestlers. Heat stroke is usually preceded by prolonged strenuous physical exercise in individuals who are poorly acclimatized, or in situations in which evaporation of perspiration is blocked. During exercise, metabolic heat continues to rise. Decreased blood plasma volume causes the heart to beat faster and work harder to pump blood through the circulatory system. The thermoregulatory system is overloaded, and the body's cooling mech-

anisms fail to dissipate the rising core temperature. The hypothalamus shuts down all heat-control mechanisms, including the sweat glands, to conserve water loss. This creates a vicious circle: as temperature increases, the metabolic rate increases, which in turn increases heat production. The skin becomes hot and dry. As the temperature continues to rise, permanent brain damage may occur. Core temperature can rise to 40.6°C (105°F) and has been known to reach 41.7 to 42.2° C (107 to 108°F). If untreated, death is imminent. Mortality is directly related to magnitude and duration of hyperthermia.

The level of mental status impairment differentiates heat stroke from heat exhaustion. Initial symptoms include a feeling of burning up with a moderate level of confusion, disorientation, agitation, profuse sweating, and an unsteady gait. As the condition deteriorates, sweating ceases. The skin is hot and dry, and appears reddened or flushed **(Fig. 2-3B)**. The individual breathes deeply and has dilated pupils (a "glassy" stare). As core temperature rises, the pulse becomes rapid and strong, as high as 150 to 170 beats per minute. The individual may become hysterical or delirious. Tissue damage by excessive body heat leads to vasomotor collapse, shallow breathing, decreased blood pressure, and a rapid and weak pulse. Muscle twitching or seizures may occur just before the individual lapses into a coma.

The on-site emergency responder should immediately activate EMS. Move the athlete to a cool place, remove all equipment and unnecessary clothing, and rapidly cool the body **(Table 2-1)**. The most effective cooling method is ice water immersion.[6] If ice water immersion is not available, other cooling methods should be used. These methods include immersing in cool water; wrapping in cool, wet towels; using fans; and applying crushed ice packs to the neck, axilla, and groin. Fans and cool mist machines, however, have limited use in humid conditions. After the athlete is transported to the nearest medical center, the athlete should not resume physical activity until he or she has returned to the pre-dehydrated state and has been cleared by a physician.

Dizzy

Headache

Profuse sweating

Rapid, shallow breathing

Cool, clammy skin

Ashen or gray skin

Body temperature normal or slightly elevated

Rapid, weak pulse

Uncoordinated gait

A

Disoriented

Unconscious

Initially profuse sweating; no sweat in later stages

Shallow breathing

Hot, dry skin

Reddish skin

Body temperature increased markedly

Rapid, strong pulse

B

➤ **FIGURE 2-3.** Signs and symptoms of heat exhaustion and heat stroke. **A.** Heat exhaustion. **B.** Heat stroke.

COLD-RELATED CONDITIONS

Hypothermia, or reduced body temperature, occurs when the body is unable to maintain a constant core temperature. In cold weather, three primary heat-promoting mechanisms attempt to maintain or increase core temperature. The initial response is cutaneous vasoconstriction to prevent blood from shunting to the skin. Because the skin is insulated with a layer of subcutaneous fat, heat loss is reduced. The second response is to increase metabolic heat production by shivering, which is involuntary contraction of skeletal muscle, or to increase physical activity. During vigorous exercise, skeletal muscles can produce 30 to 40 times the amount of heat produced at rest. During gradual, seasonal changes, more of the hormone thyroxine is released by the thyroid gland, which serves as the third avenue to increase metabolic rate.

Preventing Cold-Related Injuries

During cold weather, body heat is lost through respiration, radiation, conduction, convection, and evaporation. Although the body attempts to generate heat through heat-producing mechanisms, they may be inadequate to main-

tain a constant core temperature. Several steps that can be taken to prevent heat loss are summarized in **Box 2-10**.

Cold Conditions

People tend to adapt less readily to cold than to heat. Even inhabitants of cold regions show only limited evidence of adaptation, such as a higher metabolic rate. Like heat illness, cold injuries range from minor frostbite to the more severe general systemic cooling, or hypothermia, which can be life threatening. Cold emergencies occur in two ways. In one, the core temperature remains relatively constant but the shell temperature decreases. This results in localized injuries from frostbite. The second cold emergency occurs when both core temperature and shell temperature decrease, leading to general body cooling. All body processes slow down and systemic hypothermia results. If left unabated, death is imminent.

FROSTBITE INJURIES

Frostbite is caused by freezing soft tissue, and it is classified on a continuum of three degrees **(Table 2-2)**. In superficial frostbite, the area may feel firm to touch, but

➤ ➤ BOX 2-10

Reducing the Risk of Cold Injuries

- Check weather conditions and consider possible deterioration.
- Identify individuals who may be susceptible to cold and observe closely.
- Dress in several light layers.
- Wear windproof, dry, well-insulated clothing that allows for water evaporation; wool, polypropylene, or polyesters such as Capilene or Thermastat are recommended.
- Carry windproof pants and jacket if conditions warrant; keep your back to the wind.
- Wear well-insulated, windproof mittens, gloves, hats, and scarves.
- Wear well-insulated footwear that keeps feet dry.
- Avoid dehydration. Do not drink alcoholic beverages or snow because these worsen hypothermia.
- Carry nutritious snacks that predominantly contain carbohydrates.
- Eat small amounts of food frequently.
- Do not stand in one position for extended periods. Wiggle your toes and keep moving to bring warm blood to various areas of the body.
- Stay dry by wearing appropriate rain gear or protective clothing. If you get wet, change into dry clothing as soon as possible.
- Breathe through your nose, rather than your mouth, to minimize heat and fluid loss.
- Watch the face, ears, and fingers for signs of frostbite.

the tissue beneath is soft and resilient. The skin initially appears red and swollen, and the individual complains of diffuse numbness that may or may not be preceded by an itchy or prickly sensation. If the frostbite extends into the subcutaneous or deep layers, the skin feels hard because it is actually frozen tissue. The area then turns white with a yellow or blue tint that looks waxy.

A person with superficial frostbite should be removed from the cold and taken indoors immediately and treated with careful, rapid warming of the area. Remove clothing, jewelry, or rings, and immerse the injured area in water heated to 39 to 42°C (102 to 108°F) for 30 to 45 minutes.[7] A whirlpool is ideal, but if this is unavailable, use a basin large enough so the skin does not touch the sides of the container. Hot water may cause burns and should be avoided. When the part is com-

pletely rewarmed, the affected area should be dried and a sterile dressing applied to the injured area. If fingers or toes are involved, sterile dressings should be placed between the digits before covering. The entire area can be covered with towels or a blanket to keep it warm, and the individual should be transported to the nearest medical center with the affected limb slightly elevated. Deep frostbite is best rewarmed under controlled conditions in a hospital. EMS should be activated to transport the individual.

SYSTEMIC BODY COOLING (HYPOTHERMIA)

Hypothermia is a danger to athletes exposed to cold for long periods, such as long distance runners and Nordic ski racers, especially those who are slowing down late in a race because of fatigue or injury. Any injured or ill athlete who has been exposed to cold weather or cold water, however, is suspected of having hypothermia until proven otherwise.

Exposed surfaces on the hands, face, head, and neck lose most of the body heat through radiation. Air movement coupled with cold produces a wind chill factor that causes heat loss from the body much faster than in still air. The faster the wind, the higher the wind chill factor (Fig. 2-4).

When core temperature falls below 34.4°C (94°F), essential biochemical processes begin to slow. Heart and respiration rates slow, cardiac output and blood pressure fall, and, as the skin and muscles cool, shivering increases violently. Numbness sets in, and even the simplest task becomes difficult to perform. If core temperature continues to drop below 32°C (90°F), shivering ceases and muscles become cold and stiff. **Cold diuresis** (polyuria) occurs as blood is shunted away from the shell to the core in an effort to maintain vascular volume. This leads to excessive excretion of urine by the kidneys. If intervention is not initiated, death is imminent.

In mild hypothermia, the individual is still shivering. The individual may appear clumsy, apathetic, or confused and may slur speech, stumble, and drop things. In more severe cases, an individual does not feel any sensation or pain, and shivering ceases to occur. Movements become jerky, and the individual becomes unaware of his or her surroundings.

With mild hypothermia, EMS should be activated immediately while the individual is carefully moved into a warm shelter. Rewarming of the individual can be

TABLE 2.2	SIGNS AND SYMPTOMS OF FROSTBITE
First degree:	Skin is soft to touch and appears initially red, then white, and is usually painless. The condition is typically noticed by others first.
Second degree:	Skin is firm to touch, but tissue beneath is soft and appears initially red and swollen. Diffuse numbness may be preceded by an itchy or prickly sensation. White or waxy skin color may appear later.
Third degree:	Skin is hard to touch and totally numb, and appears blotchy white to yellow-gray or blue-gray.

Ambient temperature, °F															
40	35	30	25	20	15	10	5	0	-5	-10	-15	-20	-25	-30	
Equivalent temperature, °F															
Calm															Calm
40	35	30	25	20	15	10	5	0	-5	-10	-15	-20	-25	-30	Calm
37	33	27	21	16	12	6	1	-5	-11	-15	-20	-26	-31	-35	5
28	21	16	9	4	-2	-9	-15	-21	-27	-33	-38	-46	-52	-58	10
22	16	11	1	-5	-11	-18	-25	-36	-40	-45	-51	-58	-65	-70	15
18	12	3	-4	-10	-17	-25	-32	-39	-46	-53	-60	-67	-76	-81	20
16	7	0	-7	-15	-22	-29	-37	-44	-52	-59	-67	-74	-83	-89	25
13	5	-2	-11	-18	-26	-33	-41	-48	-56	-63	-70	-79	-87	-94	30
11	3	-4	-13	-20	-27	-43	-49	-60	-67	-72	-82	-90	-98		35
10	1	-6	-15	-21	-29	-37	-45	-53	-62	-69	-76	-85	-94	-101	40**

■ Little danger   ■ Danger   ■ Great danger

* °C = 0.556 (°F −32)
** Convective heat loss at wind speeds above 40 mph has little additional effect on body cooling

➤ **FIGURE 2-4.** Wind chill index. From McArdle WD, Katch FI, Katch VL. Exercise physiology: Energy, Nutrition, and Human Performance. 5th ed. Philadelphia: Lippincott Williams & Wilkins, 2001:649.

accomplished by allowing him or her to shiver until warm inside a sleeping bag, or by using external rewarming devices such as hot water bottles or heating pads. Hot tubs can be used if available. The water should be approximately 43°C (110°F).[7] Hot (preferably noncaffeinated) drinks may be useful after the individual is partly rewarmed and able to swallow. The individual should continue to be rewarmed en route to the nearest medical facility.

EXERCISING IN THUNDERSTORMS

An environmental, and seldom discussed, threat is participating under inclement weather conditions where rain, lightning, and thunderstorms are present. Most organized outdoor sport practices and competitions are held between 3 and 9 PM, peak periods for the development of thunderstorms and lightning.

Injuries Due to Lightning

Lightning poses a triple threat of injury: burns from the high temperature of the lightning strike; injury caused by the elicited mechanical forces activated by the intense levels of electricity (electromechanical forces); and resulting concussive forces that can propel objects through the air, causing blunt trauma (e.g., fracture, concussion). The most common condition associated with a lightning strike is **cardiac asystole** (cardiac standstill) and respiratory arrest. Fortunately, the heart is likely to spontaneously restart if the victim is not experiencing respiratory arrest. Surprisingly the most critical factor in determining morbidity and mortality associated with a lightning strike is the duration of **apnea** (cessation of breathing) rather than cardiac asystole. It is common for

a person to become unconscious, confused, or to develop amnesia after a lightning strike.

If the person is conscious and has normal cardiorespiratory function, a secondary assessment should be conducted to determine whether the individual has sustained burns, fractures, or other trauma. If the individual is not breathing and is in cardiac arrest, activate EMS and begin immediate rescue breathing and CPR. Unless ruled out, always suspect a cervical spine injury and treat accordingly. Any person struck by lightning should immediately be transported to the nearest medical facility.

Lightning Safety Policy

As discussed earlier, most organized outdoor sport practices and competitions are conducted between the hours of 3 and 9 PM, when the risk of thunderstorms is greatest— 70% of all lightning injuries and fatalities occur in the afternoon.[8] Thunderstorms can become threatening within 30 minutes of the first sign of thunder. All coaches, athletic trainers, athletic directors, athletic supervisors, managers, and athletes should understand how thunderstorms develop and why lightning strikes. The organization or institution should develop a policy that can be implemented when conditions are favorable for thunderstorm and lightning activity. This lightning safety policy can decrease the risk of injury and death and can protect the organization or institution from litigation if the policy is referred to and heeded **(Box 2-11)**.

PRIMARY INJURY ASSESSMENT

Occasionally, collisions occur in sport activities and more than one player is injured. **Triage** refers to assessing all injured individuals quickly, then returning to and treating the most seriously injured person immediately. The primary survey should establish the level of unresponsiveness and initiate or maintain adequate breathing and circulation until help arrives. Assessment of all injuries, no matter how minor, should always include a primary assessment. In most cases, this assessment is completed quickly when approaching injured people and observing them moving or talking. As such, one can proceed immediately to the secondary injury assessment. However, if the person is not moving or is unresponsive, initiate the primary survey. Students should enroll in an appropriate class sponsored by the American Red Cross, National Safety Council, or American Heart Association to receive CPR training. It is assumed that all students using this textbook have completed such a certification.

When approaching the individual, the emergency responder should check the surrounding area to see whether any equipment or apparatus may have contributed to the injury. Unless a possible spinal injury has been ruled out, always assume that one is present and stabilize the head and neck before proceeding. The

➤ ➤ **BOX 2-11**

Lightning Safety Policy for All Outdoor Activities Including Swimming

1. Formalize a lightning-safety emergency action plan that includes:
   - Identifying a designated weather watcher (i.e., person who monitors local weather forecasts, looks for signs of threatening weather, and notifies Command Captain [see next bullet] if situation is dangerous)
   - Identifying Command Captain who determines when individuals should be removed from the activity area
   - Identifying safe locations from lightning (for each activity area or site)
   - Creating specific criteria for suspension and resumption of activities (refer to #4, 5, and 6).
   - Identifying recommended lightning safe-strategies (refer to #7, 8, and 9).

2. Identify safe locations inside buildings. The electric and telephone wiring and plumbing aid in grounding a building. However, it is important to not be connected to these pathways while inside the structure during thunderstorms.

3. Identify secondary sources of safety (i.e., inside a vehicle with a metal roof with the windows closed). Convertible cars and golf carts are not acceptable.

4. Know how close the storm is to your location. Using the "flash-to-bang method," count the seconds between seeing a lightning flash and hearing the thunder. Divide this number by 5 (light travels approximately five times as fast as sound). This number indicates how many miles away the storm is from you. If the lightning (flash) to thunder (bang) is within thirty seconds, all outdoor activities should end, and all participants should seek shelter.

5. Postpone or suspend activity if a thunderstorm appears imminent (regardless of whether lightning is seen or thunder heard).

6. Allow 30 minutes to pass after the last sound of thunder or flash of lightning before resuming outdoor activities.

7. With extremely large athletic events, plan ahead to determine safe strategies and safe locations.

8. Avoid being near the highest point of an open field or in open water. Stay away from tall or individual trees, lone objects (poles), metal objects, standing pools of water, and open fields.

9. Avoid taking showers and using plumbing facilities (including indoor and outdoor pools) and land-line telephones. Cordless or cellular telephones are safer to use but should only be used for emergency use.

10. If you feel your hair stand on end or your skin tingle, immediately assume the lightning safe position (i.e., crouched position with only the feet in contact with ground, wrapping your arms around your knees and lowering your head to minimize body surface area; do not lie flat on the ground).

11. Follow basic first aid procedures when managing victims of a lightning strike.

12. If an individual is suspected of being struck by lightning, survey the scene for safety. Ongoing thunderstorms still pose a threat. Then perform the following steps:
    - Activate EMS
    - Move the victim carefully to a safe location, if needed.
    - Assess breathing and circulation. Treat for apnea and cardiac asystole.
    - Assess and treat for hypothermia and shock.
    - Assess and treat for possible fractures.
    - Assess and treat any burns.

13. All persons employed by the athletic/activity center should maintain current cardiopulmonary resuscitation (CPR) and first aid certification.

14. All individuals should have the right to leave an athletic site or activity, without fear of repercussion or penalty, to seek a safe structure or location if they believe they are in danger from impending lightning activity.

Adapted from Walsh KM, et. al. 2000. National Athletic Trainers' Association position statement: Lightning safety for athletics and recreation. J Ath Train, 35(4):472.

National Athletic Trainers' Association (NATA) recommends not removing athletic helmets unless individual circumstances dictate otherwise.[10] With the helmet on, the level of consciousness can still be determined, and most injuries are clearly visible. One can still perform neurologic tests, examine the eyes for movement or reactivity to light, and check the nose and ears for fluid. The helmet and shoulder pads elevate the supine athlete. If helmet and shoulder pad removal is required, a coordinated effort must be made to avoid cervical hyperextension.

SECONDARY INJURY ASSESSMENT

A secondary injury assessment involves a detailed, hands-on, head-to-toe assessment to detect conditions that may not pose an immediate threat to life but, if left unrecognized and untreated, could lead to serious complications. If the individual is moving and speaking or if the individual is unconscious and ABCs are adequate, begin the secondary injury assessment. In nearly all cases, an individual will regain consciousness in a short period and can then respond to questions. A popular methodical process used extensively in basic sports injury care is the **HOPS** format. HOPS is an acronym for:

History of the injury

Observation and inspection

Palpation

Special tests

The HOPS format uses both subjective information (history of the injury) and objective information (observation and inspection, palpation, and special tests) to recognize and identify problems contributing to the condition. In emergencies, HOPS assessment includes an overall scan of the entire body. In a nonemergency sport injury, HOPS assessment focuses on a specific injury or condition.

History of the Injury

An accurate history of the injury can help determine the extent and seriousness of injury. The individual's response, or lack of response, to verbal commands can also determine the level of consciousness. In a semiconscious or unconscious individual, information can be gathered from other players, officials, or bystanders. Remember, however, that an individual who is not fully responsive may have a head or neck injury. As such, stabilization of the head and neck must be maintained throughout the entire secondary survey. Ask the conscious individual to describe his/her perception of the problem, including the primary injury, how it happened, site and severity of pain, and any weakness or change of sensation that may have resulted from the injury.

Position yourself close to the individual and speak in a calm, confident manner. Tell the individual not to move the head or neck for any reason. Reassure the individual that you are there to help. Questions should be open-ended to allow the person to provide as much information as possible about his or her perception of the problem. Listen attentively for clues that may indicate the nature of the injury. Do not lead the individual. Let him or her describe what happened. Be professional and reassuring. **Field Strategy 2-2** lists several questions to determine a history of the injury.

Observation

In approaching the individual, observe any noticeable deformities that may indicate a possible fracture or dislocation. Is the individual breathing normally or in respiratory distress? Can the individual focus on your face and respond to commands? Is the person alert, restless, lethargic, or nonresponsive? Does he or she moan, groan, or mumble? Do the pupils of the eyes appear normal or dilated? Dilated pupils indicate shock, hemorrhage, cardiac arrest, coma, or death. Is there redness, bruising, or discoloration in the facial area or behind the ears? Note any clear fluid or bloody discharge from the ears or nose, which could be cerebrospinal fluid leaking from the cranial area because of a skull fracture. Is there visible swelling or deformity in the muscle or joint? Always do bilateral comparison whenever possible.

Because vision and eye movement are directly linked to brain function, an eye test can indicate whether the brain has been injured, as in a concussion. To test vision and eye movement, ask the individual to maintain his or her head in a fixed position and ask how many fingers you are holding up. If the individual is unable to see clearly, it is called **diplopia**, or double vision. This condition occurs when the external eye muscles do not work in a coordinated manner. Next, ask the individual to watch your fingers move to various positions. Move the fingers up and down and side to side. Watch the tracking of the eyes. Do they move smoothly and together? Test the individual's depth perception by placing a finger several inches in front of the individual and ask the person to reach out and touch the finger. Move the finger to several different locations and repeat the touch.

Palpation

Palpation involves using the pads of the fingers in small circular or side-to-side motions to detect anomalies in bony and soft tissue structures, such as skin temperature, swelling, point tenderness, **crepitus**, deformity, muscle spasm, and sensation. Palpation begins at the head and moves methodically down to the feet. **Field Strategy 2-3** lists the process commonly used in a head-to-toe assessment.

Palpation of soft tissues can detect deformity, such as an indentation, that may indicate a rupture in a musculotendinous unit. A protruding, firm bulge may indicate a joint dislocation, ruptured bursa, or **hematoma** (mass of encapsulated clotted blood). Swelling may indicate diffuse hemorrhage or inflammation in a muscle, ligament, bursa, or joint capsule. Note where point tenderness is elicited because it may indicate the injured structure.

Possible fractures can be detected with palpation, percussion, vibration, compression, and distraction **(see Fig. 4-12)**. Palpation can detect deformity, crepitus, swelling, or increased pain at the suspected fracture site. Percussion uses a tapping motion of the finger over a bony structure. For example, if an upper arm (humerus) fracture is suspected, tap lightly on the inside bony prominence at the elbow (medial epicondyle of the humerus). If the athlete reports pain in a specific region on the humerus, suspect a possible fracture. Compression is performed by gently compressing the distal end

FIELD STATEGY 2.2 DETERMINING THE HISTORY OF INJURY AND LEVEL OF CONSCIOUSNESS

Stabilize the head and neck; there may be a spinal injury!

If unconscious:

• Call the athlete's name loudly and gently touch the arm. If the athlete does not respond, pinch the soft tissue in the armpit and note any withdrawal from the painful stimuli. If no response, immediately initiate the primary survey.

• If ABCs are adequate, proceed to the secondary survey. If you did not see what happened, question other players, officials, and bystanders. Ask the following questions:

 • What happened?

 • Did you see the individual get hit or did he/she just collapse?

 • How long has the individual been unconscious? Was it immediate or gradual? If gradual, did anyone talk to the individual before you arrived? What did the person say? Was it coherent? Did the person moan, groan, or mumble?

 • Has this ever happened before to this individual?

If conscious, ask the athlete the following questions:

• What happened? (If the athlete is lying down, find out whether he or she was knocked down, fell, or rolled voluntarily into that position.)

• Did you hear any sounds or any unusual sensations when the injury occurred? Are you alert and aware of your surroundings? Is there any short- or long-term memory loss?

• Do you have a headache? Where is the pain? Can you point to the area? Is the pain getting worse or better? (If there is more than one painful area, ask which area hurts the most.)

• Can you describe the pain? Is it localized or does it radiate into other areas?

• Have you ever injured this body part before, or experienced a similar injury? When did this happen?

• How are you feeling now? Are you nauseous or sick to your stomach? Are you dizzy? Can you see clearly?

• Are you taking any medication (e.g., prescription, over-the-counter, vitamins, birth control pills)?

• Are you allergic to anything?

of the bone toward the proximal end, or by encircling the body part, such as a foot or hand, and gently squeezing, thereby compressing the heads of the bones together. Again, if a fracture is present, pain will increase at the suspected fracture site. Distraction employs a tensile force, whereby the application of traction to both ends of the fractured bone helps to relieve pain.

To determine whether any major nerve damage has occurred, run your fingernails along both sides of the arms and legs, and ask the athlete if it feels the same on both sides of the body part. Pain perception can also be tested by applying a sharp and dull point to the skin. Note whether the athlete can distinguish the difference.

Special Tests

In an emergency, special tests are usually limited to determining whether a spinal injury is present. This can be assessed by the athlete's response to verbal and motor commands. In a semiconscious or conscious athlete, the inability to move a body part may indicate seri-ous nerve damage to the central nervous system. Although initial assessment of unresponsiveness is completed in the primary survey, further assessment of muscular movement should be completed before moving the individual.

When evaluating muscle movement, avoid any unnecessary movement of the athlete. Ask the athlete to wiggle the fingers and toes on both hands and feet. If this task is completed, place your fingers in both of the athlete's hands and ask the person to squeeze the fingers. Compare grip strength in both hands. Then have the athlete move both feet and compare bilateral strength.

In an unconscious individual, a verbal or motor response is not possible. Painful stimulation, however, may produce a reaction movement. For example, pinching the soft tissue in the person's armpit may produce an eyelid flutter or involuntary movement away from the stimulus. Lack of a reaction indicates either a serious head or neck injury or a coma. This individual should not be moved until emergency personnel arrive. Monitor the ABCs, and treat for shock.

FIELD STATEGY 2.3   PROTOCOL FOR HEAD-TO-TOE PALPATION

- Stabilize the head and neck until a spinal injury is ruled out. While conducting the examination, do not move the limbs or change body position.
- Palpate the scalp and facial area for lacerations, deformities, or depressions. Discoloration over the mastoid process behind the ear (Battle's sign) or around the eyes (raccoon eyes), or presence of blood or cerebrospinal fluid from the ears or nose, may indicate a skull fracture.
- Check the eyes for any injury, presence of contact lenses, pupil size, and response to light. Both pupils may appear slightly dilated in an unconscious athlete. If the individual is conscious, check eye movement and vision.
- Check the mouth for a mouthguard, dentures, broken teeth, or blood that may have caused or could cause a possible airway obstruction. Sniff for any odd breath odor, such as a fruity smell (diabetic coma) or alcohol.
- Palpate the cervical spine for point tenderness or obvious deformity. Check the anterior neck for indications of impact or bruising.
- Inspect and palpate the chest for possible wounds, discoloration, deformities, and chest expansion upon breathing. With a conscious athlete, use sternal or lateral rib compression to determine a possible rib fracture.
- Inspect and palpate the abdomen for tenderness, rigidity, distention, spasms, or pulsations. Palpate the lower back for deformity and point tenderness.
- Inspect and palpate the upper extremities for deformity, point tenderness, swelling, muscle spasm, and discoloration. Touch the fingers and ask if the athlete can feel it. Does it feel the same on both hands? Can the athlete move the fingers and squeeze your hand? Is there bilateral grip strength?
- Inspect and palpate the pelvis and lower extremities for deformity, point tenderness, swelling, muscle spasms, and discoloration. Squeeze the gastrocnemius and pinch the top of the foot. Touch the toes and ask if the athlete can feel it. Does it feel the same on both feet? Have the athlete wiggle the toes and move the feet.
- Recheck pulse and breathing rate every 2 to 5 minutes until the ambulance arrives.
- Remember: Do no harm to the individual. If in doubt, assume the worst and treat accordingly.

DETERMINATION OF FINDINGS

After completing the secondary assessment, a decision must be made on how best to handle the situation. If EMS has already been activated, control hemorrhage, splint suspected fractures, treat for shock, and wait for the ambulance to arrive before moving the individual. An individual should be referred to the nearest trauma center if any life-threatening situation is present or if any loss of normal function occurs. Conditions that warrant activation of EMS and referral to a physician are listed in **Box 2-12**. If in doubt, always refer.

Summary

1. An emergency medical services (EMS) system is a well-developed process that jointly activates the emergency health care services of the sport facility and community to provide immediate health care to injured individuals.
2. On an annual basis, the facility and staff charged with providing emergency sports injury care to the

physically active should meet with representatives from local EMS agencies to discuss, develop, and evaluate the emergency procedures plan.
3. If an injury occurs at a sport or fitness facility, the most medically qualified individual should:
   - Assess any life-threatening condition
   - Determine whether EMS should be summoned
   - Supervise the management and stabilization of the injured party until the ambulance arrives
4. Once on the scene, EMTs or paramedics assume the major responsibility of care and will:
   - Conduct a more detailed assessment of the injury
   - Take vital signs
   - Provide additional care, as needed
   - Secure and immobilize the injured party onto an appropriate stretcher
   - Transport the individual to the nearest medical facility for advanced care
5. Emergency situations include an obstructed airway, cardiopulmonary emergencies, an unconscious athlete, serious hemorrhage, fractures, shock, anaphylaxis, hyperthermia, or hypothermia.

➤ ➤ BOX 2-12

Emergency Conditions That Should Be Referred to the Nearest Trauma Center or Physician

MEDICAL EMERGENCIES THAT REQUIRE ACTIVATION OF EMS (911)

- Respiratory arrest or any irregularity in breathing
- Severe chest or abdominal pains
- Excessive bleeding from a major artery or a significant loss of blood
- Suspected spinal injury
- Head injury with loss of consciousness
- Open fractures and fractures involving the femur, pelvis, or several ribs
- Joint fracture or dislocation with no distal pulse
- Severe signs of shock or possible internal hemorrhage
- Suspected hyperthermia or hypothermia

INJURIES THAT REQUIRE IMMEDIATE REFERRAL TO A PHYSICIAN

- Eye injuries
- Dental injuries when a tooth has been knocked loose or knocked out
- Minor or simple fractures
- Lacerations that may require suturing
- Injuries with a noticeable functional deficit
- Loss of normal sensation; diminished or absent reflexes
- Noticeable muscular weakness in the extremities
- Any injury about which you may have doubts regarding the severity or nature of the injury

6. Cardiac arrest may result from strenuous physical activity in a dehydrated state, direct trauma, electrical shock, excessive alcohol or other chemical substance abuse, suffocation, drowning, or heart anomalies. Cardiac anomalies are the most direct cause of sudden death in athletes. Hypertrophic cardiomyopathy is the most common cause of death in athletes younger than 30 years old.

7. An athlete in shock is best treated by maintaining body heat by keeping the athlete warm and by elevating the feet and legs 8 to 12 inches.

8. The body generates heat via cutaneous vasoconstriction and by increasing the metabolic heat production by shivering or physical activity. The body also generates heat through the hormone thyroxine during gradual, seasonal changes. The body loses heat through respiration, radiation, conduction, convection, and evaporation.

9. Acclimatization and proper hydration are critical for preventing heat illness. Minerals lost through sweating generally can be replaced through the diet. With prolonged exercise, a small amount of electrolytes added to a rehydration beverage replaces fluids more effectively than drinking plain water.

10. Heat cramps are caused by excessive water and electrolyte loss during and after intense exercise in the heat. Treatment involves passive stretching of the involved muscles and ice massage over the affected area.

11. Heat exhaustion is a functional illness and is not associated with organ damage. Treatment involves moving the individual to a cool place and rapidly cooling the body.

12. Heat stroke signifies significant elevated core temperature and dehydration. Immediately activate EMS because the athlete may require airway management, intravenous fluids, and, in severe cases, circulatory support. While waiting for EMS to arrive, move the athlete to a cool place and try to rapidly cool the body.

13. Frostbite occurs when the core temperature remains relatively constant but the shell temperature decreases. Hypothermia occurs when both core and shell temperatures decrease, leading to general body cooling.

14. An individual struck by lightning can receive multiple injuries, including burns from the high temperature of the lightning strike; injuries from the elicited mechanical forces activated by the intense levels of electricity; and direct trauma injuries from the concussive forces that can propel objects in the air.

15. Assessment of all injuries, no matter how minor, should always include a primary injury assessment. Primary injury assessment determines unresponsiveness and assesses the ABCs. The secondary survey includes a hands-on, head-to-toe assessment to detect medical and injury-related problems that do not pose an immediate life-threatening situation, but may do so if left untreated.

16. The HOPS format uses both subjective information (history of the injury) and objective information (observation and inspection, palpation, and special tests) to recognize and identify problems contributing to the condition.

17. As a rule, refer an individual to the nearest trauma center if any life-threatening situation is present or if the injury results in loss of normal function.

References

1. Murray R. 1996. Dehydration, hyperthermia, and athletes. Science and practice. J Ath Train, 31(3):248-252.
2. Granjean AC, and Reimers KJ. "Sports nutrition." In *The team physician's hand book*, edited by MB Mellion, WM Walsh, and GL Shelton. Philadelphia: Hanley & Belfus, 1997.
3. Shi X, and Gisolfi CV. 1998. Fluid and carbohydrate replacement during intermittent exercise. Sports Med, 25(3):157-172.
4. American College of Sports Medicine. 1996. Position Stand on Exercise and Fluid Replacement. Med Sci Sports Exerc, 28(1):i-vii.
5. Gatorade Sports Science Institute. *Dehydration & heat injuries: Identification, treatment, and prevention.* Chicago: Gatorade, 1997.
6. Armstrong LE, et al. 1996. Whole-body cooling of hyperthermic runners: comparison of two field therapies. Am J Emerg Med, 14(4):355-358.

7. Bowman WD. Safe exercise in the cold and cold injuries. In *The team physician's hand book*, edited by MB Mellion, WM Walsh, and GL Shelton. Philadelphia: Hanley & Belfus, 1997.

8. Uman MA. *All about lightning*. New York: Dover Publications, 1996.

9. Walsh KM, et. al. 2000. National Athletic Trainers' Association position statement: Lightning safety for athletics and recreation. J Ath Train, 35(4):471-477.

10. National Athletic Trainers' Association. *Position stand: Helmet removal guidelines*. Dallas: National Athletic Trainers' Association, 1998.

3

The Sports Injury Process

OBJECTIVES

1. Define compression, tension, shear, and stress, and explain how each can play a role in injury to biological tissues.

2. Describe the process of acute inflammation after injury.

3. Identify how a soft tissue wound repairs itself through the proliferative and maturation phases of tissue healing.

Participation in sport eventually leads to some type of sport-related injury. These injuries may be caused by direct trauma from collisions with another player or object; by overuse; or by abnormal twisting motions that lead to joint sprains, strains, or fractures. Regardless of the sport environment, athletes often ask their coach or fitness instructor questions about possible injuries. It is not the intent of this book to educate coaches and fitness instructors on how to evaluate and assess sports injuries. This task is in the domain of certified athletic trainers and physicians. However, in the absence of a certified athletic trainer, the coach or fitness instructor may be the only individual who has daily contact with an injured athlete. It is essential that coaches and fitness instructors have a basic understanding of how injuries occur and how they heal. Therefore, this chapter first discusses the forces that may lead to injury (mechanism of injury). Understanding how the injury occurred discloses what tissues may be injured and can facilitate the immediate care provided to the injured athlete. Next, the chapter discusses the processes by which injured tissues heal.

MECHANISMS OF INJURY

How an injury occurs is referred to as the mechanism of injury. Determining how an injury occurs is complicated by several factors. First, forces are applied to the body at different angles, over different surface areas, and over different periods of time. Second, the human body is composed of many different types of tissue that respond differently to applied forces. Finally, injury to the human body is not an all-or-none phenomenon. That is, injuries range from mild to moderate to severe.

Injury is caused by an abnormal force. Force is a push or pull acting on a body. During sport participation, athletes can apply a force to a ball, bat, racquet, or club. Conversely, athletes can absorb forces from impact with a ball, the ground or floor, or an opponent. Force is commonly categorized according to the direction from which the force acts on the affected structure. Force acting along the long axis of a structure is called **axial force**. When the opponent in fencing is touched with the foil, the foil is loaded axially. When the human body is in an upright standing position, body weight creates axial loads on the femur and the tibia, the major weight-bearing bones of the lower extremity.

Axial loading that produces a squeezing or crushing effect is called **compressive force** or compression **(Fig. 3-1)**. When a football player is sandwiched between two tacklers, the force acting on the player is compressive. Compressive forces sustained during contact sports often result in bruises or contusions if padding is insufficient.

Axial loading in the direction opposite that of compression is called **tensile force**, or tension **(Fig. 3-1)**. Tension is a pulling force that stretches the object to which it is applied. Muscle contraction produces tensile force on the attached bone, enabling movement of that bone. When the foot and ankle are inverted or rotated excessively, the tensile forces applied to the ligaments may result in an ankle sprain.

Compressive and tensile forces are directed toward and away from an object. A third category of force, termed shear, acts parallel or tangent to a plane passing through the object **(Fig. 3-1)**. **Shear force** tends to cause one part of the object to slide against, displace, or shear with another part of the object. Shear forces acting on the spine can cause spondylolisthesis, a condition involving anterior slippage of a vertebra with the vertebra below it.

When force is sustained by the human body, another important factor related to the likelihood of injury is the magnitude of the **stress** produced by that force. When a given force is distributed over a large area, the resulting stress is less than if the force were distrib-

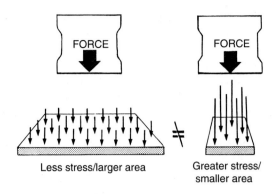

➤ **FIGURE 3-2.** Stress over a surface area. The stress produced by a force depends on the area over which the force is spread. When a given force is distributed over a large area, the resulting stress is less than if the same force were distributed over a smaller area.

uted over a smaller area **(Fig. 3-2)**. Alternatively, if a force is concentrated over a small area, the stress is relatively high. A high magnitude of stress, rather than a high magnitude of force, usually results in injury to biological tissues. One of the reasons that football and ice hockey players wear pads is that a pad distributes any force sustained across the entire pad, thereby reducing the stress acting on the player.

Injuries can result from a single traumatic force of relatively large magnitude or from repeated forces of relatively small magnitude. When a single force produces an injury, the injury is called an **acute injury**, and the causative force is termed macrotrauma. An acute injury, such as a ruptured anterior cruciate ligament or a fractured humerus, is characterized by a definitive moment of onset followed by a relatively predictable process of healing. When repeated or chronic loading over time produces an injury, the injury is called a **chronic injury** or a stress injury, and the causative mechanism is termed microtrauma. A chronic injury, such as a stress fracture, develops and worsens gradually over time, typically culminating in a threshold episode in which pain and inflammation become evident. Chronic injuries can persist for months or years.

THE HEALING PROCESS

When an injury damages tissue, the human body reacts rapidly in a predictable sequence of physiologic actions designed to repair the injured tissues. Healing of damaged tissues is a three-phase process involving acute inflammation, proliferation, and maturation.

Acute Inflammatory Phase (0–6 days)

When injury occurs, the body's response to trauma is called **inflammation**, commonly referred to as swelling. Although inflammation can be produced in response to chemical, thermal, and infectious agents, the focus here

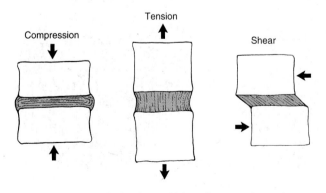

➤ **FIGURE 3-1.** Mechanisms of injury. Compression and tension are directed along the longitudinal axis of a structure, whereas shear acts parallel to a surface.

is on the inflammatory response after injury. Depending on the nature of the causative forces, inflammation can be acute or chronic. An acute inflammatory response is relatively brief and involves the creation of **exudate**, a plasmalike fluid that exudes out of tissue or its capillaries and is composed of protein and granular leukocytes (white blood cells). A chronic inflammatory response, alternatively, is prolonged and is characterized by nongranular leukocytes and the production of scar tissue.

The beginning of the acute inflammatory phase involves the activation of three mechanisms that act to stop blood loss from the wound. First, blood flow is reduced through local **vasoconstriction**, lasting from a few seconds to as long as 10 minutes. The resulting reduction in blood flow volume in the region promotes increased blood viscosity or resistance to the flow, which further reduces blood loss at the injury site. A second response to the loss of blood is the platelet reaction **(Fig. 3-3)**. The platelet reaction causes clotting as individual cells irreversibly combine with each other and with fibrin produced by the coagulation cascade, which is the result of the third response to trauma. When combined, a mechanical plug is formed that occludes the end of a ruptured blood vessel. The platelets also produce an array of chemical mediators that play significant roles in the inflammatory and proliferation phases of healing.

After vasoconstriction, **vasodilation**, or an increase in blood flow, occurs. One process activated during this phase is the attraction of neutrophils and macrophages to rid the injury site of debris and infectious agents through **phagocytosis (Fig. 3-4)**. As blood flow to the injured area slows, these cells are redistributed to the periphery, where they begin to adhere to the endothelial lining. **Mast cells** are connective tissue cells that carry **heparin**, which prolongs clotting; **histamine**, which promotes further vasodilation; and **bradykinin**, which promotes vasodilation, increases blood vessel wall permeability, and stimulates nerve endings to cause pain.

The increased blood flow to the region causes swelling or **edema**. Blood from the broken vessels and damaged tissues forms a **hematoma** that, combined with necrotic tissue, forms the **zone of primary injury**. Approximately 1 hour post-injury, as the vascular walls become more permeable and increased pressure within the vessels forces a plasma exudate out into the interstitial tissues (between the cells), swelling increases **(Fig. 3-4)**. This increased permeability of the blood vessel walls typically exists for only a few minutes in cases of mild trauma. Normal permeability usually returns in 20 to 30 minutes. More severe trauma can result in a prolonged state of increased permeability and sometimes result in delayed onset of increased permeability; swelling is not apparent until some time has elapsed since the original injury. The tissue exudate provides a critically important part of the body's defense, both by diluting toxins present in the wound and by enabling delivery of the cells that remove damaged tissue and enable reconstruction.

As the body continues to react to the inflammatory process, reparative cells in the exudate arrive at the injury site. Platelets and basophil leukocytes release enzymes that interact with other chemicals in the cell membranes to produce chemical mediators. These mediators include **prostaglandins** and leukotrienes, which attract leukocytes to the damaged area. This chain of chemical activity produces the **zone of secondary injury**, which includes all of the tissues affected by inflammation, edema, and hypoxia. After the debris and waste products from the damaged tissues are ingested through phagocytosis, the leukocytes reenter the blood stream, and the acute inflammatory reaction subsides.

The Proliferative Phase (3–21 days)

The proliferative phase involves repair and regeneration of the injured tissue. This phase takes place from approximately 3 days after the injury through the next 3 to 6

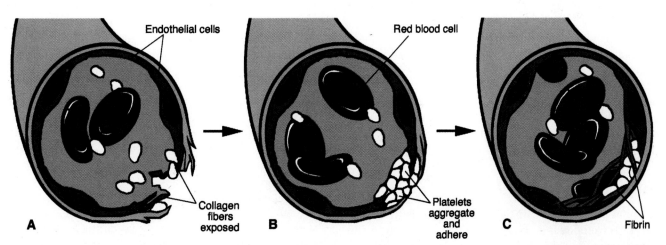

➤ FIGURE 3-3. Blood clotting mechanism. **A.** When injury occurs to a blood vessel, collagen fibers in the inner lining are exposed. **B.** As a result, the platelet reaction causes platelets to move to the area and combine with each other. **C.** As fibrin in the blood plasma combines with the platelets, a mechanical plug is formed to occlude the end of a ruptured blood vessel.

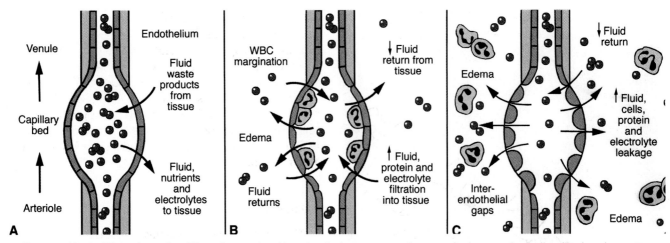

➤ F IGURE 3 - 4 . Edema formation. Edema forms when histochemical agents open the pores in the vascular walls, allowing plasma to migrate into the interstitial space between the cells. WBC—white blood cell.

weeks, overlapping the later part of the inflammatory phase. The proliferative processes include the development of new blood vessels (angiogenesis), the process of fibrous tissue formation, the generation of new epithelial tissue, and wound contraction. This stage begins when the size of the hematoma is sufficiently reduced to allow room for new tissue growth. Although skin and bone can regenerate themselves, other soft tissues replace damaged cells with scar tissue.

Healing through scar formation begins with the accumulation of exuded fluid, which contains a large concentration of protein and damaged cellular tissues. This accumulation forms the foundation for a highly vascularized mass of immature connective tissues that include **fibroblasts**, which are cells capable of generating collagen. The new connective tissue matrix is fueled by nutrients from the blood supply and the newly forming blood vessels, which depend on the mechanical support and protection from the matrix. The matrix rapidly forms crosslinks that contribute to stabilization of the wound site. The fibroblasts that have been chemically drawn to the hypoxic sites within the wound region secrete the collagen and promote angiogenesis by helping the growing blood vessels attach to the basement membrane collagen. These cells then fuse and form new vessels.

Other characteristics of the proliferation stage include an increased number of blood vessels, increased water content in the injury zone, and re-epithelialization at the surface caused by epithelial cells migrating from the periphery toward the center of the wound.

Maturation Phase (up to 1+ year)

The final phase of soft tissue wound repair is the maturation, or remodeling, phase. This phase involves the maturation of the newly formed tissue into scar tissue. The associated characteristics include decreased fibroblast activity, increased organization of the extracellular matrix, decreased tissue water content, reduced vascularity, and a return to normal histochemical activity. In soft tissue, these processes begin about 3 weeks post-injury, overlapping the proliferative phase. Because scar tissue is fibrous, inelastic, and nonvascular, it is less strong and less functional than the original tissues. The development of the scar also typically causes the wound to shrink, resulting in decreased flexibility of the affected tissues.

Although the epithelium has typically completely regenerated by 3 to 4 weeks post-injury, the tensile strength of the wound at this time is only approximately 25% of normal.[1] After several more months, strength may still be as much as 30% below preinjury strength.[2] This is partly caused by the orientation of the collagen fibers, which tends to be more vertical during this time than in normal tissue. The collagen turnover rate in a newly healed scar is also high; therefore, failure to provide appropriate support for the wound site can result in a larger scar.

Remodeling continues for a year or more as collagen fibers become oriented to the tissue's normal mechanical stress. The tensile strength of scar tissue may continue to increase for as long as 2 years post-injury. **Box 3-1** summarizes the three stages of the healing process.

Muscle fibers are permanent cells that do not reproduce or proliferate in response to either injury or training. However, some reserve cells in each muscle fiber are able to regenerate muscle fiber after injury. Severe muscle injury can result in scarring or the formation of **adhesions** within the muscle, which inhibit the potential for fiber regeneration from the reserve cells. Consequently, after severe injury, muscle may regain only about 50% of its preinjury strength.[3]

Because tendons and ligaments have few reparative cells, healing of these structures is a slow process that can take more than a year. Regeneration is enhanced by proximity to other soft tissues that can assist with supply of the required chemical mediators and building blocks. For this reason, isolated ligaments such as the anterior

> ➤ ➤ **B o x 3 - 1**

Phases of Soft Tissue Wound Healing

Inflammation (0–6 days):

Vasoconstriction promotes increased blood viscosity (thickness), reducing blood loss through bleeding.

The platelet reaction initiates clotting and releases growth factors that attract reparative cells to the site.

Coagulation of the clot is formed.

Vasodilation and increased blood vessel wall permeability facilitate the migration of neutrophils and macrophages in plasma exudate to cleanse the site through phagocytosis.

Proliferation (3–21 days):

Fibroblasts produce a supportive network of collagen.

The platelet response and the hypoxic wound environment stimulate angiogenesis.

Epithelial cells migrate from the periphery toward the center of the wound to enact re-epithelialization.

Maturation (up to 1+ years):

Fibroblast activity decreases, and habitual loading produces increased organization of the extracellular matrix.

A return to normal histochemical activity allows for reduced vascularity and water content.

The collagen fibers continue to proliferate, replacing immature collagen precursors and resulting in contracture of the wound.

Scar tissue formation results in decreased size and flexibility of the involved tissues.

Remodeling causes collagen fiber alignment along lines of habitual stress, with tensile strength increasing for up to 2 years post-injury.

bilization of the injury leads to atrophy, loss of strength, and decreased rate of healing in these tissues. The amount of atrophy is generally proportional to the time of immobilization. Thus, although immobilization may be necessary to protect the injured tissues during the early stages of recovery, strengthening exercises should be implemented as soon as appropriate during rehabilitation of the injury. The sport participant is at increased risk for reinjury as long as the affected tissues are below preinjury strength.

Summary

1. The most common mechanisms of injury include:
   - Compressive force from axial loading, which compresses or crushes an object
   - Tensile force from tension or traction on an object
   - Shearing force, which acts parallel or tangent to a plane passing through the object
2. Wound healing entails three overlapping phases: inflammation, proliferation, and maturation (remodeling).
3. During the inflammatory phase, blood loss is curtailed, clotting takes place, and histochemical reactions promote coagulation, vasodilation, and attraction of specialized cells to rid the wound site of foreign or infectious agents.
4. The proliferative phase includes the development of new blood vessels, formation of fibrous tissue, generation of new epithelial tissue, and wound contraction.
5. The maturation phase involves remodeling of the newly formed tissue.

References

1. Wong MEK, Hollinger JO, and Pinero GJ. 1996. Integrated processes responsible for soft tissue healing. Oral Surg Oral Med Oral Pathol Oral Radiol Endod, 82(5):475–492.
2. Orgill D, and Demling RH. 1988. Current concepts and approaches to wound healing. Crit Care Med, 16:899.
3. American Academy of Orthopaedic Surgeons. *Athletic training and sports medicine.* Park Ridge: American Academy of Orthopaedic Surgeons, 1991.
4. Hefti F, and Stoll TM. 1995. Healing of ligaments and tendons. Orthopade 24(3):237–245.

cruciate have poor chances for healing.[4] If tendons and ligaments undergo abnormally high tensile stress before scar formation is complete, the newly forming tissues can be elongated. If this occurs in ligaments, joint instability may result.

Because tendons, ligaments, and muscles **hypertrophy** (increase in size) and **atrophy** (decrease in size) in response to levels of mechanical stress, complete immo-

CHAPTER 4

Wound Care

OBJECTIVES

1. Identify the two main body segments, and demonstrate anatomic position.

2. Define terms relative to direction.

3. Describe the basic principles associated with the Occupational Safety and Health Administration universal safety precautions.

4. Identify what forces are best resisted by skin, muscle, tendon, ligament, and bone.

5. List common open wounds to the skin, and describe their treatment.

6. Describe the distinguishing features of a muscle, synovial joint, and a bone.

7. Describe how the signs and symptoms of a strain differ from a sprain.

8. List the general principles of acute care for closed, soft-tissue injuries.

9. Explain the various types of fractures, and describe general fracture care.

10. Describe the three methods of moving an injured athlete.

11. Explain the differences between cryotherapy and thermotherapy and explain when each is used during the injury process.

In the previous chapter, mechanisms of injury were introduced. Axial loading produces a squeezing or crushing effect, more commonly called a compressive force. A tensile force is a pulling force that stretches the object to which it is applied. Shear forces occur when one part of an object slides, displaces, or shears with respect to another part of the object. These three mechanisms of injury place stress on various body tissues. When the tissue reaches its maximal tolerance of the force, called its **yield point**, injury occurs. The resulting injuries are typically

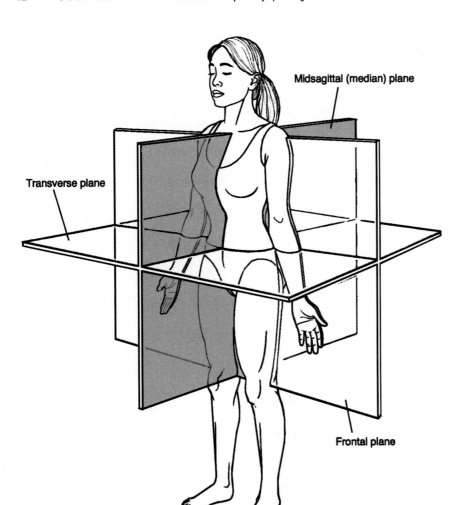

Midsagittal (median) plane

Transverse plane

Frontal plane

➤ FIGURE 4-1. Anatomic position. All directional terms are based on anatomic position. In this position, the body is erect, facing forward, with the arms at the side of the body, palms facing forward. Joint movement is based on how the body moves in relation to the planes of space along which movement occurs. These three planes split the body into equal halves of mass: midsagittal plane (right and left halves), frontal plane (anterior and posterior halves), and transverse plane (superior and inferior halves). For an individual standing in anatomic position, the three planes all intersect at a single point known as the body's center of gravity or center of mass.

divided into two main categories: soft tissue injuries and bone injuries.

This chapter first introduces medical terminology used to identify body segments, anatomic position, and directional terms used to communicate with the medical community. Discussion then focuses on soft tissue injuries to the skin, muscles, tendons, and joint structures. Because open wounds may involve the transmission of infectious diseases, universal safety precautions established by the Occupational Safety and Health Administration (OSHA) are presented. Fractures are then discussed, followed by methods to transport an injured athlete to the sideline. Finally, information is presented on the use of cold therapy (cryotherapy) and heat therapy (thermotherapy) on sports injuries as part of the injury process.

ANATOMIC FOUNDATIONS

Using correct terminology is crucial when communicating with members of the medical community. Anatomic terms, such as superior and inferior, medial and lateral, or thoracic and abdominal, help pinpoint the exact location on which to focus. Combined with basic medical terms, one can describe the site and what motions are

affected by an injury. Anatomic considerations of skin, muscle, ligaments and joint structures, and bones are discussed in specific sections of this chapter.

Anatomic Position

The human body is separated into two main segments: axial and appendicular. The axial segment relates to the head and trunk and includes the chest and abdomen. The appendicular segment relates to the extremities. Direction or position on the body is based on the **anatomic position**. In this position the body is erect, facing forward, with the arms at the side of the body, palms facing forward **(Fig. 4-1)**.

Directional Terms

Directional terms are used to describe where one body part is relative to another. For example, the elbow is superior to the wrist, the chest is on the anterior thorax, and the big toe is on the medial side of the foot. These terms are always used relative to anatomic position, regardless of the body's actual position. In speaking with the school's athletic trainer, a coach might report that one

Term	Definition	Illustration	Example
TABLE 4.1	**DIRECTIONAL TERMS**		
Superior (cranial)	Toward the head or cranium		The heart is superior to the abdomen
Inferior (caudal)	Toward the lower part of the body		The pelvic cavity is inferior to the thoracic cavity
Anterior	Toward the front of the body		The quadriceps muscles lie anterior to the femur
Posterior	Toward the back of the body		The buttock muscles lie posterior to the pelvis
Proximal	Closest to a reference point		The shoulder is proximal to the elbow
Distal	Farthest from a reference point		The wrist is distal to the elbow
Medial	Toward or at the midline of the body		The little finger is medial to the thumb
Lateral	Away from the midline of the body		The thumb is lateral to the little finger
Bilateral	Pertaining to both sides of the outer body		The ears are bilateral on the skull
Superficial	Toward or at the body surface		The skin is superficial to the muscles
Deep	Away from the body surface		The femur is deep to the skin

of the basketball players has pain on the lateral side of the ankle. In this manner, the athletic trainer can better visualize where the pain is located. Common directional terms used in injury assessment are defined and illustrated in **Table 4-1**.

SOFT TISSUE INJURIES

Skin, muscle, tendons, and ligaments are soft (nonbony) tissues, and are named collagenous tissues after their major building block, collagen. Collagen is a protein that is strong in resisting tension. It provides strength and flexibility to tissues but is relatively inelastic. Elastin, another protein, provides added elasticity to some connective tissue structures, such as the ligamentum flavum of the spine.

SKIN

Because the skin is the body's first layer of defense against injury, it is the most frequently injured body tissue. Control of bleeding and preventing infection are the primary concerns when treating skin injuries.

Anatomic Considerations

The skin is composed of two major regions. The outer region, known as the epidermis, has multiple layers containing the pigment melanin, along with the hair, nails, sebaceous glands, and sweat glands **(Fig. 4-2)**. Beneath the epidermis is the dermis, which contains blood vessels, nerve endings, hair follicles, sebaceous glands, and sweat glands. The skin is able to resist multidirectional loads, including compression, tension, and shear.

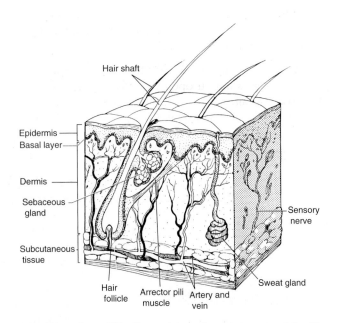

▶ **FIGURE 4-2.** Skin. Illustrated are the structures contained in the epidermis and dermis.

Open Soft Tissue Wound Classifications

There are five common open wounds seen in sports injury care **(Fig. 4-3)**:

1. **Abrasion**. Abrasions are caused by shear when the skin is scraped with sufficient force, usually in one direction, against a rough surface like the floor or artificial playing surface. The greater the applied force, the more layers of skin that are scraped away. Blood may ooze from the wound, but bleeding is usually not severe. Regardless of size, abrasions are extremely painful because of the number of nerve endings exposed. If the dermis is exposed, a primary concern is that dirt and foreign materials scraped over the wound may penetrate the exposed blood vessels, which increases the risk for infection unless the wound is properly cleansed and debrided.

2. **Incision**. Incisions are caused by a sharp, cutting object, such as broken glass; they are also caused when the impact causes the skin to be split over an underlying bone. The wound has sharp, even cuts with smooth edges that tend to bleed freely. If the incision is caused by impact over a bone, an associated contusion usually occurs (bruising due to crushing the surrounding tissues). These wounds tend to heal better than lacerations because the edges of the wound are smooth and can be approximated more easily during treatment.

3. **Laceration**. A laceration is an irregular tear in the skin that typically results from a combination of tension and shear. As such, the edges are often jagged, leading to significant bleeding, especially if an artery is cut. Skin and tissue may be torn away, increasing the risk of infection. Healing is not as good as in an incision.

4. **Avulsion**. An avulsion is a severe laceration that results in complete separation of the skin from the underlying tissues. A flap of skin may remain hanging or be torn off completely. Bleeding is profuse, and scarring is often extensive. If the avulsed skin is still attached by a flap of skin, circulation may be compromised. A primary concern with this injury is to make sure that the flap is lying flat and that it is aligned in its normal position before securing a dressing.

5. **Puncture**. A puncture wound is formed when a sharp object, such as a shoe spike or nail, penetrates the skin and underlying tissues with tensile loading. Although the opening in the skin may appear small, the wound may be extremely deep, posing a serious threat for infection. A puncture wound usually does not cause a bleeding problem; however, the object that caused the injury may remain imbedded in the wound.

Although not associated with an open skin wound, two other wounds do affect the skin. Blisters are minor skin injuries caused by repeated application of shear in

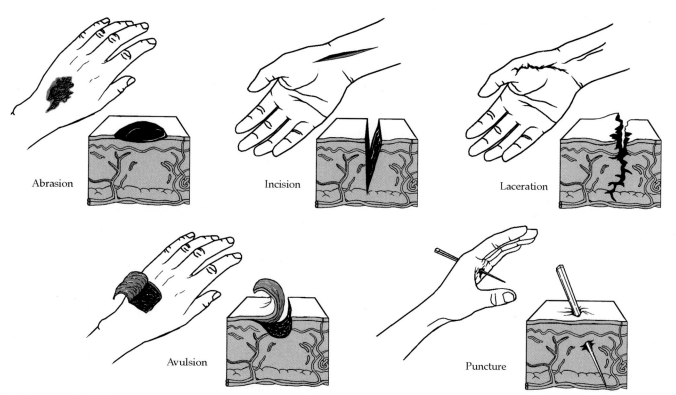

➤ **FIGURE 4-3.** Common open wounds. The five most common open wounds are abrasion, incision, laceration, avulsion, and puncture. The primary concern with each wound is to control bleeding and safeguard against infection.

one or more directions, as happens when a shoe rubs back and forth against the foot. The result is a pocket of fluid between the multiple layers of the epidermis as fluid migrates to the site of injury. If the movement is between the epidermis and dermis, there may be blood in the pocket of fluid. These wounds are generally closed unless the blister should break, so infection is not the norm. The primary concern with this injury is to prevent further irritation to the area. If the blister should break, it should be treated as an abrasion.

Skin bruises are injuries resulting from compression sustained during a blow. Damage to the underlying capillaries causes the accumulation of blood within the skin. As a closed injury, the primary concern is to control superficial bleeding within the skin and underlying tissues by applying ice and compression.

Open Soft Tissue Injury Care

In providing wound care for open soft tissue injuries, it is critical to follow the OSHA universal precautions and infection control standards **(Field Strategy 4-1)**. In addition to using safety equipment, disinfecting equipment and materials used during wound care, and properly discarding contaminated materials, the athletic trainer and coach should follow several other steps in general wound care:

- If possible, wash hands before beginning treatment.
- Apply gloves and apply direct pressure to the wound with sterile gauze or a nonstick material.

- Cleanse the wound and the area around the wound (at least twice its size) with saline water or soap and water **(Fig. 4-4)**.
- Dress and bandage the wound site securely for continued play.
- Creams or ointments may or may not be used with occlusive dressings. If used, cover dressings beyond their borders with underwrap and elastic adhesive tape where possible.
- Change the dressing daily, and look for signs of infection (local heat, swelling, redness, pain, pus, elevated body temperature).

For specific injuries, **Field Strategy 4-2** explains the basic care for common open wounds. It is assumed that the coach is already gloved. These techniques can be adapted for other open wounds.

MUSCLES AND TENDONS

Muscles are responsible for producing motion at a joint, maintaining posture, stabilizing joints, and generating heat as they contract. Injury to one or more muscles can be a major setback for a competitive athlete. However, with proper treatment and rehabilitation, athletes can return to full participation at their preinjury fitness level.

Anatomic Considerations

Muscle is a highly organized structure. Each muscle cell, or fiber, is surrounded by a sheath known as the endomy-

FIELD STATEGY 4.1   GENERAL GUIDELINES FOR PREVENTING SPREAD OF BLOODBORNE PATHOGENS

- Latex gloves should always be worn. Other protective equipment that should be worn when blood or other bodily fluids could be splashed, spurted, or sprayed include the following:
  - Eye wear or face guards
  - Masks or protective guards
  - Gowns or aprons
- After any exposure to potentially infectious material, immediately wash and disinfect hands and other skin surfaces.
- Clean large spills of bodily fluids and bloodborne pathogens by flooding the contaminated area with disinfectant before removing the spill. After removing the spill, the area should be disinfected again and thoroughly scrubbed.
- Disinfect all horizontal surfaces (i.e., treatment tables, taping tables, workspace, and floors) regularly, after each use and immediately after spills or soiling occurs. Use a scrubbing process.
- Disinfect with a cleaning solution of 1:10 to 1:100 solution (nonscented bleach to water). Exercise caution when using this solution near therapeutic modalities or skin because of caustic and corrosive properties of bleach. The solution must be mixed daily to be effective.
- Soiled linens and towels should be separated from regular laundry, handled with gloves, and placed in a leak-proof bag that is visibly designated for biohazard items.
- All items should be washed with detergent and water for 25 minutes, at a minimum of 71°C (160°F). Disinfectant solution should be added to heavily contaminated water.
- All disposable contaminated products (i.e., gauze, paper towels, cotton) should be handled with gloves and placed in leak-proof biohazard bags.
- Sharps containers should be readily available. They should be leak proof, puncture resistant, red, and visibly designated with a biohazard sign. Reusable sharp objects, such as pointed scissors or tweezers, should be sterilized after each use.
- Disposal of contaminated items and sharps containers should comply with OSHA standards.

---

sium. Small numbers of fibers are bound up into fascicles by a dense connective tissue sheath called the perimysium. A muscle is composed of a number of fascicles surrounded by the epimysium **(Fig. 4-5)**.

The structure and composition of muscle enable it to function in a viscoelastic fashion-that is, muscle is characterized by both time—dependent extensibility and elasticity. **Extensibility** is the ability to be stretched or to increase in length, whereas **elasticity** is the ability to return to normal length after either lengthening or shortening has taken place. The viscoelastic aspect of muscle extensibility enables muscle to stretch to greater lengths over time in response to a sustained tensile force. This means that a **static stretch** maintained over a period of 30 seconds is more effective in increasing muscle length than a series of short **ballistic stretches**.

Another of muscle's characteristic properties is irritability or **excitability**—the ability to respond to a stimulus. Stimuli affecting muscles can be either electrochemical, such as an action potential from the attaching nerve, or mechanical, as with an external blow to the muscle. If the stimulus is sufficient, muscle responds by developing tension.

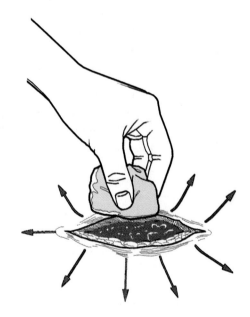

➤ FIGURE 4-4. Cleansing an open wound. When cleaning an open wound, use separate strokes and wipe away from the edge of the wound. Do not touch a clean area with a contaminated portion of the gauze.

FIELD STRATEGY 4.2 **CARE OF OPEN WOUNDS**

ABRASIONS

1. Clean and remove visible contaminants with a fluid flush with water and sweeps of gauze.

2. Clean both the wound site and area around the wound with soap and water or an antiseptic solution (see **Fig. 4-4**).

3. Dress and bandage the wound securely for continued play.

4. For dirty abrasions, or when it has been at least 5 years since the athlete has had a tetanus booster, refer for medical care.

INCISIONS AND LACERATIONS

1. Clean both the wound site and area around the wound with soap and water or an antiseptic solution.

2. Spray tape adherent on a cotton-tipped applicator and apply above and below the wound.

3. Beginning in the middle of the wound, bring the edges together and secure the Steri-Strip® below the wound. Lift up against gravity and secure above the wound. Make sure the edges of the wound are approximated.

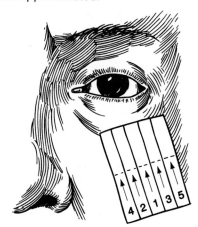

4. Apply the second Steri-Strip® immediately adjacent to one side of the original strip. Apply the third strip on the other side. Alternate sides until the entire wound is covered.

5. Dress the wound with an adhesive tincture base covering with an occlusive or nonstick sterile dressing.

6. Sutures may be desirable for any depth of laceration, especially around the face. However, any wound open to the full thickness of the dermis should be sutured within 10 hours of the injury.

7. Refer for medical care if it has been more than 5 years since the athlete has had a tetanus booster, or if signs of infection appear.

BLISTERS

1. Clean both the wound site and area around the wound with soap and water or an antiseptic solution.

2. Leave the roof of the blister intact for at least 24 hours, and cover the area with a topical antibiotic and dry sterile dressing. Do **not** aspirate a blood-filled blister.

3. Pad the nontender skin around the blister with an adhesive, soft-foam material (donut pad), New Skin®, or 2nd Skin®.

4. Dress and bandage the wound site securely for continued play.

5. If the blister is open, treat as an abrasion.

The ability to develop tension is a property unique to muscle. Although some sources refer to this ability as contractility, a muscle may or may not contract (shorten) when tension is developed. For example, isometric "contraction" involves no joint movement and no change in muscle length, and eccentric "contraction" actually involves lengthening of the muscle developing tension. Only when a muscle develops tension concentrically does it also shorten.

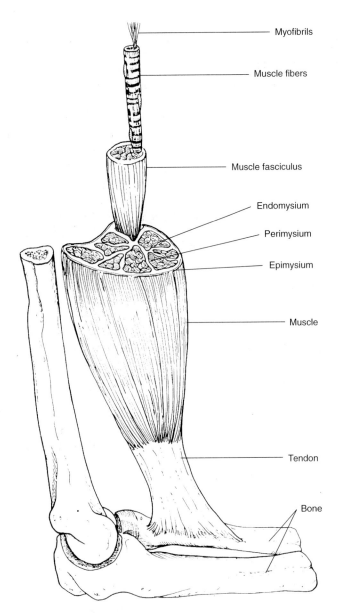

Myofibrils

Muscle fibers

Muscle fasciculus

Endomysium

Perimysium

Epimysium

Muscle

Tendon

Bone

➤ FIGURE 4-5. Muscle tissue.

When a stimulated muscle develops tension, the amount of tension present is the same throughout the muscle and tendon and at the site of the tendinous attachment to bone.

Muscles attach to bones either directly or indirectly. In direct attachments, the epimysium of the muscle fuses with the periosteum of the bone or perichondrium of a cartilage. More commonly, however, indirect attachments occur when the muscle's connective tissue extends beyond the muscle in a ropelike tendon or a flat, broad **aponeurosis**, which then attaches to the periosteum or perichondrium. Tendons can resist high, unidirectional tensile loads when the attached muscle contracts.

Muscle Injury Classification

Muscle injuries are either acute or chronic. Acute muscle conditions include contusions, cramps, spasms, and strains.

Chronic conditions include tendinitis, myositis/fasciitis, and bursitis.

1. **Contusions**. Muscle **contusions** or bruises result from a direct compressive force sustained from a heavy blow. Severity of these injuries varies according to the area and depth over which blood vessels are ruptured. **Ecchymosis**, or tissue discoloration, may be present if the hemorrhage is superficial. As blood and lymph flow into the damaged area, swelling occurs, often resulting in a hematoma—the formation of a hard mass composed of blood and dead tissue. This mass may restrict range of motion if close to a joint. Nerve compression usually accompanies such injuries, leading to pain and, sometimes, temporary paralysis. Muscle contusions are rated according to the extent of associated joint range of motion impairment.

   First degree—Little to no range of movement restriction.
   Second degree—A noticeable reduction in range of motion.
   Third degree—Severe restriction of motion. The fascia surrounding the muscle may also be ruptured, causing swollen muscle tissues to protrude.

2. **Muscle cramps and spasms**. A **cramp** is a painful involuntary contraction that is either clonic (alternating contraction and relaxation) or tonic (continued contraction over a period of time). Cramps appear to be caused by a biochemical imbalance, sometimes associated with muscle fatigue. A muscle **spasm** is a short, involuntary contraction caused by reflex action that can be biochemically derived or initiated by a mechanical blow to a nerve or muscle.

3. **Strains**. Muscle and tendon **strains** are caused by an abnormally high tensile force that produces rupturing of the tissue and subsequent hemorrhage and swelling. The likelihood of injury depends on the magnitude of the force acting and the structure's cross-sectional area. The greater the cross-sectional area of a muscle, the greater its strength, meaning the more force it can produce and the more force that is translated to the attached tendon. However, the larger the cross-sectional area of the tendon, the greater the force that it can withstand because an increased cross-sectional area translates to reduced stress. The muscle portion of the musculotendinous unit usually ruptures first because tendons, by virtue of their collagenous composition, are about twice as strong as the muscles to which they attach. Muscle strains are rated according to the extent to which associated motion is impaired **(Table 4-2)**.

4. **Tendinitis**. **Tendinitis** is a chronic condition involving inflammation of a tendon, characterized by pain and swelling with tendon movement. It is closely related to normal aging and degenerative changes within tendons. The mechanism of injury is usually overuse or repetitive overstretch or overload. Pain

TABLE 4.2 **CLASSIFICATIONS OF STRAINS**	First Degree	Second Degree	Third Degree
Damage to muscle fibers	Few fibers of muscle are torn	Nearly half of muscle fibers are torn	All muscle fibers are torn (rupture)
Weakness	Mild	Moderate to severe	Moderate to severe
Muscle spasm	Mild	Moderate to severe	Moderate to severe
Loss of function	Mild	Moderate to severe	Severe
Swelling	Mild	Moderate to severe	Moderate to severe
Palpable defect	No	No	Yes (if early)
Pain on contraction	Mild	Moderate to severe	None to mild
Pain with stretching	Yes	Yes	No
Range of motion	Decreased	Decreased	May increase or decrease depending on swelling

exists throughout the length of the tendon and increases during palpation. Crepitus may be also present. In this case, the condition is called **tenosynovitis**, or inflammation of the tendon sheath surrounding the tendon. The classic characteristic is a creaking sensation over the involved tendon.

5. **Myositis/fasciitis. Myositis** relates to inflammation of the muscle tissue, whereas **fasciitis** relates to inflammation of the fascia that supports and separates muscles. Common conditions associated with myositis are chronic groin strain and shin splints. Plantar fasciitis is one of the more common chronic inflammatory conditions of the foot.

6. **Bursitis. Bursitis** involves irritation of one or more bursae, the fluid-filled sacs that reduce friction in the tissues surrounding joints. Bursae are common in sites where muscles or muscle tendons overlie and rub against bone. The condition may also be acute or chronic, brought on either by a single traumatic compressive force or by repeated compressions associated with overuse of the joint.

JOINTS

A joint is the meeting of two bones. Joints are such a critical component of an athlete's body, any of which can be injured during sports participation. As such, detailed information is presented on the various types of joints found in the body, their functional classification, distinguishing anatomic features, and joint motion. Next, sprains and dislocations are discussed. Finally, the care of closed tissue injuries is presented.

Anatomic Considerations

Joints are classified by their structure or function. Structurally, they are grouped as fibrous, cartilaginous, or synovial joints. Fibrous joints occur when the bone ends are united by collagenic fibers, and tend to be immobile (sutures of the skull or joints around the teeth) or slightly mobile (syndesmosis at the distal tibiofibular joint). Car-

tilaginous joints exist when bone ends/parts are united by cartilage, such as the pubic symphysis (fibrocartilage). Synovial joints occur when the bone ends/parts are covered with articular cartilage and enclosed within an articular capsule lined with synovial membrane **(Fig. 4-6)**. Synovial joints are freely movable, depending on the design of the joint. All joints of the limbs fall into this class.

The functional classification is based on the amount of movement allowed at the joint. Synarthroses are immovable joints, amphiarthroses are slightly movable

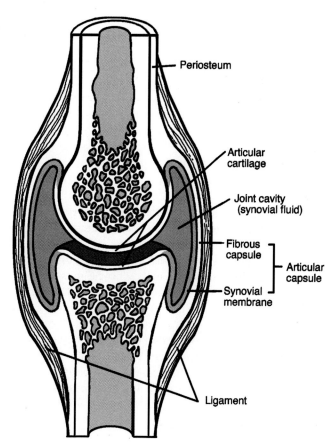

➤ **FIGURE 4-6.** Joint structures. General anatomy of a freely movable synovial joint.

joints, and diarthroses are freely movable joints. Since many of the joints of the body are freely movable synovial joints, discussion on joint structures will focus on this type of joint.

Synovial joints have five distinguishing features **(Fig. 4-6)**:

1. **Articular cartilage**. Hyaline cartilage covers the opposing bone surfaces, and serves to absorb compression placed on the joint, thereby keeping bone ends from being crushed.
2. **Joint (synovial) cavity**. The joint cavity is the space between the bones, which is filled with synovial fluid.
3. **Articular capsule**. The joint cavity is enclosed by a double-layered joint capsule. The inner layer is a synovial membrane that covers all internal joint surfaces not covered by hyaline cartilage. The outer layer is a tough, flexible fibrous capsule that is continuous with the periosteum of the articulating bones.
4. **Synovial fluid**. Synovial fluid has a viscous, egg-white consistency due to hyaluronic acid secreted by the synovial membrane, and occupies all free spaces within the joint capsule. Also found within the articular cartilage, synovial fluid provides a slippery weight-bearing film that reduces friction between the cartilages, lubricates the free surfaces, and nourishes their cells. When the joint is compressed, the synovial fluid is forced from the cartilage. Then, as joint pressure is relieved, synovial fluid seeps back into the articular cartilage like water into a sponge.
5. **Reinforcing ligaments**. Synovial joints are reinforced by numerous ligaments. Ligaments resist large tensile loads along the long axis of the ligament, but can also resist smaller tensile loads from other directions. This is because ligaments contain more elastin than tendons, and so, are somewhat more elastic than tendons. Often the ligaments are **intrinsic**, or capsular; that is, they are thickened portions of the joint capsule. In other cases, the ligament is found outside the capsule (**extrinsic** or extracapsular), such as the lateral collateral ligament at the knee, or deep to it (intracapsular), such as the cruciate ligaments of the knee. Since intracapsular ligaments are covered with synovial membrane, they do not actually lie within the joint cavity (extrasynovial).

Other than the basic structures found in synovial joints, some synovial joints have other structural components. At the hip and knee joints, for example, fatty pads lie between the fibrous capsule and the synovial membrane or bone. Other joints have wedges of fibrocartilage called menisci that separate the articular surfaces of the bones. These discs improve the fit between the adjoining bones, making the joint more stable. These can be seen in the knee, jaw, and sternoclavicular joint.

Joint Movement

Range of motion at a joint is dependent upon the muscles that cross that joint. Movement occurs when the muscles contract. Movement is described in directional terms relative to the lines, or axes, around which the body part moves and the planes of space along which the movement occurs. Planes are nothing more than a flat surface that sections the body into two parts. The most frequently used body planes are the **sagittal** or median plane, which divides the body vertically into right and left parts; the **frontal** or coronal plane, which divides the body vertically into anterior and posterior parts; and the **transverse** plane, which divides the body horizontally into superior and inferior parts **(Fig. 4-1)**.

Range of motion can be described as a nonaxial movement (slipping movement only, since there is no axis around which movement can occur), uniaxial movement (movement in one plane), biaxial movement (movement in two planes) or multiaxial movement (movement in or around all three planes). These movements can be further described as gliding, angular, or rotational. Gliding is the simplest joint movement. One flat, or nearly flat, bone glides or slips over another bone. An example of this type of joint can be found in the intercarpal or intertarsal bones of the wrist and foot, respectively. Angular movements increase or decrease the angle at a joint, and may occur along any plane of the body. These movements include flexion, extension, abduction, and adduction. Rotation involves the rotating of a bone around its own long axis. This can be seen at the hip and shoulder. For example, in medial rotation of the thigh, the anterior surface of the femur moves toward the median plane of the body; lateral rotation involves moving the anterior surface away from the median plane of the body.

Injury assessment typically focuses on freely movable joints. Although a specific joint can perform an isolated single motion, many activities, such as throwing or kicking a ball, require several simultaneous movements. In injury assessment, a single movement, such as abduction or flexion, is used to assess range of motion and muscle weakness at a specific joint. The various individual motions are defined in **Box 4-1** and illustrated in **Figure 4-7**.

Joint Injury Classification

Joint injuries may involve joint sprains, subluxations, or dislocations.

1. **Sprain**. Ligament **sprains** are caused by an abnormally high tensile force that produces rupturing of the tissue and subsequent hemorrhage and swelling. Under normal conditions, intermittent compression and tension increase strength, especially at the bony attachment. However, constant compression or tension causes ligaments to deteriorate. Like strains, sprains are also categorized as first, second, and third degree **(Table 4-3)**.

➤ ➤ B o x 4 - 1

Joint Movements

Flexion. Movement along the sagittal plane that decreases the angle of the joint; e.g., bending the elbow.

Extension. Movement along the sagittal plane that increases the angle of the joint; e.g., straightening a flexed elbow.

Dorsiflexion and plantar flexion. Because the foot joins the leg at a right angle, both up and down motions of the foot technically decrease the angle and could both be called flexion. To avoid confusion, special terms are used. Lifting the foot toward the shin is called dorsiflexion; depressing the foot away from the shin is called plantar flexion.

Abduction. Movement along the frontal plane whereby the limb moves away from the midline of the body; e.g., raising the arm.

Adduction. Movement along the frontal plane whereby the limb moves toward the midline of the body; e.g., lowering a raised arm to the side of the body. Note: abduction and adduction of the fingers relates to movement away from the midline of the body part. In this instance, the midline is the longest digit—the third finger or second toe.

Circumduction. Movement that involves flexion, abduction, extension, and adduction in succession. While the distal end of the limb moves in a circle, the point of the cone (the shoulder or hip) remains less stationary.

Rotation. Turning of a bone around its own long axis; e.g., movement between the first two cervical vertebrae.

Supination and pronation. Used at the wrist, supination refers to rotating the forearm laterally so that the palm faces anteriorly or superiorly (i.e., you can hold a cup of soup in your hand). In pronation, the forearm rotates medially and the palm faces posteriorly or inferiorly (i.e., palm lying down on a table).

Inversion and eversion. Used at the foot, inversion implies that the sole of the foot turns medially. In eversion, the sole faces laterally.

Protraction and retraction. Movement in the transverse plane. For example, the mandible is protracted when you jut out the jaw and is retracted when you move it back into its original position.

Elevation and depression. Elevation means lifting a body part superiorly, such as when you shrug your shoulders. Depression is the opposite; or, moving the elevated part inferiorly.

Opposition. Movement at the joint between the first metacarpal and carpals of the wrist, which involves touching the thumb to the tips of the other fingers of the same hand.

3. **Dislocation.** Dislocations are actually classified as third-degree joint sprains, whereby the supporting ligaments have been totally disrupted leading to a complete displacement of joint surfaces so that they no longer make normal contact. This injury produces severe pain, a major loss of tissue continuity, loss of range of motion, and complete instability of the joint.

Closed Soft Tissue Injury Care

Closed wound care focuses on immediately reducing inflammation, pain, and secondary hypoxia. Several initial steps should be followed by the athletic trainer or coach in providing general acute care. This process is commonly called the PRICE principle (protected rest, ice, compression, elevation):

- Apply crushed ice packs directly to the skin as quickly as possible following the injury.
- Do not place a towel or elastic wrap (dry or wet) between the crushed ice pack and skin. This will reduce the effectiveness of the treatment.
- Apply the crushed ice pack for 30 minutes (40 minutes for a large muscle mass such as the quadriceps).[1]
- Elevate the body part at least 6 to 10 inches above the level of the heart.
- Secure the ice pack with a wet elastic wrap. Apply the wrap in a distal to proximal direction. Check the pulse distal to the elastic wrap.
- After the initial ice treatment, remove the ice pack, replace the compression wrap, and continue elevation.
- Reapply the crushed ice pack every 2 hours (every hour if the athlete is active between applications, i.e., walking on crutches or showering) until the athlete goes to bed. This process may extend to 72+ hours postinjury.
- The compression wrap should be worn throughout the night and the mattress should be elevated.
- Maintain compression continuously on the injury until swelling is gone.

Further discussion on the importance of using ice during acute care will be discussed later in the chapter in Using Cryotherapy During the Healing Process. **Field Strategy 4-3** discusses the basic care of closed soft tissue injuries after the acute protocol has been followed. Because the severity of injuries can range from mild to severe, these steps are provided only as a general guide. Each injury must be assessed and treated on an individual basis.

BONES

Bones provide the framework to support the human body. They protect vital organs (i.e., brain, heart, and lungs), serve as a reservoir for minerals (i.e., calcium and phosphate), form the bulk of blood cells, and with the help of muscles, produce movement.

2. **Subluxation.** A subluxation is a partial displacement of the joint surfaces, and is usually transient in nature. The supporting ligaments may be torn, but have not completely ruptured.

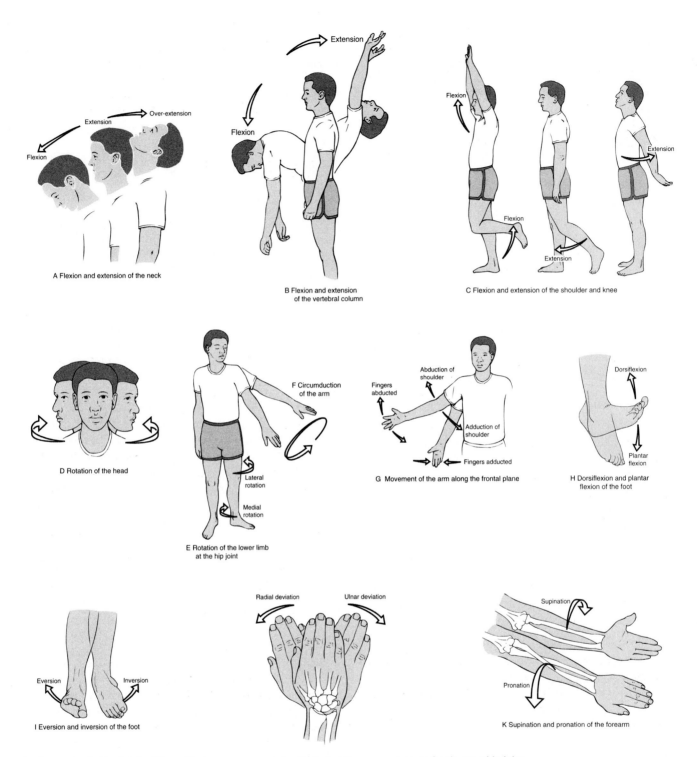

➤ **FIGURE 4-7.** Joint motions. Shown are movements allowed at the more common freely movable joints.

Anatomic Considerations

Bones are classified by their shape as long, short, flat, and irregular. As the name implies, long bones are considerably longer than they are wide, and consist of a shaft plus two ends **(Fig. 4-8)**. All bones of the limbs are considered long bones, except the patella. Short bones are typically cubelike. The bones of the wrist and ankle are examples of short bones. Flat bones, such as the ribs and sternum, are characteristically thin, flat, and usually a bit curved. Irregular bones do not fit into any of the previous categories. Examples of irregular bones are the vertebrae of the spine and the hip bones.

Nearly all long bones have the same general structure.

1. **Diaphysis**. The shaft of the bone is called the diaphysis, and is composed of compact bone that surrounds the central medullary cavity.

TABLE 4.3 CLASSIFICATIONS OF SPRAINS	First Degree	Second Degree	Third Degree
Damage to ligament	Few fibers of ligament are torn	Nearly half of fibers are torn	All ligament fibers are torn (rupture)
Distraction with stress tests	< 5 mm distraction	5 - 10 mm distraction	> 10 mm distraction
Weakness	Mild	Mild to moderate	Mild to moderate
Muscle spasm	None	None to minor	None to minor
Loss of function	Mild	Moderate to severe	Severe (instability)
Swelling	Mild	Moderate	Moderate to severe
Pain on contraction	None	None	None
Pain with stretching	Yes	Yes	No
Range of motion	Decreased	Decreased	May increase or decrease depending on swelling; dislocation or subluxation possible

2. **Epiphyses**. The epiphyses are located at the ends of the bone, and are typically larger than the diaphysis. Between the diaphysis and epiphysis of an adult long bone is an epiphyseal line. This is a remnant of the epiphyseal plate, which is a cartilaginous disc found near the ends of the long bones where longitudinal bone growth occurs. During or shortly following adolescence, the plate disappears and the bone fuses, terminating longitudinal growth. Most epiphyses close around age 18, although some may be present until about age 25.

3. **Membranes**. The outer layer of the bone is called the periosteum, which is richly supplied with nerve fibers, lymphatic vessels, and blood vessels that enter the bone via a nutrient foramen. The periosteum is secured to the underlying bone by Sharpey's fibers. The periosteum also serves as an attachment site for tendons and ligaments. At these sites, the Sharpey's fibers are exceptionally dense.

Although the most rapid bone growth occurs before adulthood, bones continue to grow in diameter throughout most of the lifespan. The internal layer of the periosteum builds new concentric layers of bone tissue on top of the existing ones. At the same time, bone is resorbed or eliminated around the sides of the medullary cavity, so that the diameter of the cavity is continually enlarged. The bone cells that form new bone tissue are called osteoblasts, and those that resorb bone are known as osteoclasts. In healthy adult bone the activity of osteoblasts and osteoclasts, referred to as bone turn-over, is largely balanced. The total amount of bone remains approximately constant until about the time that women reach their 40s and men reach their 60s, when a gradual decline in bone mass begins. Sport participants past these ages may be at increased risk for bone fractures. Regular participation in weight-bearing exercise, however, has been shown to be effective in reducing age-related bone loss.

Bone Injury Classification

A **fracture** is a disruption in the continuity of a bone **(Fig. 4-9)**. The type of fracture sustained depends on the type of mechanical loading, as well as the health and maturity of the bone at the time of injury. The high mineral content in bone allows for a high degree of stiffness and strength in the bone. As such, a bone can resist compression, and has some degree of flexibility and strength to resist tension and shear. Unlike soft tissue, when forces from opposite directions are directed at different points along a long bone, **bending** of the bone can occur. When bending is present, the structure is loaded in tension on one side and in compression on the opposite side, which can ultimately lead to fracture **(Fig. 4-10A)**. The application of torque about the long axis of a bone can cause **torsion**, or twisting of the structure, producing failure at an oblique angle to the long axis of the bone **(Fig. 4-10B)**.

The most common types of fractures include:

- **Simple (closed)**. The bone clearly fractures, but the bone ends do not break the skin.
- **Compound (open)**. At least one of the bone ends penetrates through the soft tissues and the skin.
- **Depressed**. Occurs more frequently on flat bones when the broken bone portion is driven inward.
- **Transverse**. The fracture occurs on a straight line across the bone.
- **Comminuted**. The bone fragments into several pieces.
- **Oblique**. The fracture occurs diagonally when torsion occurs on one end while the other end is fixed.
- **Epiphyseal**. Separation involves the epiphysis of the bone.
- **Spiral**. Jagged bone ends are S-shaped because excessive torsion is applied to a fixed bone.
- **Greenstick**. An incomplete fracture; as a green stick breaks. More common in children than adults.

FIELD STATEGY 4.3   CARE OF CLOSED WOUNDS

CONTUSIONS

For superficial contusions:

1. Pad with soft (open-celled) material next to the skin and more dense (closed-cell) material as an external covering.
2. Cut a hole that matches the contused area in the soft material, or keep it solid.
3. Secure the pad with elastic athletic tape or an elastic wrap.
4. After play and periodically during the next few days, apply ice, compression, and elevation to the site.
5. Repeat until pain and swelling are gone.

For deep contusions, determine disability after temporary paralysis subsides:

1. In moderate and severe cases, follow acute protocol for at least 24 hours with the muscle in a stretched position.
2. If an antalgic gait is present, fit for crutches, and instruct the athlete to use a partial- or non–weight-bearing gait.
3. Seek medical advice for complications.

MUSCLE STRAINS

Mild strains:

1. Apply a compression wrap (elastic, stockinette, or athletic tape) to muscle belly and tendon.
2. If cold is applied immediately before return to play, use a mild warm-up with a compression wrap before allowing return.
3. Apply heat after 72 hours.

Moderate to severe cases are treated by acute care protocol and referred for medical care:

1. Maintain joints above and below the strain in a neutral, lengthened position.
2. Immobilize, if necessary, and modify daily activity.
3. Apply heat when no increase in swelling has occurred within 1 to 2 days and when point tenderness and pain are minimal during active motion.

TENDON INJURIES

Mild injuries:

1. Use cold and isometric or eccentric exercise as tolerated.
2. Apply heat after 72 hours; combine strengthening with stretching in a pain-free range.

Moderate to severe cases are treated by acute care protocol and referred for medical care:

1. Maintain joints above and below the affected tendon in a neutral, lengthened position.
2. Avoid painful motions, and modify daily activities as necessary.
3. Apply heat when no increase in swelling has occurred within 1 to 2 days and when point tenderness and pain are minimal during active motion.

LIGAMENT SPRAINS

Mild injury:

1. Use protective device (brace) or athletic tape to limit joint laxity and motion at end range.
2. If ice is applied immediately before return, use a mild warm-up before allowing return to play.
3. Heat may be applied when swelling has subsided and when palpable pain upon movement is minimal.

Moderate to severe cases are treated by acute care protocol and referred for medical care:

1. In a neutral stable position, follow general guidelines for ice application and immobilize, if necessary.
2. Modify daily activity, sport activity level, or equipment.

(Continued)

FIELD STATEGY 4.3   CARE OF CLOSED WOUNDS (CONTINUED)

Dislocations:

1. Splint using standard first aid procedures and refer for medical care.

2. Assess the distal pulse, sensation, and movement; treat for shock and activate EMS, if necessary.

BURSITIS

Mild cases:

1. Pad (donut pad) the area surrounding the bursitis.

2. Apply heat after 72 hours; continue to pad until pain free.

Moderate to severe cases:

1. Limit movement by placing a compression pad over the bursa using a compression wrap.

2. Immobilize, if necessary, and modify daily activities.

3. When pain and inflammation are under control, apply heat.

INFECTED BURSA

1. Immobilize the joint and apply hot packs.

2. Refer to a physician for medical care. Antibiotics may need to be prescribed.

- **Stress**. Incomplete fractures resulting from repeated low-magnitude forces that worsen over time.
- **Avulsion**. A bone fragment is pulled off by an attached tendon or ligament.
- **Impacted**. Bone is impacted, or driven into, another piece of bone.

The bones of children and adolescents are more prone to growth-plate injuries and avulsion fractures, rather than ligament and muscle-tendon injuries, which are more common in adults. These epiphyseal injuries may involve the cartilaginous epiphyseal plate, articular cartilage, or **apophysis (Fig. 4-11)**. The apophyses are sites where a major tendon attaches onto a growing bony prominence. Both acute and repetitive loading can injure the growth plate, potentially resulting in premature closure of the epiphyseal junction and termination of bone growth. "Little league elbow," or medial epicondylitis, for example, is a stress injury to the medial epicondylar epiphysis of the humerus. Because of the potential for epiphyseal injuries, any suspected fracture or joint injury on an adolescent should be referred immediately to a physician for further evaluation and possible x-rays.

Fracture Care

Possible fractures can be detected with palpation, percussion, compression, and distraction **(Fig. 4-12)**. Palpation can detect deformity, crepitus, swelling, or increased pain at the fracture site. Percussion uses a tapping motion of the finger over a bony structure. Vibrations travel through the bone and cause increased pain at a fracture site. Compression is performed by gently compressing the distal end of the bone toward the proximal end, or by encircling the body part, such as a foot or hand, and gently squeezing, thereby compressing the heads of the bones together. Again, if a fracture is present, pain will increase at the fracture site. Distraction employs a tensile force, whereby the application of traction to both ends of the fractured bone will help relieve pain. Signs and symptoms of a fracture are summarized in **Box 4-2**.

A suspected fracture should always be referred to a physician for further evaluation and possible x-rays, par-

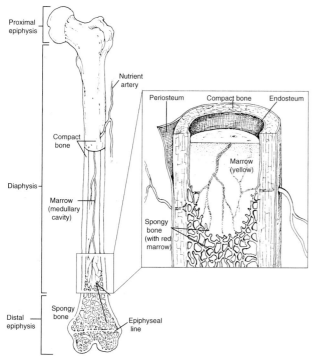

Proximal epiphysis

Nutrient artery

Periosteum Compact bone Endosteum

Compact bone

Marrow (yellow)

Diaphysis

Marrow (medullary cavity)

Spongy bone (with red marrow)

Spongy bone

Distal epiphysis

Epiphyseal line

➤ **FIGURE 4-8.** Bone structure. Note the epiphyseal growth lines at the end of the bone.

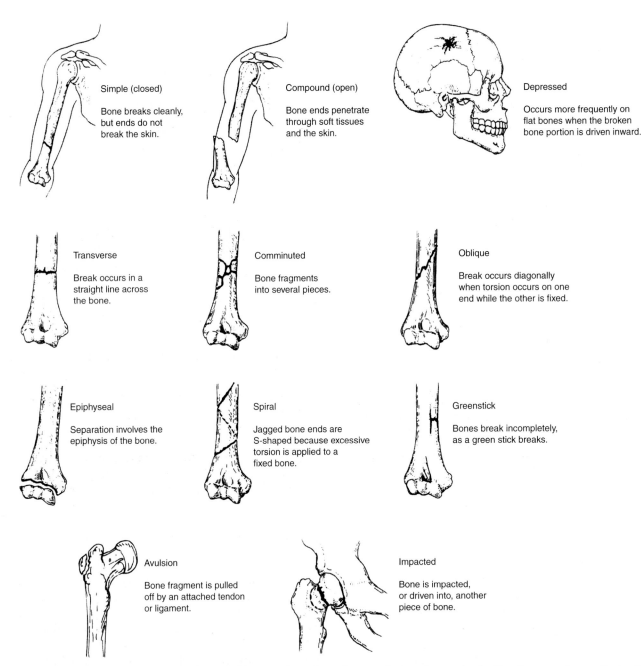

▶ FIGURE 4-9. Types of fractures. The type of fracture depends on the type of excessive mechanical loading as well as on the health and maturity of the bone at the time of injury.

ticularly with adolescents. The joint above and below the suspected fracture site should be splinted before the individual is moved to avoid damage to surrounding ligaments, tendons, blood vessels, and nerves. **Field Strategy 4-4** explains the immediate management of fractures.

MOVING THE INJURED PARTICIPANT

Once the injury has been evaluated, a decision must be made on the manner to safely remove the injured athlete from the field. These include ambulatory assistance, manual conveyance, and transporting by a spine board.

Ambulatory Assistance

Ambulatory assistance is used to provide support or aid to an injured athlete who is able to walk. This implies that the injury is minor, and no further harm will occur if the individual is ambulatory. In performing this technique, two individuals of equal or near-equal height should support both sides of the injured individual. The injured person drapes his or her arms across the shoulders of the assistants while their arms encircle the injured player's back. The assistants then escort the player off the field.

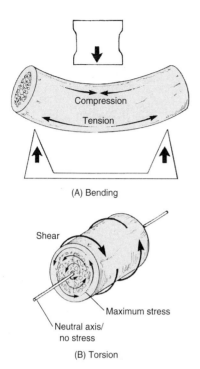

(A) Bending

Shear

Maximum stress

Neutral axis/
no stress

(B) Torsion

➤ FIGURE 4-10. Bone injury mechanisms. Bones loaded in bending are subject to compression on one side and tension on the other side. Because bone is stronger in resisting compression than tension, the side of the bone loaded in tension fractures if the bending moment is sufficiently large (A). Bones loaded in torsion develop internal shear stress, with maximal stress at the periphery and no stress at the neutral axis (B).

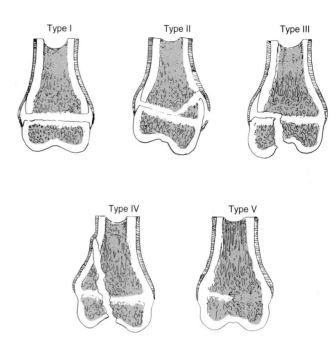

➤ FIGURE 4-11. Epiphyseal injuries. The bones of children and adolescents are more prone to growth plate injuries and avulsion fractures than to ligament and muscle-tendon injuries. Fractures may involve the cartilaginous epiphyseal plate, articular cartilage, or apophysis.

Manual Conveyance

If the individual is unable to walk or the distance is too great to walk, manual conveyance may be used. The injured person continues to drape his or her arms across the assistants' shoulders, while one arm from each assistant is placed behind the athlete's back and the other arm is placed under the athlete's thigh. Both assistants lift the legs up, placing the athlete in a seated position. The injured person is then carried off the field. Again, it is essential that the injury be fully evaluated before moving the individual in this manner.

Transporting by Spine Board

The safest method to move an individual is with a spine board. If this is necessary, EMS should be summoned. When the ambulance arrives, the EMTs or paramedics may request some help in moving the injured individual onto the spine board. Ideally, five trained individuals should roll, lift, and carry an injured person. The captain (the most medically trained individual) will stabilize the head and give commands for each person to slowly lift the injured individual onto the stretcher. The individual is then secured onto the spine board. On command, the spine board is raised to waist level. The individual should

be carried feet first so the captain can constantly monitor the individual's condition. **Field Strategy 4-5** describes how to assist in securing and moving an athlete on a spine board.

USING CRYOTHERAPY IN THE INJURY PROCESS

The extent of a sports-related injury can be significantly affected by altering the temperature of the injured tissues. Within minutes of an injury, the application of cold (**cryotherapy**) can lead to vasoconstriction at the cellular level and decreases tissue metabolism (i.e., decreases the need for oxygen), which reduces secondary hypoxia. Capillary permeability and pain are decreased, and the

➤ ➤ BOX 4-2.

Signs and Symptoms of Fracture
- Pain and tenderness directly over the fracture site
- Rapid swelling and discoloration/contusion
- Deformity or shortening of the limb (compare bilaterally)
- Grating or crepitus when bone ends rub together
- Guarding or disability
- Possible exposed bone ends if the skin is split open

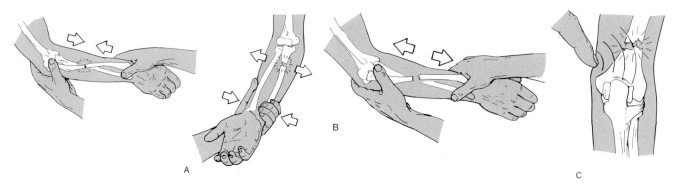

➤ FIGURE 4-12. Determining a possible fracture. **A.** Compression (axial and circular). **B.** Distraction. **C.** Percussion. If the bone is fractured, pain increases with percussion and compression but decreases with distraction.

release of inflammatory mediators and prostaglandin synthesis are inhibited. As the temperature of peripheral nerves decrease, a corresponding decrease is seen in pain perception. With nerve impulses inhibited and muscle spindle activity decreased, muscles in spasm are relaxed, breaking the pain-spasm cycle and leading to an **analgesic**, or pain-free, effect.

Because vasoconstriction leads to a decrease in metabolic rate, inflammation, and pain, cryotherapy is the modality of choice during the acute phase of an injury. Skin freezes at about 25° however, a bag of ice reaches a low temperature of only 32° so one need not be afraid of freezing the skin surface if ice is applied directly to the injury site. Cryotherapy, usually in the form of an ice bag, is applied for 20 to 30 minutes for maximum cooling of both superficial and deep tissues. Barriers used between the ice and skin can slow heat transfer. Research has shown that a dry towel or dry elastic wrap should not be used in treatment times of 30 minutes or less. Rather, the cold agent should be applied directly to the skin for optimal therapeutic effects.[1,2] A cold, wet elastic compression wrap can hold the ice bag in place, and can assist in decreasing hemorrhage and hematoma formation, yet can still expand in cases of extreme swelling. Elevation above the level of the heart uses gravity to reduce pooling of fluids and pressure inside the venous and lymphatic vessels, to prevent fluid from filtering into surrounding tissue spaces. The result is less tissue necrosis and local waste leading to a shorter inflammatory phase. The combination of protected rest, ice, compression, and elevation (**PRICE**) can significantly reduce the acute inflammatory phase of healing **(Fig. 4-13A)**.

Ice application is continued until 48 to 72 hours after injury, or until acute bleeding and capillary leakage have stopped, whichever is longer. However, compression with an elastic wrap should be maintained as long as swelling is present. Another consideration is the length of time it takes to rewarm the injured area. Knight has shown that except for the fingers, the rewarming time to approach normal body temperature is at least 90 minutes.[1] This

FIELD STATEGY 4.4   MANAGEMENT OF BONE INJURIES

1. Remove clothing and jewelry from around the injury site.
2. Clothing should be cut away with scissors to avoid moving the injured area.
3. Check the distal pulse and sensation. If either is abnormal, activate EMS.
4. Cover all wounds, including open fractures, with sterile dressings. Secure the dressings.
5. Do not attempt to push bone ends back underneath the skin.
6. Pad the splint to prevent local pressure.
7. Apply minimal inline traction and maintain it until the splint is in place and secured.
8. Immobilize the joints above and below the fracture site.
9. If pain increases with gentle traction or the limb resists positioning, splint in the position found.
10. Severely angulated fractures should **not** be straightened unless it is necessary to incorporate the limb into the splint. With such injuries, immobilize the limb in that position, moving it as little as possible during splint application.
11. Splint firmly, but do not impair circulation.
12. Recheck distal pulse and sensation after applying splint.
13. Check vital signs, treat for shock, and transport the athlete to a medical facility.

FIELD STATEGY 4.5 **TRANSPORTING AN INJURED INDIVIDUAL ON A SPINE BOARD**

1. *Unless ruled out, assume the presence of a spinal injury.* The "captain" of the team stabilizes the head and neck in the exact position in which the victim was found, regardless of the angle. Place the arms next to the body and legs straight. If the individual is lying face down, roll the individual supine. Four or five people are required to "log roll" the individual. The captain should position the arms in the cross arm technique so that, during the log roll, the arms end in the proper position.

2. Place the spine board as close as possible beside the individual. Each person is responsible for one body segment: one at the shoulder, one at the hip, one at the knees, and, if needed, one at the feet. On command, roll the individual on the board in a single motion.

3. Once the individual is on the board, the captain continues to stabilize the head and neck while another person applies support around the cervical region. The chest and then the feet are secured to the board. With a football player, *do not* remove the helmet.

4. When the individual is secured, four people lift the stretcher while the captain continues to monitor the individual's condition. Transport the individual feet first.

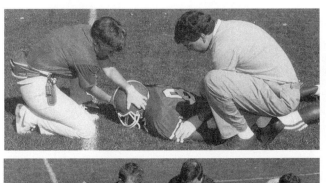

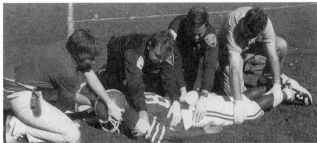

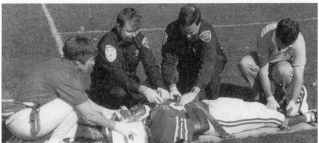

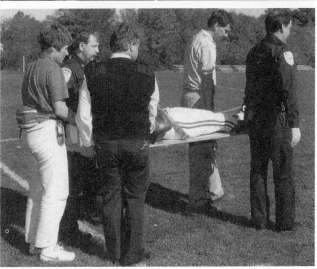

results in a treatment protocol of applying an ice pack for 20 to 30 minutes, followed by 90 minutes of rewarming. Fingers can rewarm more quickly, even following a 20- to 30-minute ice treatment, presumably due to their increased circulation. Fingers need only 20 to 30 minutes to rewarm.

Depth of cold penetration can reach 5 cm, and depends on the amount of subcutaneous insulation, vascular response to skin cooling, limb circumference, and temperature and duration of application.[3] With each method of cold application, the individual will experi-

ence four progressive sensations: cold, burning, aching, and finally analgesia. The acute care protocol for soft tissue injuries using ice packs was explained in the section on Closed Soft Tissue Injury Care.

USING THERMOTHERAPY IN THE INJURY PROCESS

Thermotherapy, or heat application, is typically used in the proliferation phase of healing to increase blood flow and promote healing in the injured area. If used during

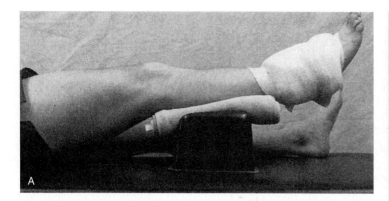

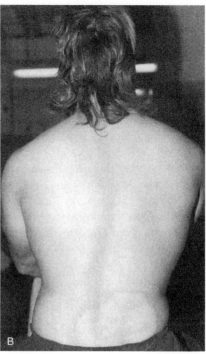

➤ **FIGURE 4-13.** Ice treatments. **A.** Ice, compression, and elevation can reduce acute inflammation. **B.** A slightly raised wheal formation may appear shortly after cold application in individuals who are sensitive to cold or have cold allergies.

the acute inflammatory stage, heat application may overwhelm the injured blood and lymphatic vessels, leading to increased hemorrhage and edema. When applied at the appropriate time, however, heat can increase circulation and cellular metabolism, produce an analgesic, or sedative effect, and assist in the resolution of pain and muscle-guarding spasms. Vasodilation and increased circulation result in an influx of oxygen and nutrients into the area to promote healing of damaged tissues. Debris and waste products are removed from the injury site. Used before stretching exercises or active exercise, thermotherapy can increase extensibility of connective tissue, leading to increased range of motion.

The greatest degree of elevated temperature occurs in the skin and subcutaneous tissues within 0.5 cm of the skin surface. In areas with adequate circulation, temperature will increase to its maximum within 6 to 8 minutes of exposure. Muscle temperature at depths of 1 to 2 cm will increase to a lesser degree and require a longer duration of exposure (15 to 30 minutes) to reach peak values.[4] After peak temperatures are reached, a plateauing effect or slight decrease in skin temperature is seen over the rest of the heat application. As mentioned earlier, fat is an insulator and has a low thermal conductivity value. Therefore, tissues under a large amount of fat will be minimally affected by superficial heating agents.

APPLICATION OF COMMON TREATMENTS

An **indication** is a condition that could benefit from a specific modality, whereas a **contraindication** is a condition that could be adversely affected if a particular modality is used. Modalities may be indicated and contraindicated for the same condition. For example, thermotherapy

(heat therapy) may be contraindicated for tendinitis during acute inflammation; however once inflammation is controlled, heat therapy may be indicated. Frequent assessment of the condition will indicate if the appropriate modality is being used. **Box 4-3** and **Box 4-4** list common indications and contraindications for cryotherapy and thermotherapy applications, respectively.

Ice Massage

Ice massage is particularly useful for relieving pain that may inhibit stretching of a muscle, and it decreases muscle soreness when combined with stretching.[5] It is commonly used before range of motion exercises and friction massage when treating chronic tendinitis and muscle strains. Treatment consists of water frozen in a cup, then rubbed over the skin in small circular motions for 7 to 10 minutes. A wooden tongue depressor frozen in the cup provides a handle for easy application.

Ice Packs

Ice packs made of flaked ice or small cubes can be safely applied to the skin for 20 to 30 minutes without danger of frostbite. Furthermore, ice packs can be molded to the body's contours, held in place by a cold compression wrap, and elevated above the heart to minimize swelling and pooling of fluids in the interstitial tissue spaces.

Chemical Packs

Chemical packs are convenient to carry in a first aid or athletic training kit. They are disposable after a single use, can conform to the body part, but can be expensive.

Cryotherapy Application

INDICATIONS	CONTRAINDICATIONS
Acute or chronic pain	Decreased cold sensitivity or hypersensitivity
Acute or chronic muscle spasm/guarding	Cold allergy
Acute inflammation or injury	Circulatory or sensory impairment
Postsurgical pain and edema	Raynaud's disease or cold urticaria
Superficial first-degree burns	Hypertension
Used with exercises to:	Uncovered open wounds
Facilitate mobilization	Cardiac or respiratory disorders
Relieve pain	Nerve palsy
Decrease muscle spasticity	Arthritis
Increase range of motion	Leukemia or systemic lupus

The packs are activated by squeezing or hitting the pack against a hard area. The chemical reaction is at an alkaline pH and can cause skin burns if the package breaks open and the contents spill **(Fig. 4-14)**. As such, the packs should never be squeezed in front of the face and, if possible, should be placed inside another plastic bag. Treatment ranges from 15 to 20 minutes; however, as the pack warms, it becomes ineffective as a cold treatment.

Whirlpools

Whirlpools combine warm or hot water with a hydromassaging effect to increase superficial skin temperature. Physiologically, warm or hot whirlpools are analgesic agents that relax muscle spasms, relieve joint pain and stiffness, provide mechanical debridement, and facilitate range of motion exercises after prolonged immobilization. Buoyancy facilitates increased range of motion, and the hydromassaging effect is controlled by the amount of air emitted through the jets. The more agitation, the greater the water movement. The jets can be directed at a specific angle; however, they should never be pointed directly at an injury site. Treatment time ranges from 20 to 30 minutes. Total body immersion exceeding 20 to 30 minutes can lead to dehydra-

tion, which in turn leads to dizziness and high body core temperature. Only the body parts being treated should be immersed.

Hot Tubs and Jacuzzis

Hot tubs and jacuzzis are readily available to athletes. Because organic contaminates, high water temperature, and turbulence reduce chlorine's effectiveness as a bacterial agent, infection with *Pseudomonas aeruginosa*, causing folliculitis, is an alarming and increasing problem. To prevent infection, these tubs must have a good filtration and chlorination system. Chlorine and pH levels should be monitored hourly during periods of heavy use, and calcium hardness should be evaluated weekly.[3] The water should be drained, superchlorinated, and refilled once every 3 months. The water temperature should not exceed 38.9°C (102°F).

SUMMARY

1. Skin is able to resist multidirectional loads, including compression, tension, and shear. Open skin injuries include abrasions, incisions, lacerations, avulsions, and puncture wounds.

Thermotherapy Application

INDICATIONS	CONTRAINDICATIONS
Subacute or chronic injuries, to:	Acute inflammation or injuries
Reduce swelling, edema, and ecchymosis	Impaired or poor circulation
Reduce muscle spasm or guarding	Subacute or chronic pain
Increase blood flow to:	Impaired or poor sensation
Increase ROM before activity	Impaired thermal regulation
Resolve hematoma	Malignancy
Facilitate tissue healing	
Relieve joint contractures	
Fight infection	

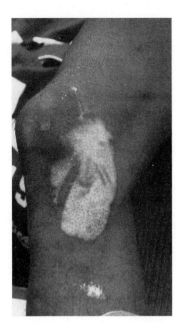

➤ FIGURE 4-14. Chemical ice packs. Although chemical ice packs are convenient to carry, this soccer player fell asleep with a chemical ice bag on his knee, unaware of a small leak in the bag. The resulting irritation led to a second-degree chemical burn to the skin.

2. Tendons connect muscle to bone and enable resistance to high, unidirectional tensile loads when the attached muscle contracts.
3. Ligaments connect bone to bone and can resist large tensile loads along the long axis of the ligament and smaller tensile loads from other directions.
4. Joint movement is described in directional terms relative to the lines, or axes, around which the body part moves and the planes of space along which the movement occurs. The three most common planes are as follows:
   • Sagittal or median plane, which splits the body vertically into right and left parts
   • Frontal or coronal plane, which splits the body vertically into anterior and posterior parts
   • Transverse plane, which divides the body horizontally into superior and inferior parts
5. Injury to the musculotendinous unit is called a strain. Injury to a ligament is called a sprain. Both strains and sprains are graded as first-degree (mild),

second-degree (moderate), or third-degree (severe) injuries.
6. Because bone is stronger in resisting compressive forces than in resisting both tension and shear forces, acute compression fractures are rare. Most fractures occur on the side of the bone placed in tension.
7. Excessive forces external to the body can produce torque about the long axis of a structure, causing torsion or twisting of the structure and leading to injury.
8. Because the bones of children contain larger relative amounts of collagen than adult bones, they are more flexible and resistant to fracture than adult bones. Children and adolescents are more prone to greenstick fractures, growth-plate injuries, and avulsion fractures. Any joint injury should be referred to a physician for further care.
9. An injured athlete can be removed from the field via ambulatory assistance, manual conveyance, or a spine board.
10. Cryotherapy is used to decrease pain, inflammation, muscle guarding, and spasm. It is also used to facilitate early movement.
11. Thermotherapy is used to treat nonacute or chronic injuries to reduce swelling, edema, discoloration, and muscle spasm; to increase blood flow and range of motion; to facilitate tissue healing; to relieve joint contractures; and to fight infection.

References

1. Knight KL. *Cryotherapy in sport injury management.* Champaign: Human Kinetics, 1995.
2. Tsang KKW, et al. 1997. The effects of cryotherapy applied through various barriers. J Sport Rehab, 6(4):343–354.
3. Walsh MT. Hydrotherapy: The use of water as a therapeutic agent. In *Thermal agents in rehabilitation,* edited by SL Michlovitz. Philadelphia: FA Davis, 1996.
4. Rennie FA, and Michlovitz SL. Biophysical principles of heating and superficial heating agents. In *Thermal agents in rehabilitation,* edited by SL Michlovitz. Philadelphia: FA Davis, 1996.
5. Myrer JW, Draper DO, and Durrant E. 1994. Contrast therapy and intramuscular temperature in the human leg. J Ath Train, 29(4):318–322.

Care of Specific Injuries

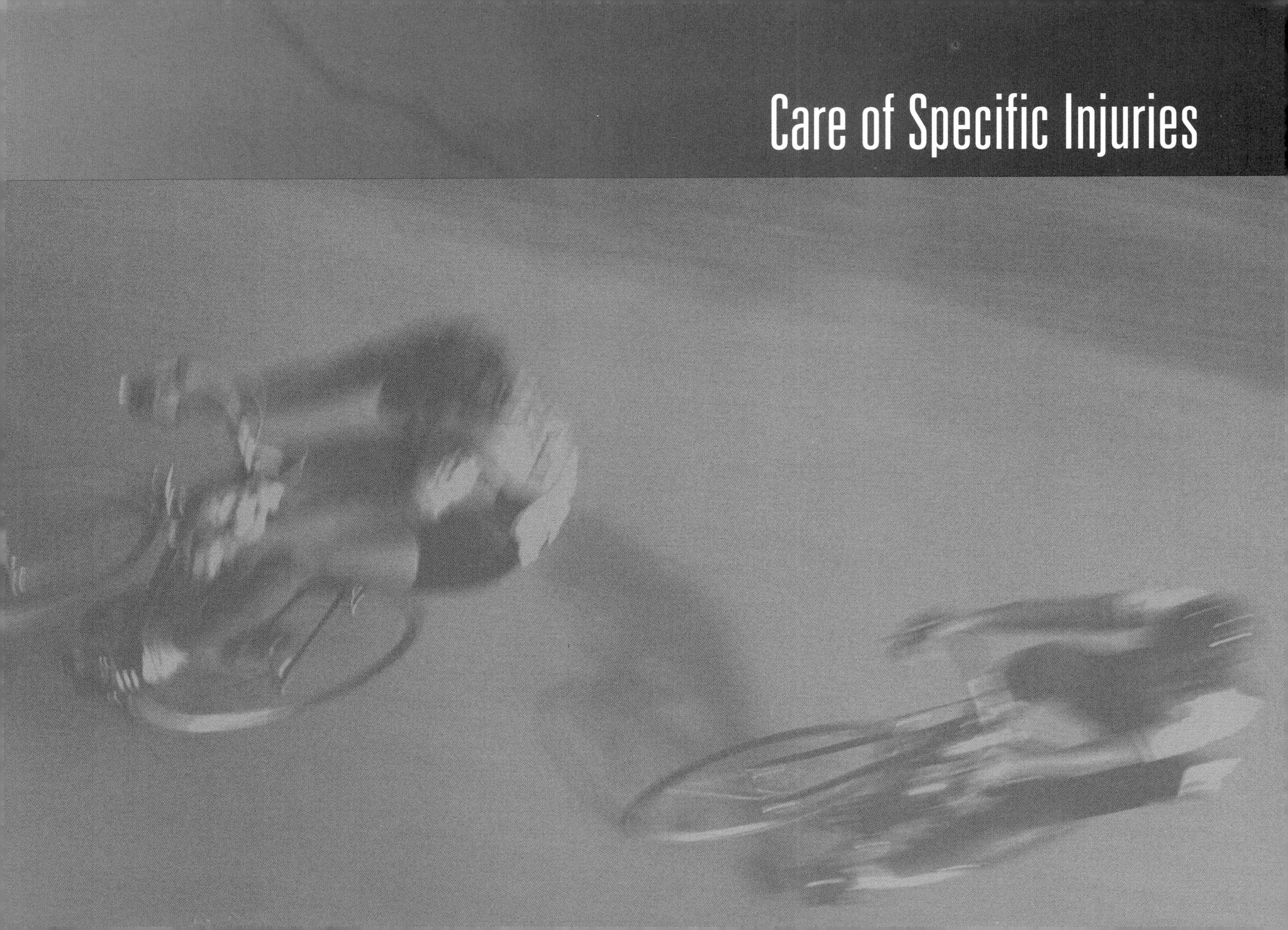

Section II

CHAPTER 5

Cranial and Facial Conditions

KEY TERMS

Anterograde amnesia

Battle's sign

Blowout fracture

Cauliflower ear

Concussion

Conjunctivitis

Contrecoup-type injury

Coup-type injury

Detached retina

Diffuse injuries

Diplopia

Dural sinuses

Epistaxis

Extruded tooth

Focal injuries

Hyphema

Intruded tooth

Malocclusion

Meninges

Meningitis

Nystagmus

Otitis externa

Periorbital ecchymosis

Photophobia

Postconcussion syndrome

Raccoon eyes

Retrograde amnesia

Tinnitus

OBJECTIVES

1. Locate the important bony and soft tissue structures of the head and facial region.

2. Recognize the importance of wearing protective equipment to prevent injury to the head and facial region.

3. Identify forces responsible for cranial injuries.

4. Recognize important signs and symptoms that indicate a skull fracture or intracranial injury.

5. Demonstrate a basic assessment of a cranial injury.

6. Identify common facial injuries as well as their assessment and management.

The head and facial areas are frequent sites for minor injuries, including lacerations, contusions, and mild concussions. Although intracranial injuries have been associated with sport-related fatalities, measures such as increased standards in protective equipment, rule changes that prohibit leading with the head for contact, and the development and use of the face mask have significantly decreased the incidence of these injuries. The number of eye, ear, and dental injuries significantly decreases when protective equipment is worn. This chapter begins with information on cranial injuries, their management, and protocol for a basic assessment of a head injury. Finally, common injuries to the facial area and their management are presented.

CRANIAL ANATOMY

This review of anatomy focuses on the bones of the skull, the brain and its coverings, the twelve cranial nerves that emerge from the brain stem, and the arterial blood vessels that nourish the skull. A basic understanding of this anatomy can help the coach understand why certain signs and symptoms occur with damage to the specific anatomic structures of the region.

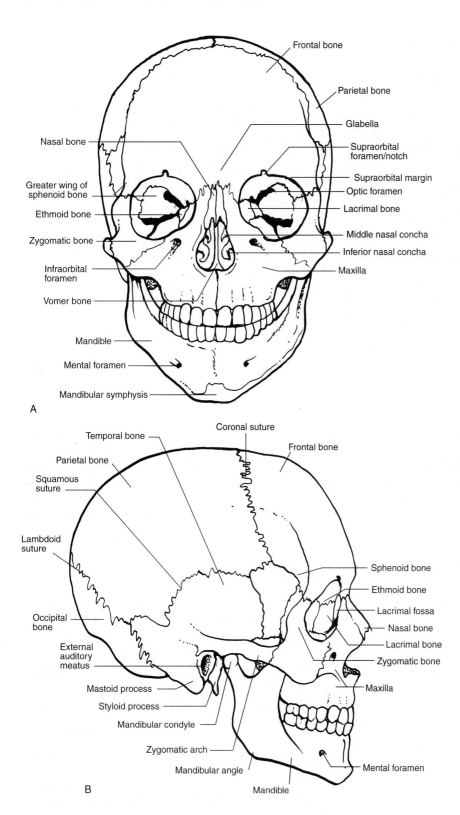

A

B

➤ **F I G U R E 5 - 1 .** The bones of the skull.
A. Frontal view. **B.** Lateral view.

Bones of the Skull

The skull is primarily composed of flat bones that inter-lock at immovable joints called sutures **(Fig. 5-1)**. The bones that form the portion of the skull known as the cranium protect the brain. The facial bones provide the structure of the face and form the sinuses, orbits of the eyes, nasal cavity, and mouth. The large opening at the base of the skull that sits atop the spinal column is called the foramen magnum.

The Brain

The four major regions of the brain are the cerebral hemi-spheres, diencephalon, brainstem, and cerebellum. The entire brain and spinal cord are enclosed in three layers

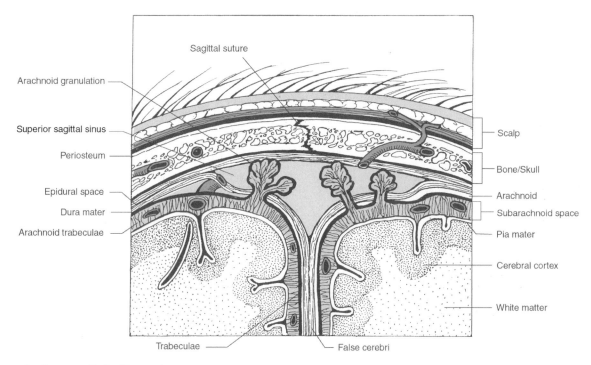

Sagittal suture

Arachnoid granulation

Superior sagittal sinus

Periosteum

Epidural space

Dura mater

Arachnoid trabeculae

Scalp

Bone/Skull

Arachnoid

Subarachnoid space

Pia mater

Cerebral cortex

White matter

Trabeculae

False cerebri

➤ FIGURE 5-2. The meninges.

of protective tissue known collectively as the **meninges (Fig. 5-2)**. The outermost membrane is the dura mater, a thick, fibrous tissue containing **dural sinuses** that act as veins to transport blood from the brain to the jugular veins of the neck. The arachnoid mater is a thin membrane internal to the dura mater, separated from the dura mater by the subdural space. Beneath the arachnoid mater is the subarachnoid space, which is filled with cerebrospinal fluid (CSF). This space contains the largest of the blood vessels supplying the brain. The arachnoid mater is connected to the inner pia mater by weblike strands of connective tissue. The dura mater and arachnoid mater are rather loose membranes, but the pia mater is in direct contact with the cerebral cortex. The pia mater contains several small blood vessels.

Nerves of the Head and Face

Twelve pairs of cranial nerves emerge from the brain, some with motor functions, some with sensory function, and some with both. Knowledge of their function is critical in assessing a cranial injury. The cranial nerves are numbered and named according to their functions **(Table 5-1).**

Blood Vessels of the Head and Face

The major vessels supplying the head and face are the common carotid and vertebral arteries **(Fig. 5-3)**. The common carotid artery ascends through the neck on either side to divide into the external and internal carotid artery just below the level of the jaw. The external carotid arteries and their branches supply most regions of

the head external to the brain. The middle meningeal artery supplies the skull and dura mater; if this artery is damaged, serious epidural bleeding can result. The internal carotid arteries send branches to the eyes and portions of the brain. The left and right vertebral arteries and their branches supply blood to the posterior region of the brain.

PROTECTIVE EQUIPMENT FOR THE HEAD AND FACE

Many head and facial injuries can be prevented with regular use of properly fitted helmets and facial protective devices, such as face guards, eye wear, ear wear, mouthguards, and throat protectors. Helmets, in particular, are required in football, ice hockey, men's lacrosse, baseball, softball, whitewater sports (kayaking), amateur boxing, and bicycling. Helmets must be fitted properly to disperse impact forces.

Football Helmets

Football helmet designs are typically single- or double-air bladder, closed-cell padded, or a combination of the two. Air bladders are excellent at absorbing shock, but they must be inspected daily by the players to ensure that adequate inflation is maintained for a proper fit. Helmet shells can be constructed of plastic or a polycarbonate alloy. Polycarbonate is a plastic used in making jet canopies and police riot gear and is lightweight, scratch-resistant, and impact-resistant. The life expectancy of helmets varies. Coaches should closely adhere to manufacturers' recommendation for replacements of old helmets.

TABLE 5.1	**THE CRANIAL NERVES**			
Number	**Name**	**Sensory**	**Motor**	**Function/Assessment**
I	Olfactory	X		Sense of smell
II	Optic	X		Test visual field (blurring or double vision)
III	Oculomotor		X	Test pupillary reaction to light
				Perform upward and inward gazes
IV	Trochlear		X	Perform downward and lateral gaze
V	Trigeminal	X	X	Touch face to note difference in sensation
				Clench teeth; push down on chin to separate jaws
VI	Abducens		X	Perform lateral and medial gaze
VII	Facial	X	X	Close eyes tight
				Smile and show the teeth
VIII	Vestibulocochlear	X		Identify the sound of fingers snapping near the ear
	(Acoustic)			Balance and coordination (stand on one foot)
IX	Glossopharyngeal	X	X	Gag reflex; ask the athlete to swallow
X	Vagus	X		Gag reflex; ask the athlete to swallow or say "Ahh"
XI	Accessory		X	Resisted shoulder shrug
XII	Hypoglossal		X	Ask athlete to stick out the tongue, note any
				deviation to one side

Helmets must be approved by the National Operating Committee on Standards for Athletic Equipment (NOCSAE). The NOCSAE mark on a helmet indicates that it meets minimum impact standards and can tolerate forces applied to several different areas of the helmet.

Always follow manufacturers' guidelines when fitting a football helmet. Before the helmet is fitted, athletes should have haircuts in the style that will be worn during the athletic season and should wet their heads to simulate game conditions. **Field Strategy 5-1** shows how to fit a football helmet. Once fitted, the helmet should be checked daily for proper fit. Fit can be altered by hair length, deterioration of internal padding, loss of air from cells, and spread of the face mask. Fitting is performed by inserting a tongue depressor between the pads and face. When the depressor is moved back and forth, a firm resistance should be felt. A snug-fitting helmet should not move in one direction when the head moves in another. In addition, the helmet should be checked weekly to ensure proper fit and compliance with safety standards **(Box 5-1)**.

Each helmet should have the purchase date and tracking number engraved on the inside. Detailed records should be kept that identify the purchase date, use, reconditioning history, and certification seals. Each athlete should be instructed on the proper use, fit, and care of the helmet. In addition, each athlete should sign a statement that confirms he or she has read the NOCSAE seal and has been informed of the risks of injury through improper use of the helmet or facemask when striking an opponent. This statement should be signed, dated, and kept as part of the player's medical files.

Other Helmets

Ice hockey helmet standards are monitored by the American Society for Testing and Materials (ASTM) and the Hockey Equipment Certification Council (HECC). These helmets are required to carry the stamp of approval from the Canadian Standards Association (CSA). Proper fit is achieved when a snug-fitting helmet does not move in one direction when the head is turned in another direction.

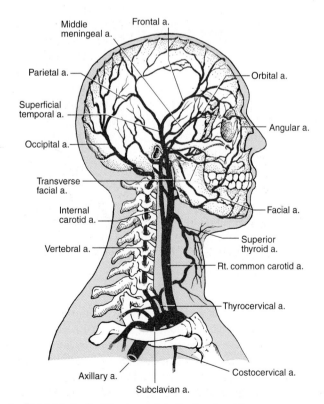

Middle meningeal a.
Frontal a.
Parietal a.
Orbital a.
Superficial temporal a.
Occipital a.
Angular a.
Transverse facial a.
Internal carotid a.
Facial a.
Vertebral a.
Superior thyroid a.
Rt. common carotid a.
Thyrocervical a.
Axillary a.
Costocervical a.
Subclavian a.

➤ FIGURE 5-3. Blood supply to the head and face.

FIELD STATEGY 5.1   PROPER FITTING OF A FOOTBALL HELMET

1. The player should have a haircut in the style that will be worn during the competitive season and should wet his or her hair to simulate game conditions. Measure the circumference of the head above the ears, using the tape measure supplied by the manufacturer. The suggested helmet size is listed on the reverse side of the tape.

2. Select the proper sized shell and adjust the front and back sizers and jaw pads for a proper fit.

3. Inflate the air bladder by holding the bulb with an arch in the hose; to deflate, the hose is in a straight position.

4. Ensure that the helmet fits snugly around the player's head and covers the base of the skull but does not impinge the cervical spine when the neck is extended. The ear holes should match up with the external auditory ear canal.

5. Check that the four-point chin strap is of equal tension and length on both sides, placing the chin pad an equal distance from each side of the helmet **(Figure A)**.

6. Check that face mask allows for a complete field of vision and that the helmet is one to two fingerwidths above the eyebrows and extends two fingerwidths away from the forehead and nose **(Figure B)**.

7. Check that the helmet does not move when the athlete presses forward on the rear of the helmet and when he or she presses straight down on top of the helmet **(Figure C)**.

8. Check the helmet does not slip when the athlete is asked to "bull" his or her neck while you grasp the face mask, pulling left then right **(Figure D)**.

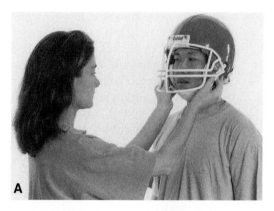
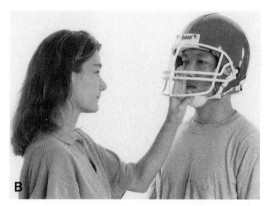
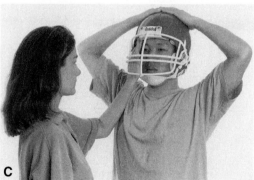
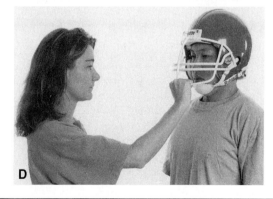

Batting helmets used in baseball and softball require the NOCSAE mark and must be a double ear-flap design. The helmets should have a thick layer of foam between the primary energy absorber and head to allow the shell to move slightly and deform. This maximizes its ability to absorb missile kinetic energy from a ball or bat and prevents excessive pressure on the cranium. The helmet should not move or fall off during batting and running bases.

Lacrosse helmets are mandatory in the men's game, optional in the women's game, and are worn by field hockey goalies. The helmet is made of a highly resistant plastic or fiberglass shell and must meet NOCSAE standards. The helmet, wire face guard, and chin pad are

➤ ➤ BOX 5-1

Weekly Helmet Inspection Checklist

❏ Check proper fit according to manufacturer's guidelines.

❏ Examine the shell for cracks, particularly around the holes. Replace the shell if any cracks are detected.

❏ Examine all mounting rivets, screws, Velcro®, and snaps for breakage, sharp edges, or looseness. Repair or replace as necessary.

❏ Replace the face guard if bare metal is visible, has a broken weld, or is grossly misshapen.

❏ Examine and replace any parts that are damaged, such as jaw pads, sweatbands, nose snubbers, and chin straps.

❏ Examine the chin strap for proper shape and fit; inspect the hardware to see if it needs replacement.

❏ Inspect shell according to the National Operating Committee on Standards for Athletic Equipment and the manufacturer's standards: only approved paints, waxes, decals, or cleaning agents are to be used on any helmet. Severe or delayed reaction to the substances may permanently damage the shell and affect its safety performance.

❏ If air- and fluid-filled helmets are used and the team travels to a different altitude, recheck the fit prior to use.

secured with a four-point chin strap. The helmet should not move in one direction when the head moves in another.

Face Guards

Face guards protect and shield the facial region from flying projectiles and come in many sizes and styles. NOC-SAE has set standards for strength and deflection for football face guards worn at the high school and college levels. Football face guards are made of heavy-gauge, plastic-coated steel rod and are designed to withstand impacts from blunt surfaces, such as the turf or another player's knee or elbow. The effectiveness of a football face guard depends on the strength of the guard itself, the helmet attachments, and the four-point chin strap on the helmet. When properly fitted, the face mask should extend two finger widths away from the forehead and allow for complete field of vision (see **Field Strategy 5.1**). No face protection should be less than two bars. If needed, eye shields made of Plexiglas or polycarbonate can be attached to the face mask.

Ice hockey face guards are made of clear plastic (polycarbonate), steel wire, or a combination of the two, and they must meet HECC and ASTM standards. Hockey face guards primarily prevent penetration of the hockey stick but are also effective against flying pucks and collisions with helmets, elbows, side boards, and the ice. The use of full-coverage face masks in amateur ice hockey has greatly reduced facial trauma. A single chin strap, however, still allows the helmet to ride back on the head when a force is directed to the frontal region, thus exposing the chin to lacerations. The guard stands away from the nose approximately 1 to 1 1/2 inches. If a wire mesh is used, the holes should be small enough to prevent penetration by a hockey stick.

Lacrosse face guards must meet NOCSAE standards. The wire mesh guard stands away from the face, but the four-point chin strap has a padded chin region in case the guard is driven back during a collision with another player. Face masks used by catchers and the home plate umpire in baseball and softball should fit snugly to the cheeks and forehead but should not impair vision. These devices can be used on players in the field and must meet ASTM standards.

CRANIAL INJURY MECHANISMS

A fracture or intracranial injury of the skull depends on the material properties of the skull, thickness of the skull in the specific area of impact, magnitude and direction of the sustained force, and size of the impact area. When the head is struck by another object such as a baseball, two phenomena occur—deformation and acceleration. The bone deforms and bends inward, placing the inner border of the skull under tensile strain, whereas the outer border is placed in compression **(Fig. 5-4A)**. If the force of impact is sufficient and the skull is thin in the region of impact, a skull fracture can occur where tensile loading occurs. In contrast, if the skull is thick and dense enough at the area of impact, it may sustain inward bending without fracture. Fracture may then occur some distance from the impact zone where the skull is thinner **(Fig. 5-4B)**.

If the force is not sufficient to lead to a skull fracture, an intracranial injury can still occur. The impact causes a shock wave to pass through the skull to the brain, causing the impact to accelerate. This acceleration can lead to shear, tensile, and compression strains within the brain substance. Shear is the most serious type of strain. If the brain is traumatized at the point of impact, it is called a **coup-type injury (Fig. 5-5A)**. The brain can be injured further as the full force of the brain's weight accelerates and hits the opposite side of the skull, leading to **contrecoup-type injury**, or an injury away from the actual impact site. In this type of injury, the head is typically moving and strikes a stationary object or a more slowly moving object. In an acceleration-deceleration injury, such as whiplash, the head is hurled forward, traumatizing the brain by the accelerated skull **(Fig. 5-5B)**. The brain is then smashed against the halted skull, which leads to further rebounding within the confines of the skull.

Cerebral trauma may lead to **focal injuries** involving only localized damage (i.e., epidural, subdural, or

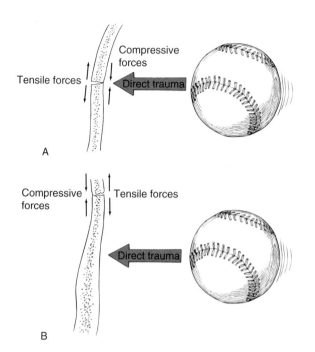

➤ FIGURE 5-4. Mechanical failure in bone. When a blow impacts the skull, the bone deforms and bends inward, placing tensile stress on the inner border of the skull. **A.** If impact is of sufficient magnitude and the skull is thin in the region of impact, a skull fracture occurs at the impact site. **B.** If the skull is thick and dense enough at the area of impact, it may sustain bending without fracture. However, the fracture may occur some distance from the impact zone in a region where the skull is thinner.

intracerebral hematomas), or **diffuse injuries** that involve widespread disruption and damage to the function or structure of the brain, such as a cerebral concussion. Although diffuse injuries account for only 25% of fatalities caused by head trauma, they are the most prevalent cause of long-term neurologic deficits in individuals.

SKULL FRACTURES

Skull fractures can be *linear* (in a line), *comminuted* (in multiple pieces), *depressed* (fragments are driven internally toward the brain), or *basilar* (involving the base of

the skull) **(Fig. 5-6)**. If there is a break in the skin adjacent to the fracture site and a tear to the underlying dura mater, the risk of bacterial infection into the intracranial cavity is high and can result in septic **meningitis**. Whenever a severe blow to the head occurs, a skull fracture should always be suspected.

Signs and Symptoms

Depending on the fracture site, different signs may appear **(Box 5-2)**. For example, a fracture at eyebrow level may lead to discoloration around the eyes (**raccoon eyes**). Blood or CSF may leak from the nose. Bony fragments may damage the optic or olfactory cranial nerves, leading to blindness or loss of smell. A basilar fracture above and behind the ear may lead to **Battle's sign**, a discoloration that can appear within minutes behind the ear. In addition, blood or CSF may leak from the ear canal, and a hearing loss or facial paralysis may be present. A fracture to the temple region may damage the meningeal arteries, causing epidural bleeding between the dura mater and skull (epidural hematoma). This can be life threatening and is discussed in more detail in the later section on focal cerebral injuries.

Management

A suspected skull fracture requires immediate action. Immediately initiate the emergency care plan and summon an ambulance. If fluids from the ears (otorrhea) or nose (rhinorrhea) are present, do not apply any pressure bandage or attempt to restrict the flow—this may increase intracranial pressure, complicating the injury. Cover open wounds with a sterile dressing, but do not apply pressure. Stabilize the neck region, which may also be injured. Initiate any emergency procedures (artificial ventilation or CPR), and treat for shock until help arrives. **Field Strategy 5-2** suggests management of a suspected skull fracture.

FOCAL CEREBRAL INJURIES

Focal cerebral injuries usually result in a localized collection of blood or hematoma. The skull has no room for

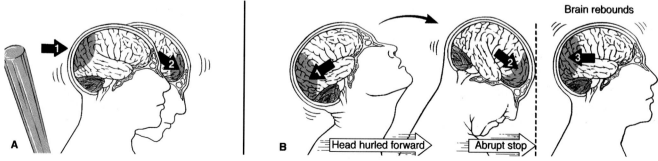

➤ FIGURE 5-5. Injury mechanisms to the head. **A.** Direct trauma can produce a coup-type injury or a contrecoup-type injury **B.** If acceleration and deceleration are involved, more extensive damage to the brain can occur.

➤➤ BOX 5-6

Information Sheet on Follow-up Care for a Head Injury

_____ has recently received a head injury during sport participation, but at this time it does not appear to be serious. Often, many signs and symptoms from a head injury do not become apparent until hours after the initial trauma. As such, we want to alert you to appropriate guidelines to follow for the next 24 hours.

For the rest of the day _____ should:

- Rest quietly for at least 24 hours
- Consume a liquid diet for the next 8 to 24 hours
- Apply ice to the head for 15 to 20 minutes every hour to relieve discomfort and swelling.
- Not use aspirin or other medication for 24 hours without a physician's approval; however, acetaminophen (normal dose only) may be used
- Not consume alcohol or drive a vehicle

Have someone wake the individual every 2 hours during the next 24 hours. If any of the following signs or symptoms are observed, seek medical help **immediately**:

- Persistent or increasing headache, particularly if it becomes localized or persists after 48 hours
- Persistent or increasing nausea or vomiting
- Mental confusion, disorientation, irritability, or forgetfulness that gets progressively worse (number or word recall)
- Loss of appetite
- Drowsiness, lethargy, sleepiness, or difficulty waking
- Any visual difficulties, dizziness, or ringing in the ears
- Unequal pupil size; slow or no pupil reaction to light
- Bleeding or clear fluid from the nose or ears
- Progressive or sudden impairment of consciousness
- Alterations in breathing pattern or irregular heartbeat
- Difficulty speaking or slurring of speech
- Convulsions or tremors

She or he should not participate or play again without medical clearance by a doctor.

Emergency Phone Numbers:
Ambulance   911

Hospital _____

Remember: If any of the symptoms or signs listed above become apparent, do not delay seeking medical treatment.

---

shield can be tinted to reduce glare from the sun; however, the plastic can become scratched and may fog up in cold weather.

Spectacles (eye glasses) contain the lenses, frame, and side shields commonly seen in industrial eye protective wear. The lenses should be 3 mm thick and be made from CR 39 plastic or polycarbonate, both of which can be incorporated with prescription lenses. CR 39 plastic lenses are generally less expensive, but they scratch more easily, are often thicker and heavier than polycarbonate, and are not impact resistant. In contrast, polycarbonate is lightweight, scratch resistant, has greater impact resistance, and can have an antifog and ultraviolet inhibitor incorporated into the lens.

The frame should be constructed of a resilient plastic, with reinforced temples, hinges, and nose piece. Adequate cushioning should protect the eyebrow and nasal bridge from sharp edges. Only polycarbonate eye protectors and eye frames that meet ASTM and parallel CSA standards offer enough protection for a sport participant.

Any individual with monocular vision or vision in only one eye should consult an ophthalmologist before participating in any sport because of the reduced visual fields and depth perception. If a decision is made to participate, the individual should wear maximum eye protection during all practices and competitions. Sport participants should wear a sweatband to keep sweat out of

FIELD STATEGY 5.3   CRANIAL INJURY EVALUATION

1. Stabilize head and neck

2. Determine initial level of consciousness

3. Check ABCs (if a helmet is worn, remove the face mask but do not remove the helmet or chin strap)

4. Activate EMS if necessary

5. History and mental status testing

6. Orientation (time, place, person, situation)

7. Concentration (digits backward, months of the year in reverse order)

8. Memory (names of teams in prior contests, recall of three words and three objects, recent newsworthy events, details of the contest)

9. Symptoms (headache, nausea, tinnitus)

10. Observe and inspect for:
    - Leakage of cerebrospinal fluid
    - Signs of trauma (deformity, body posturing, discoloration around the eyes and behind the ears)
    - Loss of emotional control (irritability, aggressiveness, or uncontrolled crying)

11. Palpate for:
    - Bony and soft tissue structures for point tenderness, crepitus, depressions, elevations, swelling, blood, or changes in skin temperature

12. Neurologic examination
    - Cranial nerve assessment
    - Pupil abnormalities (pupil size, response to light, eye movement, nystagmus, blurred or double vision)
    - Strength
    - Coordination (finger-to-nose test—eyes open, gait)
    - Sensation (finger-to-nose test—eyes closed, Romberg test, one-legged stork stand)

13. Functional tests
    - Five knee bends
    - Five sit-ups
    - Five push-ups
    - 40-yard sprint

the eye guard, and they should remove the eye guard when not participating.

Although sport participants often wear contact lenses because they improve peripheral vision and astigmatism and do not normally cloud during temperature changes, they do not protect against eye injury. Contact lenses come in two types: hard, or corneal type, that covers only the iris of the eye; and soft, or scleral type, which covers the entire front of the eye. Hard contact lenses often become dislodged and are associated more frequently with irritation from foreign bodies (corneal abrasions). Dust and other foreign matter may get underneath the lens and damage the cornea, or the cornea can be scratched while inserting or removing the lens.

Hemorrhage into the Anterior Chamber

Hemorrhage into the anterior chamber (**hyphema**) usually results from blunt trauma from a small ball (squash or racquetball), hockey puck, stick (field hockey or ice hockey), or swinging racquet (squash or racquetball). The small size of the object can fit within the confines of the eye orbit, thereby inflicting direct damage to the eye.

SIGNS AND SYMPTOMS

Initially, a red tinge in the anterior chamber may be present, but within a few hours, blood begins to settle into the anterior chamber, giving a characteristic meniscus appearance (**Fig. 5-13**).

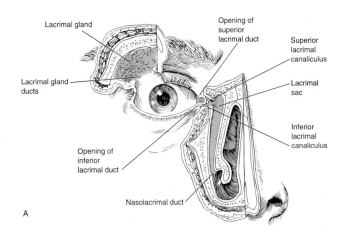

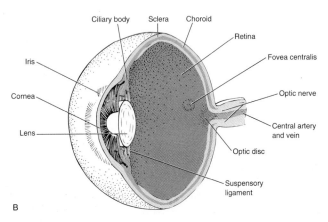

➤ FIGURE 5-12. The eye. **A.** Lacrimal structures of the eye. **B.** Internal structures of the eye globe.

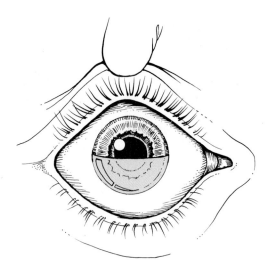

➤ FIGURE 5-13. Hyphema. Blood in the anterior chamber of the eye signals a serious eye injury.

MANAGEMENT

If a hemorrhage is present, immediately activate EMS—the individual must be transported to the nearest medical facility in a semireclining or seated position. The condition requires hospitalization, bed rest, bilateral patching of the eyes, and sedation.

Detached Retina

Damage to the posterior segment of the eye can occur with or without trauma to the anterior segment. A **detached retina** occurs when fluid seeps into the retinal break and separates the neurosensory retina from the retinal epithelium. This can occur days or even weeks after the initial trauma.

SIGNS AND SYMPTOMS

The individual frequently describes the condition with phrases like, "A curtain fell over my eye," or "I keep seeing flashes of light going on and off." Floaters and light flashes are early signs that the retina is damaged.

MANAGEMENT

Immediately refer this person to an ophthalmologist because surgery is often necessary.

Orbital "Blowout" Fracture

Direct trauma to the eye from an object, usually larger than the eye orbit, can lead to a **blowout fracture**. Upon impact, forces drive the orbital contents posteriorly against the orbital walls. This sudden increase in intraorbital pressure is released in the area of least resistance, typically the orbital floor. The globe descends into the defect in the floor.

SIGNS AND SYMPTOMS

Examination may reveal diplopia (double vision), absent eye movement, numbness on the side of fracture below the eye, and a recessed, downward displaced globe. The lack of eye movement becomes evident when the individual is asked to look up and only one eye is able to move **(Fig. 5-14)**.

MANAGEMENT

The coach should apply ice to the area to limit swelling but not add additional compression or pressure over the suspected fracture site. The individual should immediately be referred to the nearest medical facility.

Conjunctivitis (Pinkeye)

Conjunctivitis is an inflammation or bacterial infection of the conjunctiva, the membrane between the inner lining of the eyelid and anterior eyeball.

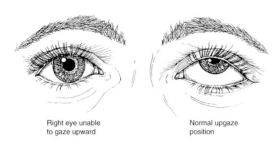

➤ FIGURE 5-14. Orbital "blowout" fracture. An orbital fracture can entrap the inferior rectus muscle, leading to an inability to elevate the eye.

Right eye unable to gaze upward

Normal upgaze position

SIGNS AND SYMPTOMS

The infection leads to itching, burning, and watering of the eye, causing the conjunctiva to become inflamed and red, giving a pinkeye appearance.

MANAGEMENT

This condition can be highly infectious. Therefore, the individual should be referred immediately to a physician for medical treatment.

Subconjunctival Hemorrhage

SIGNS AND SYMPTOMS

Because of direct trauma to the globe, several small capillaries rupture, making the white sclera of the eye appear red, blotchy, and inflamed. The condition looks much worse than it is.

MANAGEMENT

This relatively harmless condition requires no treatment and resolves spontaneously in 1 to 3 weeks. If blurred vision, pain, limited eye movement, or blood in the anterior chamber are present, however, immediate referral to an ophthalmologist is warranted.

Periorbital Ecchymosis (Black Eye)

SIGNS AND SYMPTOMS

Impact forces can cause significant swelling and hemorrhage into the surrounding eyelid. The discoloration is called **periorbital ecchymosis**.

MANAGEMENT

Treatment involves controlling the swelling and hemorrhage by using crushed ice or ice water in a latex surgical glove. It is essential that the glove does not have rosin or other powdered substances on it. Because of possible leakage, chemical ice bags should not be used. This condition requires referral to an ophthalmologist for further examination to rule out an underlying fracture or injury to the globe.

Foreign Bodies

SIGNS AND SYMPTOMS

Dust or dirt in the eyes can lead to intense pain and tearing. Tearing and photophobia (sensitivity to light) indicate a corneal abrasion.

MANAGEMENT

The individual may resist any attempt to open the eyelids to view the eye. The foreign body, if not embedded or on the cornea, should be removed with sterile gauze and the eye inspected for any visible abnormalities. If the foreign object is impaled or embedded, however, do not touch or attempt to remove the object. Activate EMS.

Assessment

Field Strategy 5-4 lists a suggested protocol for evaluating an eye injury. **Box 5-7** identifies general signs and symptoms of eye conditions that necessitate further examination by a physician.

NASAL INJURIES

The nose is composed of bone and hyaline cartilage **(Fig. 5-15)**. The roof is formed by the cribriform plate of the ethmoid bone. The nasal bones form the bridge of the nose. Inferiorly, the lateral walls are shaped by the superior and middle conchae of the ethmoid bone, the vertical plates of the palatine bones, and the inferior nasal conchae. The nasal cavity is separated into right and left halves by the nasal septum. The septum is made of cartilage that can be fractured if struck by a blunt object. This can complicate soft tissue injury assessment and treatment.

Fractures

Fractures to the nasal bone are the most common facial fracture in sport. Blunt trauma is the leading mechanism of injury with lateral forces producing the greatest amount of visible deformity.

SIGNS AND SYMPTOMS

Bleeding is usually profuse, and the nose may appear flattened and lose its symmetry, particularly if a lateral force caused the fracture. Swelling is rapid. The nasal airway can be obstructed with bony fragments, or the fracture can extend into the cranial region and cause a loss of cerebrospinal fluid. There may be crepitus over the nasal bridge and ecchymosis under the eyes. Severity can range from a slightly depressed greenstick fracture (seen in adolescents) to total displacement or disruption in the bony and cartilaginous parts of the nose.

2. Signs that indicate a possible skull fracture include:
   - Deformity
   - Unequal pupils
   - Discoloration around both eyes or behind the ears
   - Bleeding or CSF leaking from the nose or ear
   - Any loss of sight or smell
3. Signs or symptoms of increasing intracranial pressure after head trauma include:
   - Severe headache
   - Pupil irregularity or irregular eye tracking
   - Confusion, or progressive or sudden impairment of consciousness
   - Rising blood pressure and falling pulse rate
   - Drastic changes in emotional control
4. Signs and symptoms of a concussion include:
   - Headache, dizziness, or vertigo
   - Lack of awareness of surroundings
   - Nausea and vomiting
   - Deteriorating level of consciousness
   - Diminished alertness with heightened distractibility
   - Inability to maintain coherent thought patterns
   - Inability to carry out a sequence of goal-directed movements
5. Injuries that indicate increasing intracranial pressure, memory dysfunction, or gross observable incoordination require immediate referral to a physician. Activate EMS.
6. Direct trauma to the eye can lead to a black eye, hemorrhage into the anterior chamber, detached retina, or orbital fracture. Loss of visual acuity, abnormal eye movement, diplopia, numbness below the eye, or a downward displacement of the globe signals a serious condition. The individual should be referred immediately to an ophthalmologist.
7. A foreign body in the eye, if not embedded or on the cornea, should be removed and the eye inspected for any scratches, abrasions, or lacerations.
8. The nose is particularly susceptible to lateral displacement from trauma. Simultaneously, the trauma may also lead to a concussion.
9. Fractures to the facial bones often result in malocclusion.
10. When a loose tooth has been displaced outwardly or laterally, the athletic trainer or coach should try to place the tooth back into its normal position without forcing it. Teeth that are intruded should be left alone; any attempt to move the tooth may result in permanent loss of the tooth. The individual should be referred to a dentist immediately.
11. A dislocated tooth should be located, rinsed in milk or saline solution, and replaced intraorally within the tooth socket. The individual should be seen by a dentist within 30 minutes to replace the tooth.
12. Cauliflower ear is common in wrestlers and is completely preventable by wearing proper headgear at all times when on the mat.

References

1. Colorado Medical Society. Report of the Sports Medicine Committee: Guidelines for the management of concussion in sports (rev). Denver: Colorado Medical Society, 1991.
2. Quality Standards Subcommittee of the American Academy of Neurology. 1997. Practice parameter: The management of concussion in sports. Neurology, 48(3):581–585.
3. Cantu RC, and Voy R. 1995. Second impact syndrome: A risk in any contact sport. Phys Sportsmed, 23(6):27–34.
4. Kelly JP, and Rosenberg JH. 1997. Diagnosis and management of concussion in sports. Neurology, 48(3)575–580.

FIELD STATEGY 6.1   EXERCISES TO PREVENT SPINAL INJURIES (CONTINUED)

STRENGTHENING EXERCISES

G. **Angry cat stretch (posterior pelvic tilt)**. Kneel on all fours with knees hip-width apart. Tighten the buttocks, and arch the back upward while lowering the chin and tilting the pelvis backwards. Relax the buttocks and allow the pelvis to drop downward and forward.

H. **Crunch curl-up**. In a supine position with the knees flexed, flatten the back and curl up to elevate the head and shoulders from the floor. Alternate exercises include diagonal crunch curl-ups and hip crunches.

I. **Prone extension**. In a prone position, raise up on the elbows. Progress to raising up onto the hands.

J. **Alternate arm and leg lift**. In a fully extended prone position, lift one arm and the opposite leg off the surface at least three inches. Repeat with the opposite arm and leg.

K. **Double arm and leg lift**. In a fully extended prone position, lift both arms and legs off the surface at least three inches. Hold and return to starting position.

L. **Alternate arm and leg extension on all fours**. Kneel on all fours, raise one leg behind the body while raising the opposite arm in front of the body. Ankle and wrist weights may be added for additional resistance.

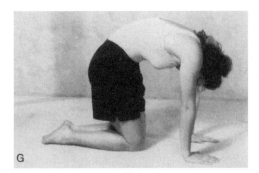
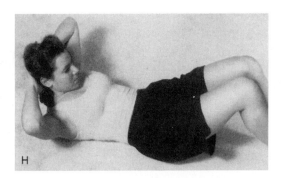
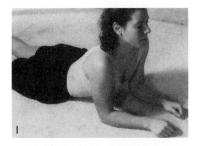
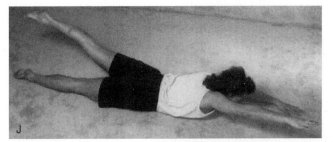
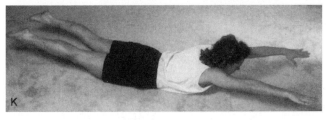
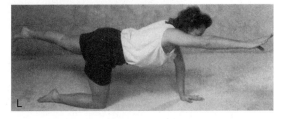

cal facet joints, makes the cervical spine the most mobile region of the spinal column. As such, this area is especially vulnerable to injury. Because the range of motion in the cervical spine is greatest in flexion, a head position of extreme flexion generates the largest bending moment. When combined with axial compressional load-ing, this generates the leading mechanism of injury for severe cervical spine injuries. For example, when a football tackle is executed with the head in a flexed position, the cervical spine is aligned in a segmented column and subjected to both large compressional forces, generated by the cervical muscles, and axial impact forces **(Fig. 6-**

FIELD STRATEGY 6.2   PELVIC STABILIZATION AND ABDOMINAL STRENGTHENING EXERCISES

A. **Stabilization in neutral position**. With the back in a neutral position, slowly shift forward over the arms adjusting pelvic position as you move. There will be a tendency to "sag" the back, so progressively tighten and relax the abdominal muscles during forward movement and backward movement, respectively.

B. **Stabilization in "two point" position**. Balance on the right leg and left arm. Slowly move forward and back without losing neutral position. Switch to the opposite arm and leg.

C. **Leg exercise**. Without arching the back, lift one leg out behind you. Do not lift the foot more than a few inches from the floor. A variation is to move a flexed knee sideways away from the body, then back to the original position.

D. **Half-knee to stand (lunges)**. Move to a standing position while maintaining neutral hip position. Push evenly with both legs. Repeat several times, then switch the forward leg.

E. **Pelvic tilt**. With the hips and knees bent and feet on the floor, do an isometric contraction of the abdominal muscles (posterior pelvic tilt) and hold. Using the phase "tuck the stomach in" may convey the correct motion. Then, arch the back, doing an anterior pelvic tilt. Alternate between the two motions until you can control pelvic motion.

F. **Bridging**. Keeping the back in neutral position, raise the hips and back off the floor (contract the abdominal muscles to hold the position). Hold for 5 to 10 seconds, drop down, and relax. Repeat. Variations include adding pelvic tilt exercises, lifting one leg off the floor (keep the back in neutral position), and combining pelvic tilts and one leg lift with bridging.

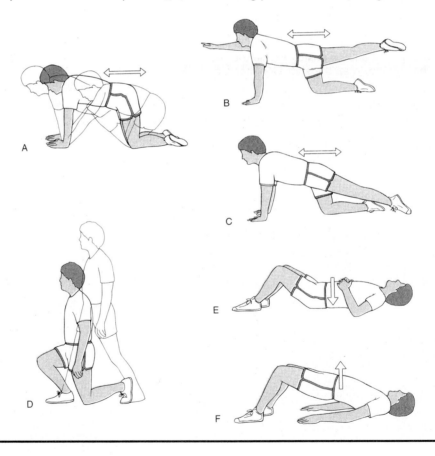

10). Impact causes loading along the longitudinal axis of the cervical vertebrae, leading to compression deformation. The intervertebral discs can initially absorb some energy; however, as continued force is exerted, further deformation and buckling occurs, leading to failure of the intervertebral discs, cervical vertebrae, or both **(Fig. 6-11)**. This results in subluxation, disc herniation, facet dislocation, or fracture-dislocation at one or more spinal levels.

Strains

Cervical strains usually involve the sternocleidomastoid or upper trapezius, although other muscles may be involved.

Preventing Low Back Injuries in Activities of Daily Living

SITTING
- Sit on a firm, straight-backed chair.
- Place the buttocks as far back into the chair as possible to avoid slouching.
- Sit with the feet flat on the floor.
- Avoid sitting for long periods, particularly if the knees are fully extended.

DRIVING
- Place the seat forward so the knees are level with the hips and reaching for the pedals is not required.
- If the left foot is not working the pedals, place it flat on the floor.
- Keep the back of the seat in a nearly upright position to avoid slouching.

STANDING
- If you must stand in one area for an extended time, do the following:
  - Shift body weight from one foot to the other.
  - Elevate one foot on a piece of furniture to keep the knees flexed.
  - Do toe flexion and extension inside the shoes.
- Hold the chin up, keep the shoulders back, and relax the knees.

LIFTING AND CARRYING
- Use a lumbosacral belt or have assistance when lifting heavy objects. To lift an object:
  - Place the object close to the body.
  - Bend at the knees, not the waist, and keep the back erect.
  - Tighten the abdominal muscles and inhale before lifting the object.
  - Exhale during the lift.
  - Do not twist while lifting.
- To carry a heavy object:
  - Hold the object close to the body at waist level.
  - Carry the object in the middle of the body not to one side.

SLEEPING
- Sleep on a firm mattress. If needed, place a sheet of 3/4-inch plywood under the mattress
- Sleep on your side and place pillows between the legs.
- If you sleep supine, place pillows under the knees. Avoid sleeping in the prone position
- Because waterbeds support the body curves evenly, they may relieve low back pain. However, avoid waterbeds if you have an acute injury.

Strains typically occur at the extremes of motion or in association with a violent muscle contraction, an external force, or weakness caused by poor posture.

SIGNS AND SYMPTOMS

Symptoms include pain, stiffness, and restricted range of motion. Palpation reveals muscle spasms, and increased

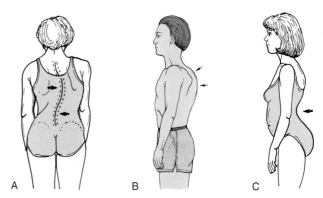

➤ FIGURE 6-7. Spinal anomalies. **A.** Scoliosis. **B.** Thoracic kyphosis. **C.** Lordosis.

pain occurs during active contraction or passive stretching of the involved muscle. Generally, symptoms subside within 3 to 7 days.

MANAGEMENT

Initial treatment includes rest, cryotherapy, prescribed nonsteroidal anti-inflammatory drugs (NSAIDs), and use of a cervical collar for support, if needed. Return to sports participation should not occur until the individual is free of neck pain and until range of motion and neck strength are normal. If the condition does not rapidly improve, referral to a physician is warranted to rule out a possible spinal fracture, dislocation, or disc injury.

Sprains

The same mechanisms that cause cervical strains also lead to cervical sprains. Both injuries often occur simultaneously. Minor activity, such as maintaining the head in an uncomfortable posture or sleeping position, can also produce sprains of the neck. Injury can occur to any of the major ligaments traversing the cervical spine, as well as to the capsular ligaments surrounding the facet joints. Severe forces, which are great enough to cause a cervical dislocation, may also lead to a cervical fracture. These injuries are discussed in the next section.

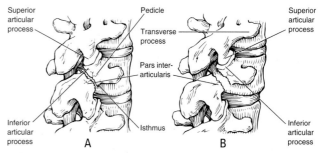

➤ FIGURE 6-8. Spondylolysis and spondylolisthesis. **A.** Spondylolysis is a stress fracture of the pars interarticularis. **B.** Spondylolisthesis is a bilateral fracture of the pars interarticularis accompanied by anterior slippage of the involved vertebra.

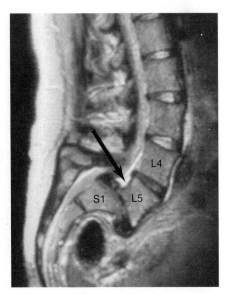

➤ FIGURE 6-9. Spondylolisthesis. In this magnetic resonance imaging scan of spondylolisthesis, note the anterior shift of the L5 vertebra.

SIGNS AND SYMPTOMS

Symptoms include pain, stiffness, and restricted range of motion, but no neurologic or bony injury usually exists. Unlike cervical strains, the symptoms of a sprain can persist for several days.

MANAGEMENT

Initial management for a cervical sprain is the same as for a muscle strain. If the condition does not rapidly improve, referral to a physician is warranted to rule out a more serious underlying condition.

Fractures and Dislocations

Unsafe practices, such as diving into shallow water, spearing in football, or landing on the posterior neck during gymnastics or trampoline activities, can lead to cervical fractures and dislocations from the axial loading and violent neck flexion. In sports, these serious injuries commonly occur at the fourth, fifth, and sixth cervical vertebrae.

SIGNS AND SYMPTOMS

Because neural damage can range from none to complete severance of the spinal cord, there is a range of accompanying symptoms (Box 6-2). Painful palpation over the spinous processes, muscle spasm, or a palpable defect indicates a possible fracture or dislocation. Radiating pain, numbness, muscle weakness, paralysis, or loss of bladder or bowel control are all critical signs of neural damage.

MANAGEMENT

Because spinal cord damage can lead to paralysis or death, any suspected unstable neck injury should be treated as a medical emergency. An unstable neck injury should be suspected in an unconscious athlete, an athlete who is awake but has numbness or paralysis, or a neurologically intact athlete who has neck pain or pain with neck movement.

Without moving the head or neck, the coach should stabilize the neck, assess the ABCs (airway, breathing, and circulation), and manage any life-threatening situations. The coach should activate Emergency Medical Services (EMS) and help the technicians immobilize the injured athlete on a spine board.

THORACIC SPINE INJURIES

The protective rib cage limits movement in the thoracic area. The thoracolumbar junction, however, is a region of potentially high stress during flexion-extension movements of the trunk. Direct blows to the back during contact sports frequently yield contusions to the muscles in the thoracic region. Such injuries range in severity but are generally characterized by pain, ecchymosis, spasm, and limited swelling.

Strains and Sprains

Thoracic sprains and strains result from either overloading or overstretching muscles in the region through violent or sustained muscle contractions.

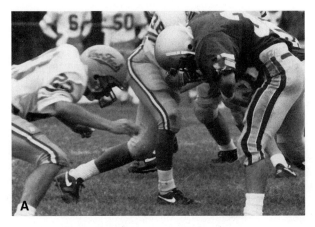

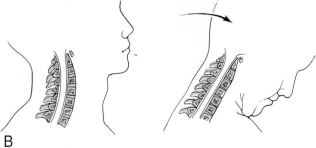

➤ FIGURE 6-10. Axial loading. In a normally erect position, the cervical spine is slightly extended. **A.** When a football tackle is executed with the head flexed at about 30°, **B.** the cervical vertebrae are aligned in a column and subjected to compressional forces (generated by the cervical muscles) and to axial loading.

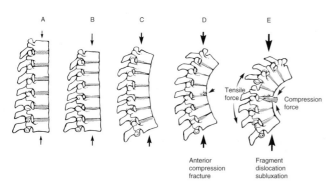

➤ FIGURE 6-11. Deformation of the intervertebral discs. **A,B.** Axial loading on the vertebral column causes compressive deformation of the intervertebral discs. **C.** As load continues and maximum compression deformation is reached, angular deformation and buckling occurs. **D,E.** Continued force results in an anterior compression fracture, subluxation, or dislocation.

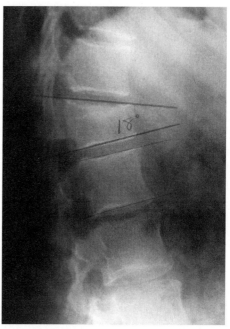

➤ FIGURE 6-12. Thoracic fracture. This radiograph shows a compression wedge fracture in the thoracic region caused by several compressed motion segments.

SIGNS AND SYMPTOMS

Painful spasms of the back muscles serve as a protective mechanism to immobilize the injured area, and they may develop as a sympathetic response to a sprain. The presence of such spasms, however, makes it difficult to determine whether the injury is actually a strain or sprain.

MANAGEMENT

Standard acute care helps diminish pain and muscle spasm. Dramatic improvement in a thoracic sprain can occur in 24 to 48 hours. Severe strains, however, may require 3 or 4 weeks to heal.

Fractures

Large compressive loads, such as those sustained during heavy weightlifting, head-on contact in football or rugby, or landing on the buttock area during gymnastics or cheerleading dismounts, can fracture the vertebral end

plates or lead to a **wedge fracture**, named after the shape of the deformed vertebral body **(Fig. 6-12)**. These fractures tend to be concentrated at the lower end of the thoracic spine in the transition region between the thoracic and lumbar curvatures. Females with **osteopenia**, a condition of reduced bone mineralization, are particularly susceptible to these fractures. More commonly, compressive stress during small, repetitive loads in an activity, such as running, leads to a progressive compression fracture of a weakened vertebral body. In addition, repeated flexion-extension of the thoracic spine, which occurs during the butterfly and breast strokes, can inflame the apophyses, or the growth centers of the vertebral bodies. **Apophysitis** is a progressive condition characterized by local pain and tenderness.

SIGNS AND SYMPTOMS

Localized pain and discomfort can be palpated over the spinous processes of the involved vertebrae. Muscle spasm and guarding are also present. Increased pain can be elicited with forward flexion and lateral flexion of the thoracic spine.

MANAGEMENT

Initial treatment for soft tissue injuries consists of cryotherapy, prescribed NSAIDs, and activity modification, such as eliminating repeated flexion-extension activities. If symptoms persist or are at the level where normal function is compromised, referral to a physician is necessary to rule out more serious conditions, such as a fracture or apophysitis.

➤ ➤ BOX 6-2

Red Flags Indicating a Possible Cervical Spine Injury

- Mechanism of injury involving violent axial loading, flexion, or rotation of the neck
- Pain over the spinous process, with or without deformity
- Unrelenting neck pain or muscle spasm
- Abnormal sensations on the head, neck, trunk, or extremities
- Muscular weakness in the extremities
- Loss of coordinated movement
- Paralysis or inability to move a body part
- Absent or weak reflexes
- Loss of bladder or bowel control

NERVE AND VASCULAR CONDITIONS

Nerve and vascular conditions in the cervical and thoracic region are typically caused by compression of soft and bony tissue into the spinal canal or intervertebral foramen. These conditions can be frightening for the athlete, particularly if abnormal neurologic signs are present.

Spinal Cord Injury

The spinal cord is well protected within the spinal column. However, when acute trauma such as a vertebral fracture or dislocation occurs, or when degenerative changes are present, neurologic complications may result. These injuries can range from a simple contusion of the cord to complete severance of the cord.

SIGNS AND SYMPTOMS

Compression on the spinal cord may result in transient **neurapraxia**, which can lead to mild bilateral sensory changes, such as burning, tingling, or numbness. Motor changes in the upper or lower extremity may range from mild weakness to temporary paralysis. These symptoms usually subside in a few minutes but may linger for 1 to 2 days.

MANAGEMENT

Any bilateral sensory changes or muscle weakness in an athlete signals a serious injury, and the athlete should be immediately referred for further evaluation by a physician.

Brachial Plexus Injury

The brachial plexus (C5 to T1) innervates the upper extremity. The plexus is typically damaged in two ways

(**Fig. 6-13**). A "stretch injury" can occur when the head is forced laterally away from the shoulder while the shoulder is simultaneously forced downward, such as when an individual is tackled and subsequently rolls onto the shoulder with the head turned to the opposite side. A stretch injury can also occur when the arm is forced into excessive external rotation, abduction, and extension. The other mechanism of injury involves a "pinching injury" when the head is rotated, laterally flexed, and compressed or extended to the same side of the shoulder, compressing the intervertebral foramen and impinging the nerve root. The fixed plexus can also be pinched between the football shoulder pad and the superior medial scapula, where the brachial plexus is most superficial. This site, called **Erb's point**, is located 2 to 3 cm above the clavicle at the level of the transverse process of the C6 vertebra.

SIGNS AND SYMPTOMS

This injury usually affects the upper trunk (C5, C6) of the brachial plexus and leads to a sensory loss or **paresthesia** in the appropriate dermatome: the lateral arm, or the thumb and index finger, respectively. Acute symptoms involve an immediate, severe, burning pain that radiates from the clavicular area down the arm into the hand, hence the nickname "burner" or "stinger." Pain is usually transient and subsides in 5 to 10 minutes, but tenderness over the supraclavicular area and shoulder weakness may persist for hours or days after the injury. The individual often tries to shake the arm to "get the feeling back." Muscle weakness is evident in shoulder abduction and external rotation. Unlike cervical cord compression, in which symptoms are always bilateral, symptoms from a brachial plexus injury are unilateral, meaning the symptoms only affect the involved side of the body.

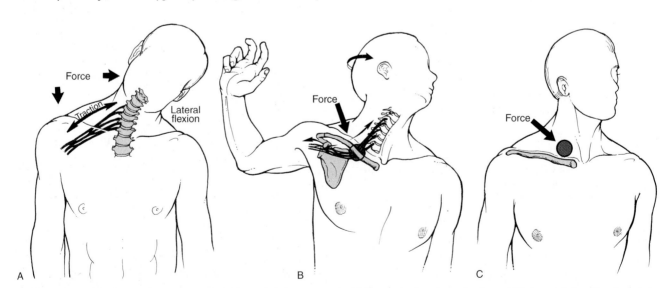

➤ **FIGURE 6-13.** Common mechanisms of a brachial plexus stretch. A blow to the head causing lateral flexion and shoulder depression may lead to a traction injury to the upper trunk of the brachial plexus **A**. An injury can also occur when a blow to the supraclavicular region causes lateral flexion with rotation and extension of the cervical spine away from the blow **B**. Compression over Erb's point, the most superficial passage of the brachial plexus, can also lead to a "pinching injury," whereby pain and paresthesia radiate into the upper extremity **C**.

TABLE 6.1 CLASSIFICATION OF "BURNERS"

Grade	Injury	Signs	Prognosis
I	Neurapraxia injury	Temporary loss of sensation or loss of motor function	Recovery within days to a few weeks
II	Axonotmesis injury	Significant motor and mild sensory deficits	Deficits last at least 2 weeks Regrowth is slow, but full or normal function is usually restored
III	Neurotmesis injury	Motor and sensory deficits persist for up to 1 year	Poor prognosis Surgical intervention is often necessary

Burners are graded in three levels **(Table 6-1)**. Grade I burners represent **neurapraxia**, the mildest lesion, whereby only a temporary loss of sensation or loss of motor function occurs. Recovery usually occurs within days to a few weeks. Grade II burners are **axonotmesis** injuries that produce significant motor and mild sensory deficits that last at least 2 weeks, but full or normal function is usually restored. Grade III burners are **neurotmesis** injuries, which cause actual damage to the nerves. These severe injuries have a poor prognosis; motor and sensory deficits persist for up to 1 year.

MANAGEMENT

When weakness is present, the individual should be removed from competition. If strength and function return completely in 1 to 2 minutes, the athlete can return to play. If any neurologic symptoms persist after this time, the athlete should not be allowed to return to play until evaluated by a physician. Return to play should occur only when full strength, range of motion, and sensation are restored in the cervical spine and extremity.

LUMBAR SPINE INJURIES

The lumbar spine must support the weight of the head, trunk, and arms, plus any load held in the hands. In addition, the two lower lumbar segments (L4-L5, L5-S1) provide a large range of motion in flexion-extension. It is not surprising, then, that mechanical abuse often results in episodes of low back pain, or that the lower lumbar discs are injured more frequently than any others in the spine.

Low Back Pain

An estimated 80% of the population experiences low back pain (LBP) at some time. Although LBP typically strikes individuals between the ages of 25 and 60 years, with frequency peaking at about age 40, it also occurs in as many as 25% of adolescents and children, ranging down to age 10.[4] Males and females appear to be equally susceptible. Although several known pathologies may cause LBP, reduced spinal flexibility, weak core musculature, repeated stress, and activities that require maximal extension of the lumbar spine are most associated with chronic LBP.

SIGNS AND SYMPTOMS

Low back pain is common in running activities because many runners have muscle tightness in the hip flexors and hamstrings. Tight hip flexors tend to produce a forward body lean, leading to anterior pelvic tilt and hyperlordosis of the lumbar spine. Because the lumbar muscles develop tension to counteract the forward bending moment of the entire trunk when the trunk is in flexion, these muscles are particularly susceptible to strains. This, coupled with tight hamstrings, can lead to a shorter stride.

MANAGEMENT

Treatment centers on avoiding excessive flexion activities and a sedentary posture **(Box 6-3)**. Ice, rest, and prescribed NSAIDs or muscle relaxants can reduce pain and inflammation. If symptoms do not improve within a week, refer the individual to a physician to rule out a more serious underlying condition. To decrease the incidence of LBP, training techniques should allow for adequate pro-

➤ ➤ **BOX 6-3**

Reducing Low Back Pain in Runners

- Wear properly fitted shoes that control heel motion and provide maximum shock absorption.
- Increase flexibility at the hip, knee, ankle plantar flexors, and trunk extensors.
- Increase strength in the abdominal and trunk extensor muscles.
- Avoid excessive body weight.
- Warm up and stretch thoroughly before and after running.
- Run with an upright stance rather than a forward lean.
- Avoid excessive side-to-side sway.
- Run on even terrain and limit hill work. Avoid running on concrete and on crowned roads.
- Avoid overstriding to increase speed because it increases leg shock.
- Gradually increase distance, intensity, and duration. Do not increase any parameter more than 10% in 1 week.
- If orthotics are worn and pain persists, check for wear and rigidity.
- Consider alternatives to running, such as cycling, rowing, or swimming.

gression of distance, speed, and hill work and should include extensive flexibility exercises for the hip and thigh region.

Disc Injuries

Prolonged mechanical loading of the spine can lead to microruptures in the annulus fibrosus, resulting in degeneration of the disc. When the nucleus of the disc works its way through the fibers of the annulus, it is called a **prolapsed disc**. It is called an **extruded disc** when the material moves into the spinal canal, where it runs the risk of impinging on adjacent nerve roots. The most commonly herniated discs are the lower two lumbar discs between L4 to L5 and L5 to S1. Most ruptures move in a posterior or posterolateral direction as a result of torsion and compression, not just compression.

SIGNS AND SYMPTOMS

Because the intervertebral discs are not innervated, the sensation of pain does not occur until the surrounding soft tissue structures are impinged. Symptoms include sharp pain and muscle spasms at the site of the herniation that often shoot down the sciatic nerve into the lower extremity. This common symptom may also be linked to **sciatica**, an inflammatory condition of the sciatic nerve. Although sciatica may result from a muscle-related or facet joint disease, or from compression of the nerve between the piriformis muscle, it is more commonly caused by a herniated disc. The resulting radiating leg pain is greater than back pain and increases with sitting and leaning forward, coughing, sneezing, and straining. The individual may walk in a slightly crouched position, leaning away from the side of the lesion.

Radiating pain can also be elicited by a **Valsalva maneuver**. The athlete holds his or her breath and bears down (as if having a bowel movement), or the athlete can blow into a closed fist. If the space has been reduced by swelling or a herniated disc, this increase in intrathecal pressure causes pain to radiate down the distribution of the involved nerve root.

MANAGEMENT

Immediate treatment involves the use of ice to reduce lumbar pain and muscle spasm. In mild cases, it may be helpful to minimize load on the spine by avoiding activities that involve impact, lifting, bending, twisting, and prolonged sitting and standing. Painful muscle spasms can be eliminated with ice or heat, administration of prescribed NSAIDs or muscle relaxants, passive exercise, and gentle stretching. Significant signs indicating the need for immediate referral to a physician include muscle weakness, sensory changes, diminished reflexes in the lower extremity, and abnormal bladder or bowel function.

Fractures

As mentioned earlier, compression fractures, although rare, more commonly involve the L1 vertebra at the thoracolumbar junction. Hyperflexion, or jack-knifing of the trunk, results in compression or crushing of the anterior aspect of the vertebral body. The primary danger with this injury is the possibility of bony fragments moving into the spinal canal to damage the spinal cord or spinal nerves.

SIGNS AND SYMPTOMS

Symptoms include immediate localized pain over the vertebrae, crepitus, and an unwillingness to move the back. Palpable pain may radiate down the nerve root if a bony fragment compresses a spinal nerve.

MANAGEMENT

Because the spinal cord ends at about the L1 or L2 level, fractures of the lumbar vertebrae below this point do not pose a serious threat, but they should still be handled carefully to minimize potential nerve damage to the cauda equina. Confirmation of a possible fracture is made with a radiograph or computed tomography scan.

SACRUM AND COCCYX INJURIES

Because the sacrum and coccyx are essentially immobile, the potential for mechanical injury to these regions is dramatically reduced. Sprains of the sacroiliac joint may result from a single traumatic episode involving bending or twisting, repetitive stress from lifting, a fall on the buttocks, excessive side-to-side or up-and-down motion during running and jogging, running on uneven terrain, suddenly slipping or stumbling forward, or wearing new shoes or orthoses. Direct blows to the region can produce contusions and fractures of the coccyx.

SIGNS AND SYMPTOMS

Symptoms include unilateral dull pain in the sacral area that extends into the buttock and posterior thigh. Muscle spasm is not common. Standing on one leg or climbing stairs may also increase the pain. If a coccygeal fracture is present, severe pain is present when sitting and may last for several months.

MANAGEMENT

Treatment for sacroiliac sprains includes cryotherapy, prescribed NSAIDs, and gentle stretching to alleviate stiffness. Treatment for coccygeal pain includes analgesics and use of padding for protection and a ring seat to alleviate compression during sitting.

ASSESSMENT OF THE SPINE

Injury assessment of the spine is complex and cannot be rushed. To review assessment guidelines for an unconscious individual with a suspected spinal injury, refer to Chapter 2.

When approaching the athlete, assess the ABCs. If the athlete is conscious, place a hand on the shoulder to calm and reassure the athlete that you are there to help. Do not remove the helmet or move the individual's head, neck, or spine. If possible, have an assistant stabilize the head while you conduct the initial assessment. A brief neuromuscular assessment should be immediately conducted to detect any motor or sensory deficits that may indicate a spinal injury. Ask the individual if he or she is experiencing any burning, numbness, or tingling in any extremity. Is there any difficulty breathing or swallowing? Can the individual wiggle the fingers and toes? Without moving the individual, ask him or her to perform a submaximal bilateral hand-squeeze test and ankle dorsiflexion. These two actions assess the cervical and lumbar spinal nerves, respectively. To test for cutaneous sensory changes, run the open hand and fingernails over the head, neck, back, thorax, abdomen, and upper and lower extremities (front, back, and sides). Ask the person if the sensation feels the same on one body segment as compared to the other. Muscle weakness or diminished sensation over the hands and feet indicate a serious injury. If any deficits are noted, initiate the emergency care plan and activate EMS.

If a fully conscious person is not experiencing severe pain, spasm, or tenderness, the individual has probably not sustained a significant spinal injury. It is more likely that the individual has experienced a minor injury, such as a muscular strain or sprain. Even if symptoms are minor, all precautions should be taken until a serious spinal injury is ruled out by qualified medical personnel. Once a significant physical finding indicates possible nerve involvement, immobilization and immediate transportation to the nearest medical facility are warranted. **Box 6-4** identifies several signs and symptoms that, if present, necessitate activating EMS.

If the individual is walking but reports neck or back pain, it is relatively safe to assume that a serious spinal injury is not present. This section focuses on a basic spinal assessment of a conscious athlete. Specific information related to an acute injury is included where appropriate.

History

A history of the injury should include information on the primary complaint; mechanism of injury; extent of pain or numbness; and knowledge of any previous injuries to the area. Ask about the location of pain (localized or radiating), type of pain (dull, aching, sharp, or burning), presence of sensory changes (numbness, tingling, or absence of sensation), and possible muscle weakness or

➤ ➤ **BOX 6-4**

Red Flags That Warrant Immobilization and Immediate Referral to a Physician
- Severe pain, point tenderness, or deformity along the vertebral column
- Loss or change in sensation anywhere in the body
- Paralysis or inability to move a body part
- Diminished or absent reflexes
- Muscle weakness in a myotome
- Pain radiating into the extremities
- Trunk or abdominal pain that may be referred from the visceral organs
- Any injury in which you are uncertain about its severity or nature

paralysis. With a neck injury, questions should be asked to determine both long- and short-term memory loss that may indicate an associated concussion or subdural hematoma. Note the length of time it takes the athlete to respond to the questions. General questions related to a spinal injury can be seen in **Field Strategy 6-3**.

Observation and Inspection

Observation should begin as soon as the individual enters the room. Body language can signal pain, disability, and muscle weakness. Note the individual's willingness or ability to move, general posture, ease in motion, and general attitude. The position of the head and neck should be observed. Is the head held erect or carried in a forward position? Are any abnormal spinal curvatures present? Are there any noticeable asymmetries, such as discrepancies in shoulder or scapula height, hip height, or patella height? Is the trunk rotated so that one shoulder is forward? Are the ribs more prominent on one side? Local inspection at the injury site should include observation for deformity, swelling, discoloration, and muscle spasm.

Palpation

In injuries that do not involve neural damage, fracture, or dislocation, palpation can proceed in the following manner. Bony and soft tissue structures are palpated to detect swelling, point tenderness, deformity, crepitus, muscle spasm, and cutaneous sensation. Any pain directly over a bony prominence should signal a potential fracture. Pain in the soft tissue area may indicate either a joint sprain or muscle strain. Muscle spasms may indicate dysfunction of the specific spinal region.

Special Tests

Because injuries to the spinal region can be complex, coaches need only assess the potential for a serious injury. If significant pain is present directly over a bony

---

FIELD STATEGY 6.2   DEVELOPING A HISTORY FOR A SPINAL INJURY

CURRENT INJURY STATUS

1. Were you knocked out or unconscious?

2. How did the injury occur (mechanism)? Did the injury involve twisting of the trunk, a violent stretch, or a jack-knife maneuver?

3. Where is the pain located? Did it come on suddenly or gradually? How severe is the pain? Describe the pain (sharp, aching, burning, radiating, deep, or superficial). Does the severity of symptoms change when you change position?

4. Do you have any muscle spasms, numbness, or change in sensation anywhere in the body?

5. Can you move your fingers and toes?

6. Do you have equal muscle strength in the hands? (Perform a bilateral hand squeeze)

7. Are there certain activities you cannot perform because of the pain?

8. What different activities have you been doing in the last week? (Look for activities such as lifting or carrying heavy objects, or positions involving bending over for long periods.)

9. Is there a certain position that alleviates the pain?

PAST INJURY STATUS

1. Have you ever injured your back before? When? How did that occur? What was done for the injury?

2. Have you had any medical problems recently? (Look for possible referred pain from visceral organs, heart, and lungs.)

3. Are you on any medication?

4. Do you have any musculoskeletal problems elsewhere in the body? (These problems may result in changes in gait or technique that transfer abnormal forces to structures in the spinal region.)

5. Has anyone in your family had a similar problem?

---

prominence, movement leads to increased acute pain or change in sensation, or the individual resists moving the spine, assume that a significant injury is present and activate EMS. When there is no potential spinal injury but the athlete continues to report pain, the coach can perform certain special tests to determine whether the injury is a minor muscle strain or ligament sprain. Again, if any pain or change in sensation occurs, stop the evaluation and immediately refer the individual to a physician for further care.

JOINT RANGE OF MOTION

Active movements, or those movements performed totally by the athlete, should not be performed when pain is present over the vertebrae or when motor/sensory deficits are present. Look for the individual's willingness to execute the movement. Is the movement fluid and complete? Does pain, spasm, or stiffness block the full range of motion? With movements to the left and right, always compare bilaterally. Spinal movements include the following:

• Cervical flexion and extension
• Cervical lateral flexion (left and right)
• Cervical rotation (left and right)
• Trunk forward flexion
• Trunk extension
• Trunk lateral flexion (left and right)
• Trunk rotation (left and right)

RESISTED MANUAL MUSCLE TESTING

Resisted manual muscle testing is used to determine whether muscle weakness is present. Stabilize the hip and trunk during cervical testing to avoid muscle substitution. With the individual seated, use one hand to stabilize the shoulder or thorax while applying manual overpressure with the other hand. When you test the thoracic and lumbar region, the weight of the trunk stabilizes the hips in a seated position. Inform the individual not to allow you to move the body part being tested.

CERVICAL COMPRESSION TEST

The compression test can detect pressure on a cervical nerve root from degeneration or narrowing of a neural foramen. Carefully compress straight down on the individual's head while the person is sitting on a stable chair or table (**Fig. 6-14**). Increased pain or altered sensation

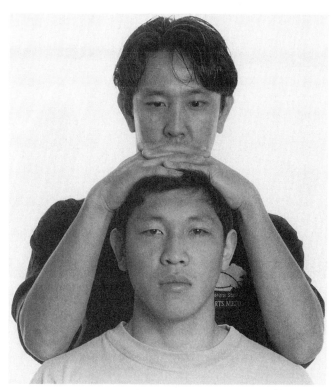

➤ **FIGURE 6-14.** Compression test. With the neck in neutral position, carefully push straight down on the individual's head. Increased pain or altered sensation is a positive sign indicating pressure on a nerve root. The test can also be performed with the neck slightly flexed to one side.

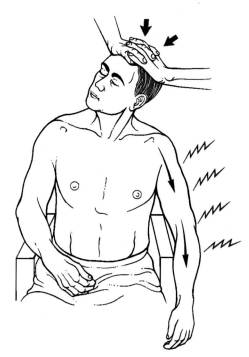

➤ **FIGURE 6-15.** Spurling test. Have the athlete extend, rotate, and laterally bend the neck. Carefully apply downward pressure on the individual's head. Increased pain indicates cervical nerve root involvement.

is a positive sign, indicating pressure on a nerve root. The distribution of the pain and altered sensation can indicate which nerve root is involved.

SPURLING TEST (FORAMINAL COMPRESSION TEST)

The Spurling test is a variation of the cervical compression test. The individual extends the neck, then rotates and laterally bends the head to the same side while the examiner applies downward pressure to the top of the head **(Fig. 6-15)**. If this position, with or without pressure, reproduces radiating pain into the upper limb, a nerve root impingement caused by a narrowing of the neural foramina is suggested. The distribution of the pain and altered sensation can indicate which nerve root is involved.

CERVICAL DISTRACTION TEST

This test is performed by placing one hand under the individual's chin and the other around the occiput, and then slowly lifting the head **(Fig. 6-16)**. The test is positive if pain decreases or is relieved as the head is lifted, indicating that pressure on the nerve root is relieved. If pain increases with distraction, it indicates ligamentous injury.

BRACHIAL PLEXUS TRACTION TEST

This test should not be performed until the possibility of bony trauma has been ruled out. While standing behind the athlete, passively flex the athlete's head to one side while applying a downward pressure on the opposite shoulder **(Fig. 6-17)**. If pain increases or radiates into the upper arm being depressed, stretching of the brachial plexus is indicated. If pain increases on the side toward the lateral bending, it indicates irritation or compression of the nerve roots between two vertebrae.

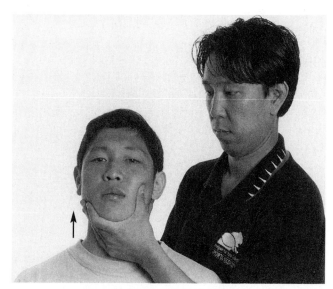

➤ **FIGURE 6-16.** Distraction test. Lift the head slowly. The test is positive if pain is decreased or relieved as the head is lifted, indicating that pressure on the nerve root is relieved. If pain increases with distraction, it indicates ligamentous injury.

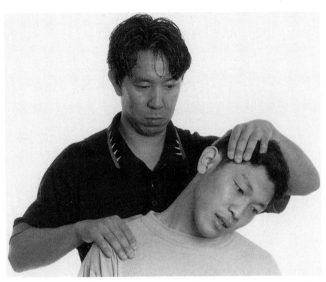

➤ FIGURE 6-17. Brachial plexus traction test. Passively apply downward pressure by doing lateral bending away from the involved shoulder and simultaneously depressing the involved shoulder. Radiating pain or a burning sensation indicates injury to the brachial plexus. If pain increases on the side toward the lateral bending, it indicates irritation or compression of the nerve roots between two vertebrae.

➤ FIGURE 6-18. Straight leg raising test. Passively flex the individual's hip while keeping the knee extended until pain or tension is felt in the hamstrings. Slowly lower the leg until the pain or tension disappears. Then, dorsiflex the foot, have the individual flex the neck, or do both simultaneously. If pain does not increase with dorsiflexion of the ankle or flexion of the neck, it indicates tight hamstrings.

STRAIGHT LEG RAISING TEST

This test is used to assess sacroiliac joint pain, irritation of the sciatic nerve, or tight hamstrings. The individual is placed in a relaxed supine position with the hip medially rotated and knee extended. Grasp the individual's heel with one hand and place the other on top of the patella to prevent the knee from flexing. The leg is slowly raised until the individual reports pain or tightness. The leg is then lowered until the pain is relieved. The individual is then asked to flex the neck onto the chest, or dorsiflex the foot, or do both actions simultaneously **(Fig. 6-18)**.

FUNCTIONAL TESTING

If any of these tests produce increased pain or neurologic changes, the individual should be referred immediately to a physician. If no serious injury exists but the individual still reports pain or discomfort when moving, he or she should not be allowed to return to participation until he or she can walk, bend, lift, jog, run, and perform sport-specific skills pain-free and with no limited movement.

Summary

1. The spine is a linkage system that transfers loads between the upper and lower extremities, enables motion in all three planes, and protects the delicate spinal cord.
2. The spinal cord extends from the brainstem to the level of the first or second lumbar vertebrae. Thirty-

one pairs of spinal nerves emanate from the cord. The distal bundle of spinal nerves is known as the cauda equina.
3. Anatomic variations that can predispose an individual to spinal injuries include kyphosis, scoliosis, lordosis, and par interarticularis fractures, which can lead to spondylolysis or spondylolisthesis.
4. Signs and symptoms that indicate a serious cervical spine injury include:
   • Pain over the spinous process, with or without deformity
   • Unrelenting neck pain or muscle spasm
   • Abnormal sensations on the head, neck, trunk, or extremities
   • Muscular weakness in the extremities
   • Paralysis or inability to move a body part
   • Absent or weak reflexes
5. A brachial plexus injury is a stretch injury commonly caused by tensile forces that lead to forceful downward traction of the clavicle while the head is distracted in the opposite direction. The injury usually affects the upper trunk (C5,C6) of the brachial plexus, leading to a sensory loss or paresthesia in the thumb and index finger.
6. Thoracic fractures tend to be concentrated at the lower end of the thoracic spine. Large compressive loads can lead to a wedge fracture.
7. Runners are particularly prone to low back pain because of tight hip flexors and hamstrings. Symptoms include localized pain that increases with active and resisted back extension. Radiating pain and neurologic deficits are usually not present.

8. The most commonly herniated discs are between the L4-L5 and L5-S1 vertebrae. Most ruptures move in a posterior or posterolateral direction because of torsion and compression.

9. Significant signs that indicate a lumbar disc condition needing immediate referral to a physician include:
   • Muscle weakness
   • Sensory changes
   • Diminished reflexes in the lower extremity
   • Abnormal bladder or bowel function

10. In a traumatic spinal injury, always complete a brief neuromuscular assessment to detect any motor or sensory deficits before moving the individual.

11. When assessing a nontraumatic spinal injury, always begin with a thorough history of the injury, and include general observations of the individual's body language, ability to move, general posture, ease in motion, and general attitude.

12. If an individual reports acute pain in the spine, reports a change in sensation anywhere on the body, or resists moving the spine, assume that a significant injury is present and activate EMS.

References

1. Zachazewski JE, Geissler G, and Hangen D. Traumatic injuries to the cervical spine. In *Athletic injuries and rehabilitation*, edited by JE Zachazewski, DJ Magee, and WS Quillen. Philadelphia: WB Saunders, 1996.
2. Hall SJ. 1985. Effect of attempted lifting speed on forces and torque exerted on the lumbar spine. Med Sci Sports Exerc, 17(4): 440–444.
3. Wilhite JM. Thoracic and lumbosacral spine. In *The team physician's handbook*, edited by MB Mellion, WM Walsh, and GL Shelton. Philadelphia: Hanley & Belfus, 1997.
4. Kujala UM, et al. 1997. Lumbar mobility and low back pain during adolescence: A longitudinal three-year follow-up study in athletes and controls. Am J Sports Med, 25(3)363–368.

7

Throat, Thorax, and Abdominal Conditions

KEY TERMS

Appendicitis

Cyanosis

Dyspnea

Hematuria

Hemothorax

Hernia

Hypertrophic
cardiomyopathy

Hypoxia

Infectious
mononucleosis

Kehr's sign

Marfan's syndrome

McBurney's point

Mitral valve prolapse

Pericardial tamponade

Peritonitis

Pneumothorax

Solar plexus punch

Stitch in the side

Sudden death

Tension pneumothorax

OBJECTIVES

1. Identify the important anatomic structures of the throat, thorax, and abdomen.

2. Recognize and manage specific injuries of the throat, thorax, and abdomen.

3. Describe life-threatening conditions that can occur from direct trauma to the throat, thorax, and abdomen.

4. Demonstrate a basic assessment of the throat, thorax, and abdomen.

Torso injuries occur in nearly every sport, particularly those involving collision into a solid object or another player. Although protective equipment and padding is available to protect the anterior throat, thorax, and viscera, only football, lacrosse, hockey, fencing, baseball, and softball require specific safety equipment for this vital region. Most injuries are superficial and easily recognized and managed. Some injuries, however, may involve the respiratory or circulatory system, leading to a life-threatening situation.

PREVENTION OF INJURIES TO THE THROAT, THORAX, AND VISCERA

In sports involving high-velocity projectiles, throat and chest protectors are required only for specific players' positions, such as a catcher or goalie. Protective equipment, together with a well-rounded physical conditioning program, can reduce the risk of injury. Although proper technique can prevent some injuries, it is not a major factor in this body region.

Protective Equipment

Facemasks with throat protectors are required only for fencing, baseball or softball catchers, and for goalies in field hockey, ice hockey, and lacrosse. Nearly all lacrosse and ice hockey players wear an optional extended pad attached to the mask to protect the throat region. Many sport participants in collision and contact sports also wear full chest and abdominal protection, such as in fencing, ice hockey, catchers in baseball or softball, and goalies in field hockey and lacrosse. In young baseball and softball players (younger than 12 years), it has been suggested that all infield players should wear chest protectors. Adolescent rib cages are less rigid, placing the heart at greater risk of direct impact. In this age group, more baseball and softball deaths occur from impacts to the chest than to the head. Shoulder pads can protect the upper thoracic region, and rib protectors can provide protection from rib, upper abdominal, or low-back contusions. Bodysuits made of mesh with pockets can hold rib and hip pads to protect the sides and back. For women, sport bras provide added support to reduce excessive vertical and horizontal breast motion during exercise. Abdominal binders may also be used to reduce the discomfort from hernias. The male genitalia are more susceptible to injury than female genitalia. Protective cups can protect the penis and scrotum from injury and are required for baseball catchers and ice hockey goalies.

Physical Conditioning

Flexibility and strengthening of the torso muscles should not be an isolated program, but should include a well-rounded conditioning program for the back, shoulder, abdomen, and hip regions. Range-of-motion and strengthening exercises should include both open and closed kinetic-chain activities. Exercises for the thorax and abdominal region are included in the chapters on the hip, shoulder, and spine, and are not repeated here. The reader should review the appropriate Field Strategies in those chapters to develop a conditioning program for the torso.

ANATOMY OF THE THROAT

The throat includes the pharynx, larynx, trachea, esophagus, a number of glands, and several major blood vessels **(Fig. 7-1)**. The laryngeal prominence on the thyroid cartilage that shields the front of the larynx is known as the "Adam's apple." The epiglottis covers the superior opening of the larynx during swallowing to prevent food and liquids from entering the upper respiratory tract. If a foreign body does slip past the epiglottis, the cough reflex is initiated, and the foreign body is normally ejected back into the pharynx. The trachea is formed by C-shaped rings of hyaline cartilage joined by fibroelastic connective tissue. Smooth muscle fibers of the trachealis muscle form the open side of the C and allow for expansion of the posteriorly adjacent esophagus as swallowed food passes through. When empty, the esophagus tube is collapsed.

The largest blood vessels coursing through the neck are the common carotid arteries **(Fig. 7-2)**. At the level

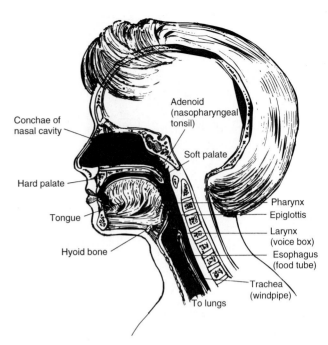

➤ **FIGURE 7-1.** Throat region. Lateral cross-sectional view.

of the Adam's apple, the common carotid arteries divide into external and internal carotid arteries, which provide the major blood supply to the brain, head, and face.

THROAT CONDITIONS

Throat injuries may include lacerations, contusions, or fracture to the trachea, larynx, and hyoid bone.

Lacerations

Although uncommon, lacerations to the neck may be caused by a skate blade. More commonly, however, lacerations occur when an athlete wears a necklace and it becomes entangled with another player or piece of equipment and subsequently is violently pulled. Because of this, it is essential that all coaches prohibit athletes from wearing jewelry during sports participation.

SIGNS AND SYMPTOMS

Bleeding can be profuse and, if sufficiently deep, can damage the jugular vein or carotid artery that pass deep on the lateral side of the neck.

MANAGEMENT

Immediate control of hemorrhage involves direct pressure over the laceration. If a major vein is severed, in addition to blood loss, air may be sucked into the vein and carried to the heart as an air embolism, which can be fatal. If the would appears severe and bleeding is profuse, Emergency Medical Services (EMS) should be acti-

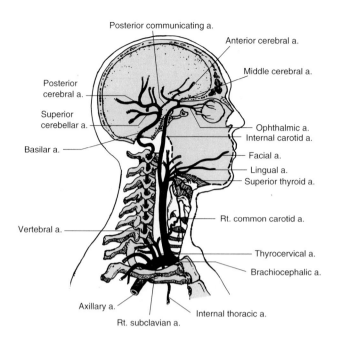

➤ **FIGURE 7-2.** The arterial supply to the neck and throat region.

vated to immediately transport the athlete to the nearest medical facility.

Contusion and Fractures

Contusions and fractures to the trachea, larynx, and hyoid bone frequently occur during hyperextension of the neck, when the thyroid cartilage (Adam's apple) becomes prominent and vulnerable to direct impact forces. A hockey cross-check or slash, a clothesline tackle in football, or a hit or blow to the neck can injure the cartilage or cause an associated injury to the cervical spine.

SIGNS AND SYMPTOMS

Immediate symptoms include hoarseness, **dyspnea** (difficulty breathing), coughing, difficulty in swallowing, and laryngeal tenderness **(Box 7-1)**. Often, the person becomes agitated and avoids any assistance.

MANAGEMENT

Immediately reassure the athlete that you are there to help. Maintaining an open airway is a priority. **Field Strategy 7-1** summarizes management of throat conditions.

ANATOMY OF THE THORAX

The thoracic cavity, or chest cavity, lies anterior to the spinal column and extends from the level of the clavicle down to the diaphragm. The bones of the thorax, includ-

ing the sternum, ribs and costal cartilages, and thoracic vertebrae, form a protective cage around the heart and lungs **(Fig. 7-3)**. The costal cartilages of the first seven pairs of ribs attach directly to the sternum, and the costal cartilages of ribs 8 to 10 attach to the costal cartilages of the immediate superior ribs. The last two rib pairs are known as floating ribs because they do not attach anteriorly to any structure. The rib cage protects the heart and lungs.

The thoracic cavity is lined with a thin, double-layered membrane called the pleura. The pleural cavity, a narrow space between the pleural membranes, is filled with a pleural fluid secreted by the membranes, which enables the lungs to move against the thoracic wall with minimal friction during breathing. The primary bronchial tubes branch obliquely downward from the trachea, then branch into approximately 25 subsequent levels until the terminal bronchioles are reached **(Fig. 7-4)**. These tiny air sacs, called alveoli, serve as diffusion chambers where oxygen from the lungs enter adjacent capillaries, and where carbon dioxide from the venous blood is returned to the lungs.

The major respiratory muscle is the diaphragm, a powerful sheet of muscle that separates the thoracic and abdominal cavities. During relaxation, the diaphragm is dome-shaped. During contraction, it flattens, thereby increasing the size of the thoracic cavity. This increase in cavity volume causes a decrease in intrathoracic pressure, resulting in inhalation of air into the lungs. The diaphragm is assisted by the intercostal muscles, both internal and external, which lift the rib cage and assist with breathing.

The heart and lungs have an intimate relationship, both physically and functionally. The right side of the heart pumps blood to the lungs, where it is oxygenated and where carbon dioxide is given off. The left side of the heart receives the freshly oxygenated blood from the lungs and pumps it out to the systemic circulation. The vessels interconnecting the heart and lungs are

1. Talk calmly to the individual. Loosen any restrictive clothing or equipment. To reduce panic and anxiety, reassure the individual that you are there to help.
2. If severe anterior throat trauma has occurred, assume that a possible cervical spinal injury may be present, and treat accordingly.
3. Activate EMS.
4. Assess the ABCs.
5. Ensure an open airway and apply ice to control swelling.
6. If a major laceration is present, control hemorrhage with firm, manual pressure and maintain the pressure during the assessment.
7. If an obvious deformity is present in the pharynx, manually straighten the airway.
8. Treat for shock and monitor vital signs until the ambulance arrives.

known as the pulmonary circuit, and the vessels that supply the body are known as the systemic circuit **(Fig. 7-5)**.

THORACIC CONDITIONS

Thoracic injuries are frequently caused when an athlete runs into an object or another player, leading to sudden compression and deformation of the rib cage. The extent of damage depends on the direction, magnitude of force, and point of impact. For example, a glancing blow may contuse the chest wall, whereas a baseball that directly impacts the ribs may fracture a rib. Several conditions can alter breathing and cardiac function. Recognizing the potential for serious underlying problems is vital to providing emergency care to an injured individual. When these problems occur, EMS should be immediately activated.

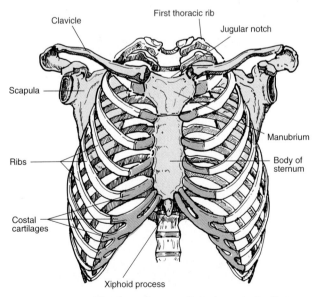

➤ FIGURE 7-3. The thoracic cage. Note that only the first seven pairs of ribs articulate anteriorly with the sternum through the costal cartilages.

(Labels in figure: Clavicle, First thoracic rib, Jugular notch, Scapula, Ribs, Costal cartilages, Xiphoid process, Manubrium, Body of sternum)

Stitch in the Side

A "**stitch in the side**" refers to a sharp pain or spasm in the chest wall, usually on the lower right side, during exertion. Potential causes include trapped colonic gas bubbles, localized diaphragmatic **hypoxia** with spasm, liver congestion with stretching of the liver capsule, and poor conditioning.

MANAGEMENT

Although the frequency of a stitch usually diminishes as the individual becomes more fit, most individuals can run through the sharp pain by doing one or more of the following:

- Forcibly exhaling through pursed lips
- Breathing deeply and regularly
- Leaning away from the affected side
- Stretching the arm on the affected side over the head as high as possible

Breast Injuries

Excessive breast motion during activity can lead to soreness, contusions, and nipple irritation.

SIGNS AND SYMPTOMS

Contusions to the breast produce localized pain and discomfort. As the condition heals, a fat necrosis or hematoma may form, both of which are painful and may result in a localized breast mass. On a mammogram, these lesions may be indistinguishable from a malignant tumor.

Nipple irritation is commonly seen in distance runners when the shirt rubs over the nipples. The resulting friction can lead to abrasions, blisters, or bleeding (runner's nipples). This condition can be prevented by applying petroleum-based products and bandaids over the nipples to reduce irritation.

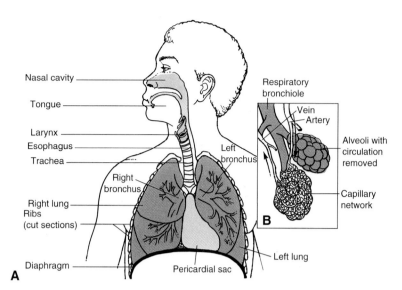

➤ **Figure 7-4.** The respiratory system. **A.** The trachea, bronchi, and lungs. **B.** The terminal ends of the bronchial tree are alveolar sacs where oxygen and carbon dioxide are exchanged.

MANAGEMENT

Although immediate management of contusions to the breast involves ice and support, direct trauma should always be recorded on a woman's permanent medical records. Treatment of injury to the nipple area involves cleansing the wound, applying an antibiotic ointment, and covering the wound with a nonadhering sterile gauze pad. Infection, secondary to the injury, may involve the entire nipple region and may necessitate referral to a physician.

Strain of the Pectoralis Major Muscle

Pectoralis major muscle strains may occur in power lifting, water skiing, football, boxing, wrestling, and basketball, or in sudden violent deceleration maneuvers, such as when punching in boxing or blocking with an extended arm in football. If the muscle ruptures, the usual mechanism involves an actively contracting muscle overburdened by a load or extrinsic force that exceeds tissue tolerance. A higher incidence of this injury is seen with anabolic steroid abuse.[1,2] Steroid use causes muscle hypertrophy and an increase in power secondary to rapid strength gain not accompanied by a concomitant increase in tendon size.

SIGNS AND SYMPTOMS

An audible pop, snap, or tearing sensation is usually accompanied by immediate, marked pain and weakness. The pain is often described as an aching or fatigue-like, rather than a sharp, pain. The tear usually occurs in the musculotendinous junction, and a defect can often be palpated with the arm abducted and externally rotated. Resisted horizontal adduction and internal rotation of the shoulder are limited.

MANAGEMENT

Initial treatment involves ice, compression, and rest. If function is limited, the individual should be referred to a physician.

Costochondral Injury

Costochondral sprains can occur during a collision with another person or during a severe twisting motion of the thorax. This action can sprain or separate the costal cartilage where it attaches to the rib or sternum **(Fig. 7-6)**.

SIGNS AND SYMPTOMS

The individual may hear or feel a pop, but the initial localized sharp pain may be followed by intermittent

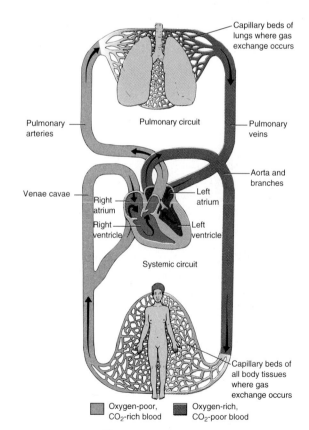

➤ **Figure 7-5.** The pulmonary and systemic circuits.

➤ FIGURE 7-6. Undisplaced costochondral separation.

stabbing pain as the displaced cartilage overrides the bone. A visible deformity and localized pain can be palpated at the involved joint. More severe sprains produce pain during deep inhalation.

MANAGEMENT

This individual should be referred to a physician. Under most conditions, the discomfort usually resolves itself with 3 or 4 weeks of rest and anti-inflammatory medication; however, the discomfort may persist for more than 6 weeks.

Fractures

Direct blows or compression of the chest can lead to a fracture of the sternum or ribs. If ribs are fractured, it rarely involves more than one or two ribs. The fifth through ninth ribs are the most commonly fractured.

SIGNS AND SYMPTOMS

With a sternal fracture, loss of breath is immediate. Severe pain is aggravated with deep inspiration if the fracture is incomplete, but pain occurs during normal respiration if the fracture is complete. With a rib fracture, intense localized pain over the fracture site is aggravated by deep inspiration, coughing, or chest movement (Box 7-2). Often, the individual takes shallow breaths and leans toward the fracture site, stabilizing the area with a hand to prevent excessive movement of the chest to ease the pain. The coach should look for any coughing up of blood, especially a bright red or frothy blood—this may indicate internal lung damage.

MANAGEMENT

If any signs of respiratory distress, **cyanosis**, or shock appear, immediately initiate the emergency care plan to have the individual transported to the nearest medical facility. **Field Strategy 7-2** summarizes the management of rib fractures.

➤ ➤ BOX 7-2

Signs and Symptoms Indicating Possible Sternal or Rib Fracture

- Signs of shock (rapid, weak pulse and low blood pressure are present when there are multiple fractures, fractures that involve damaged intercostal vessels and nerves, or when the lung or pleural sac has been penetrated)*
- History of direct blow, compression of the chest, or violent muscle contraction
- Individual may lean toward the fractured side, stabilizing the area with a hand to prevent movement of the chest
- Localized discoloration or swelling over the fracture site
- Slight step deformity
- Palpable pain and crepitus at fracture site that increases with deep inspiration
- Increased pain on manual compression of the rib cage in an anteroposterior direction

*Indicates "red flags" that necessitate the activation of EMS.

Hyperventilation

Hyperventilation is often linked to excessive pain, psychological stress, or trauma in sport participation. During activity, the respiratory rate increases. Rapid, deep inhalations draw more oxygen into the lungs. Conversely, long exhalations result in too much carbon dioxide being exhaled.

SIGNS AND SYMPTOMS

The athlete may experience an inability to catch his or her breath, numbness in the lips and hands, spasm of the hands, chest pain, dry mouth, dizziness, and, occasionally, fainting.

MANAGEMENT

Immediately calm the individual because panic and anxiety can complicate the condition. Have the athlete concentrate on slowly inhaling through the nose and exhaling through the mouth until the symptoms have stopped. An alternative treatment is to have athletes cup their hands over their own mouth and nose and breathe into their hands to restore the carbon dioxide balance.

Pneumothorax, Hemothorax, and Tension Pneumothorax

Three lung conditions—pneumothorax, hemothorax, and tension pneumothorax—can lead to a life-threatening situation (Box 7-3). In pneumothorax, a fractured rib is the leading cause. When lung tissue is lacerated, air escapes into the pleural cavity with each inhalation and prevents the lung from fully expanding (Fig. 7-7).

FIELD STRATEGY 7.2   MANAGEMENT OF RIB FRACTURES

1. Assess the ABCs.
2. Rule out underlying internal complications:
   - Look for coughing up of any bright red or frothy blood (indicates internal lung damage).
   - Listen for abnormal, or absent breathing sounds (indicates internal lung damage).
   - Record rate and depth of respirations (rapid, shallow breathing indicates shock).
   - Record strength and pulse rate (rapid, weak pulse indicates shock).
   - Note pupillary response to light (lackluster, dilated pupils indicates shock).
3. Apply a pad over the suspected fracture site.
4. Apply a sling and swathe to use the individual's arm as a splint and support; the forearm of the injured side should be supported across the chest

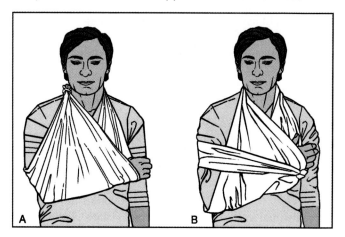

5. Do not:
   - Tape the ribs.
   - Use continuous strapping with an elastic bandage over the fracture site.
   - Wrap the chest if a deformity is present or the individual has frothy blood coming from the mouth.
5. Monitor the ABCs, watching for signs of internal bleeding that could lead to shock.
6. Treat for shock and transport the individual to the nearest medical facility.

If the fractured rib tears lung tissue and blood vessels in the chest or chest cavity, it is called a hemothorax. In tension pneumothorax, air progressively accumulates in the pleural space around the injured lung during inspiration and cannot escape on expiration. The pleural space expands with each breath, resulting in the mediastinum (the partition in the thoracic cavity that separates the right and left lungs) being displaced to the opposite side, compressing the uninjured lung and thoracic aorta.

SIGNS AND SYMPTOMS
Severe pain during breathing, hypoxia, cyanosis, and signs of shock become immediately apparent. If a hemothorax is present, coughing up frothy blood may also be seen.

MANAGEMENT
Each type of lung condition is a true emergency. The individual should be referred immediately to the nearest medical facility to prevent total lung collapse. Monitor the ABCs (airway, breathing, circulation), control any bleeding from an external wound, and treat for shock until EMS arrives.

Heart Conditions

BLUNT TRAUMA
Blunt trauma can compress the heart between the sternum and spine and lead to a myocardial contusion. Red blood cells and fluid leak into the surrounding tissues, decreasing circulation to the heart muscle. Blunt trauma may also lead to **pericardial tamponade**, the leading cause of traumatic death in youth baseball. Blunt trauma

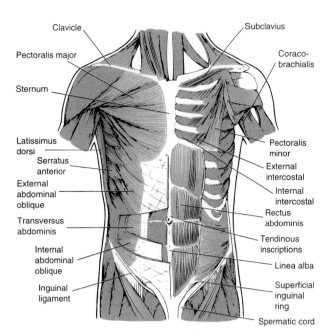

➤ FIGURE 7-9. Anterior muscles of the trunk.

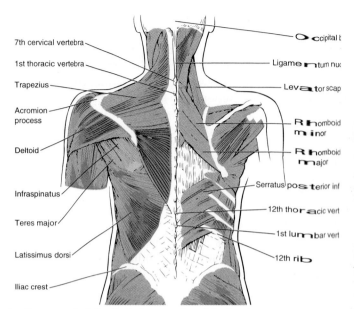

➤ FIGURE 7-10. Posterior muscles of the trunk.

SIGNS AND SYMPTOMS

Localized pain and muscle spasm in the involved muscle may be present. Any attempt to do a sit-up, straight-leg raise, or hyperextension of the back significantly increases muscle pain.

MANAGEMENT

Treatment consists of ice, rest, and early use of non-steroidal anti-inflammatory drugs (NSAIDs) for the first 36 to 48 hours. Activities such as twisting, turning, or sudden stretching should be avoided until painful symptoms subside.

SOLAR PLEXUS PUNCH

A blow to the abdomen with the muscles relaxed is referred to as a "**solar plexus punch**," and it results in an immediate inability to catch one's breath. Fear and anxiety complicate the condition.

MANAGEMENT

Immediately check that the individual is breathing. Remove any mouthguard or partial plates. Loosen any restrictive equipment and clothing around the abdomen, and have the individual flex the knees toward the chest. As paradoxical as it may seem, asking the athlete to take a deep breath and hold it, and to repeat this several times, often restores the athlete's breath more quickly. Because a severe blow may lead to an intra-abdominal injury, rib fracture, or spleen injury, rule out these injuries before the individual returns to participation.

HERNIA

A **hernia** is a protrusion of abdominal viscera through a weakened portion of the abdominal wall, and it typically occurs in or just above the groin **(Fig. 7-11)**. Many hernias are asymptomatic until the preparticipation examination, when the physician palpates the protrusion by invaginating the scrotum with a finger. Protrusion of the hernia increases with coughing. The danger of a hernia lies in continued trauma to the weakened area during falls, blows, or increased intra-abdominal pressure exerted during activity. The hernia can twist on itself and produce a strangulated hernia, which can become gangrenous.

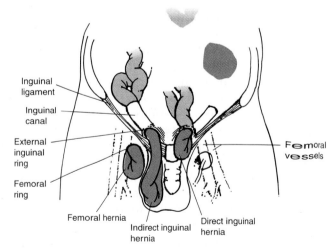

➤ FIGURE 7-11. Hernias. A hernia is classified as either an indirect hernia, where the small intestine extends into the scrotum; a direct hernia, where the small intestine extends through a weakening in the internal inguinal ring; or a femoral hernia, where the small intestine protrudes posterior to the inguinal ligament and medial to the femoral artery.

SIGNS AND SYMPTOMS

Symptoms vary, but for most hernias, the first sign is a visible tender swelling and an aching feeling in the groin. If the hernia ruptures, symptoms may include a sharp, stinging pain or a feeling of something giving way at the site of the rupture, as well as nausea and vomiting.

MANAGEMENT

If a ruptured hernia is suspected, initiate the emergency care plan and position the individual on his or her back. Place a rolled blanket under the knees to reduce tension in the abdominal area, monitor the ABCs, and treat for possible shock until EMS arrives.

Intra-abdominal Injuries

Trauma to the abdomen can lead to severe internal hemorrhage if organs or major blood vessels are lacerated or ruptured. The solid organs are more commonly injured in sport participation. Hollow viscera, if damaged, can leak the contents into the abdominal cavity. Although rarely injured in sport participation, certain systemic disorders, such as **infectious mononucleosis**, can enlarge the spleen, making it vulnerable to injury. The spleen is the most commonly injured abdominal organ and is the most frequent cause of death due to abdominal blunt trauma in sport.[4] The spleen can splint itself and stop hemorrhage, only to produce delayed hemorrhage days, weeks, or months later after a seemingly minor jarring motion,

---

> ➤ ➤ B O X 7 - 4

Red Flags Indicating A Serious Intra-abdominal Condition

- Rapid, weak pulse, low blood pressure, or cyanosis (shock)*
- Abdominal pain, often starting as mild, then rapidly increasing in severity*
- Absence of bowel sounds*
- Coughing up or vomiting blood that looks like used coffee grounds*
- Localized tenderness and rigidity over the injured organ*
- Rebound pain with release of deep palpation*
- Referred pain to the shoulder tip, back, or groin*
- Diffuse hemorrhage or distention of the abdomen*
- Nausea, weakness, and thirst
- Individual may lean forward and bring the knees to the chest to reduce tension in the abdominal muscles
- Cramps or muscle guarding (splinting)
- Shallow breathing. Abdominal respiratory motion may be absent
- Blood in the urine or stool

*Necessitates the activation of EMS.

---

such as a cough. As with the spleen, systemic diseases, such as hepatitis, can enlarge the liver, making this organ more susceptible to injury.

The vermiform appendix is a pouch extending from the cecum (*see* **Fig. 7-8**). If it becomes obstructed (for example, with hardened fecal material), venous circulation may be impaired, leading to an increase in bacterial growth and the formation of pus. The resulting inflamed appendix, called **appendicitis**, can lead to ischemia and gangrene. Serious injury to the kidney often occurs when the body is extended and the abdominal muscles are relaxed, such as when a receiver leaps to catch a pass. Suspicion should be high if impact is to the midback region, especially if persistent back or significant flank pain is present. Individuals may report blood in the urine (**hematuria**), although this may not be indicative of the severity of injury.

Damage to the bladder is rare, although hematuria may occur. Most sport participants void before running and competition. Running with an empty bladder increases the risk of gross hematuria (visible blood in the urine) because no fluid cushion exists between the posterior wall and base of the bladder. This condition is commonly seen in long-distance runners, hence the name "runner's bladder." Hematuria caused by running rapidly resolves within 24 to 48 hours of rest.

SIGNS AND SYMPTOMS

Many signs and symptoms of intra-abdominal injury are similar regardless of the organ involved; they include severe internal hemorrhage, **peritonitis** (inflammation of the peritoneum that lines the abdomen), and shock (**Box 7-4**). Variations arise in the area of palpable pain and the site of referred pain. For example, indications of a splenic rupture include a history of blunt trauma to the left upper quadrant and a persistent dull pain in the left upper quadrant, left lower chest, and left shoulder. This dull pain is called **Kehr's sign**. Pain in the upper right quadrant may indicate a liver injury. Appendicitis is indicated by acute abdominal pain in the lower right quadrant, loss of appetite, nausea, vomiting, and low-grade fever. Persistent back or flank pain may indicate injury to the kidneys.

MANAGEMENT

Acute management of suspected intra-abdominal injuries is similar regardless of the injured organ. Initially, keep the individual relaxed while a primary survey is completed, and activate the emergency care plan. Place the individual face up (supine) and flex the knees. This position relaxes the low back and abdominal muscles. Monitor the ABCs regularly and treat for shock. If external bleeding is present, control bleeding and apply an absorbent sterile dressing. **Field Strategy 7-3** summarizes acute management of intra-abdominal injuries. Athletes diagnosed with infectious mononucleosis or mono-

---

FIELD STRATEGY 7.3　　**MANAGEMENT OF SUSPECTED INTRA-ABDOMINAL INJURIES**

1. Activate EMS.
2. Lay the individual supine with the knees flexed to relax the abdominal muscles. *Do not* extend the legs or elevate the feet.
3. Assess vital signs:
   - Record the rate and depth of respiration (rapid, shallow breathing indicates shock).
   - Record pulse strength and rate (rapid, weak pulse indicates shock).
   - Record blood pressure (a marked drop in both systolic and diastolic indicates shock).
   - Note pupillary response to light (lackluster, dilated pupils indicates shock).
4. Control any external hemorrhage with a sterile dressing.
5. If the individual vomits, roll the person on the side to allow for excretion, making certain the airway remains open.
6. Treat for shock and monitor vital signs until the ambulance arrives. Give nothing by mouth.

---

like symptoms should avoid participating in collision sports until cleared by a physician.

ASSESSMENT OF THE THROAT, THORAX, AND ABDOMINAL REGIONS

Injury assessment should focus on the primary survey and history of the injury. Chest or abdominal trauma, although initially appearing superficial and minor, can mask internal hemorrhage and swelling that can seriously compromise function of the vital organs. In addition, the individual's condition can slowly deteriorate, leading to a life-threatening condition. Although general observations and palpation can confirm the possibility of a serious underlying condition, a good history of the injury and constant monitoring of vital signs are stronger assessment tools.

While approaching the individual, assess consciousness, respirations, and circulation. If the individual is having difficulty breathing, anxiety and panic may make the task more difficult. After ruling out possible spinal injury, place the athlete in a comfortable position. This position varies depending on the injury: semi-reclining if the indi-

vidual is having difficulty breathing, supine with the feet elevated if shock is present, or supine with the hip and knees flexed if an abdominal injury is present. Make sure the airway is open and clear of any blood or vomitus. Speak in a slow, calm, and confident manner. If breathing does not return to normal in a minute or two, or if any of the signs and symptoms listed in **Box 7-5** are present, activate the emergency care plan. It is always better to have EMS en route during the assessment than to wait and see if the condition gets any better. Several conditions intensify with time, thereby seriously compromising the health of the injured party. Never give any water or food to an individual with an acute abdominal injury. Food or water can aggravate the condition, and, if surgery is needed, any food or fluid in the gastrointestinal tract makes the surgery more dangerous.

History

The mechanism of injury and the extent and location of pain is critical to identify. Flank and back pain may indicate injury to the kidneys. Left upper quadrant or lower thoracic pain may indicate splenic injury. Right upper quadrant or lower thoracic pain may signal liver injury. Spleen and liver injuries may also refer pain to the left or right shoulder, respectively **(Box 7-6)**. Ask the individual what aggravates the pain. If coughing, sneezing, rapid movements, and walking down stairs aggravate the condition, the individual may have a peritoneal irritation, while musculoskeletal pain is often relieved by changing body position. Disability caused by the injury, previous injuries to the area, and family history may have some bearing on the specific condition. Specific questions that can be asked for chest and abdominal injuries are listed in **Field Strategy 7-4**.

Observation and Inspection

Observation of body position can indicate the site, nature, and severity of injury. For example, in an acute

---

➤ ➤ **BOX 7-5**

Red Flags Indicating When to Activate EMS

- Rapid, weak pulse
- Wet, cyanotic, or weak appearance
- Sudden, sharp chest pain aggravated with deep inspiration
- Shortness of breath, shallow breathing, or difficulty in breathing
- Deviated trachea or trachea that moves during breathing
- Abnormal chest movement on affected side
- Coughing up bright red or frothy blood
- Coughing up or vomiting blood that looks like used coffee grounds
- Localized abdominal pain or rigidity, often starting as mild, then rapidly increasing in severity

> ➤ ➤ B O X 7 - 6

Common Sites of Referred Pain

ORGAN	LOCALIZATION OF PAIN
Appendicitis	Lower right quadrant
Bladder	Lower pelvic region over pubic bone
Heart	Left shoulder, down medial left arm, or it can extend into neck and jaw
Kidneys	Posterior lumbar region radiating to flanks and groin
Liver and gallbladder	Upper right quadrant or right shoulder
Lung and diaphragm	Upper shoulders and neck
Spleen	Left shoulder or proximal third of left arm (Kehr's sign)

thoracic injury, the individual may lean toward the injured side, using an arm or hand to stabilize the region. In an acute abdominal injury, the individual may lie on the injured side and bring the knees toward the chest to relax the abdominal muscles. If the chest area is the location of concern, observe the position of the trachea. The trachea should be in the middle of the throat and should not move during respirations. Look for any noticeable deformity, edema, bruising, ecchymosis, and change in skin color. Deformity may indicate a sternal or rib fracture or costochondral separation. Coughing up bright blood or frothy blood indicates a severe lung injury. Diffuse bruising in the axilla and chest wall may indicate a ruptured pectoralis major. Distention in the abdomen or flank ecchymosis may indicate bleeding in the abdomen. Pale, cold, and clammy skin is associated with shock. Cyanosis indicates a lack of oxygen caused by internal pulmonary or cardiac problems.

Observe the rate and depth of respirations, and note any difficulty in catching the breath. If the condition is only transitory (i.e., the wind has been knocked out), breathing and color should return to normal quickly. If

---

FIELD STRATEGY 7.4   DEVELOPING A HISTORY FOR A THORACIC OR ABDOMINAL INJURY

CURRENT INJURY STATUS

1. How did the injury occur? What position were you in, and from what direction was the force (glancing, direct, or violent muscle contraction)? Does it hurt to take a deep breath?

2. Where is the pain located? How severe is it? When did it begin (sudden or gradual)? Can you describe the pain (sharp, aching, burning, radiating)? Did the pain disappear, then gradually increase (spontaneous pneumothorax, ruptured spleen)? Are you nauseous, lightheaded, or weak?

3. Did you hear any sounds during the incident (rib fracture, costochondral separation)? Have you had any muscle spasms or cramps with the injury?

4. What motions aggravate the symptoms? In what position are you most comfortable?

5. Have you noticed blood in the urine? Does it occur after long distance running? Is it painful when you urinate? Have you had any recent problems with diarrhea or constipation (bowel obstruction)?

PAST INJURY STATUS

1. Have you ever been injured in this area before? When? What was done for the injury?

2. Do you have a history of diabetes mellitus, rheumatic fever, Marfan's syndrome, low or high blood pressure, or high cholesterol?

3. Do you have a history of cardiovascular disease, congenital coronary artery anomalies, heart murmurs, heart palpitations, chest pains, or shortness of breath? Have you ever fainted before? Have any of these previous conditions occurred after strenuous exercise? Has anyone in your family had a history of any of these conditions?

4. Have you had any medical problems recently? (Look for problems that may be related to referred pain from the visceral organs, heart, and lungs. Remember that some injuries, such as a ruptured spleen, can splint themselves and produce delayed hemorrhage). Do you have any allergies? Are you on any medication?

FIELD STRATEGY 7.5   OBSERVATION AND INSPECTION OF THE THORAX AND VISCERA

1. Is the individual pale, cold, clammy, lethargic (in shock)?

2. In what position is the individual (standing, leaning to one side, knees drawn to the chest, hands stabilizing an area)? Do the facial expressions indicate pain, anxiety, or panic? Is cyanosis present?

3. Is the individual stabilizing an area with the hand (this may indicate where the pain is, or where the pain is being referred to).

4. Is the trachea centered or deviated to one side (tension pneumothorax)? Does the trachea move during breathing?

5. Does the symmetry of both shoulders appear well rounded with no prominent bony structures? The pectoralis major, anterior axillary fold, and abdominal muscles should look symmetrical.

6. Is there any bruising, ecchymosis, deformity, or muscular atrophy?

7. Does the rib cage look symmetrical and move symmetrically with each breath? Is shallow breathing present? Is the individual coughing up a bright red or frothy blood?

8. Are abrasions, blisters, or bleeding present at the nipples? Are the nipples and breasts bilaterally the same size?

9. Is any bruising or ecchymosis present in the abdomen (bruising in the umbilical area indicates intraperitoneal bleeding)? Is the discoloration localized or diffuse? Are there any soft tissue protrusions in the lower abdomen or groin (hernia)?

---

breathing does not return to normal quickly or if the individual's condition rapidly deteriorates, the injury is significant and the emergency plan should be activated. Note the symmetrical rise and fall of the chest. **Field Strategy 7-5** provides specific observations that can help determine the extent and severity of thoracic or abdominal injuries.

Palpation

Palpate the chest and abdominal region beginning away from the painful area, so that pain cannot be carried over into other areas. Begin with gentle circular motions, and feel for deformity, crepitus, swelling, rigidity, muscle guarding, or tenderness. Palpate the clavicle, ribs, costochondral cartilage, and sternum for deformity and crepitus. Possible fractures are assessed with gentle pressure applied to the sternum and vertebrae in an anteroposterior direction **(Fig. 7-12A)**. This action causes the rib cage to bow out laterally, leading to increased pain over the suspected fracture site. Lateral compression on the sides of the rib cage causes strain on the costochondral junctions **(Fig. 7-12B)**. Begin compression superiorly and move down in an inferior direction until the entire area is covered. Pain at a specific site indicates a positive sign.

Palpate the abdomen with the hips flexed to relax the abdominal muscles. Use the flat part of several fin-

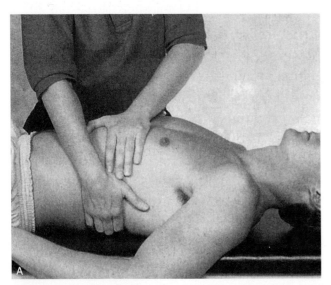 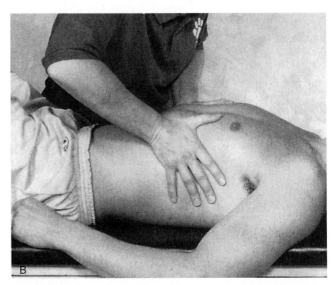

➤ **FIGURE 7-12.** Compression of the rib cage in a supine position. **A.** Anteroposterior compression of the rib cage can determine a possible rib fracture. **B.** Lateral compression of the rib cage can determine a possible costochondral separation.

gers, and move both hands in small, circular motions. Move across the abdomen in a straight line. Palpate for tenderness, muscle resistance, muscle guarding, and superficial masses or deficits in the continuity of the abdominal wall. Deeper palpation can detect rigidity, swelling, or masses. If the individual seems to be apprehensive or overreacts to palpation, ask the person questions during palpation. It is difficult to talk and voluntarily guard at the same time. If the pain is genuine, the individual will stop talking during guarding. Rebound pain, indicative of appendicitis, can be elicited at **McBurney's point**, which is located one third the distance between the anterior superior iliac spine and the umbilicus. Push the fingers gently into the abdomen at this point, then release the pressure. The rebounding pain is caused when the inflamed appendix is impacted by the viscera returning to their normal position.

Special Tests

Very few special tests exist for the thorax and visceral area. Many of these tests are too advanced for discussion and demonstration at this fundamental level. Therefore, most of the information on a thoracic or abdominal injury must be gathered during the primary survey, history, observation, and palpation phase of the assessment. If a muscular strain is suspected, active, passive, and resisted muscle testing can be performed.

Summary

1. Severe blunt trauma to the anterior neck region, thorax, and viscera can have devastating effects leading to serious ventilatory and circulatory compromise.
2. Blows to the throat may result in severe pain, laryngospasm, and acute respiratory distress.
3. A "stitch in the side" is a sharp pain or spasm in the chest wall, usually on the lower right side. Most individuals, however, can run through the pain.
4. Severe blunt trauma to the breast should be documented on a woman's permanent medical record to avoid misreading a mammogram.
5. A pectoralis major muscle strain involves an actively contracting muscle overburdened by a load or extrinsic force that exceeds tissue tolerance. Resisted horizontal adduction and internal rotation of the shoulder will be weak and accentuate the deformity if muscle fibers have been ruptured.
6. Signs and symptoms indicating a possible internal thoracic condition include the following:
   - Shortness of breath or difficulty in breathing
   - Severe chest pain aggravated with deep inspiration
   - Abnormal chest movement
   - Abnormal or absent breath sounds
7. A hernia is a protrusion of abdominal viscera through a weakened portion of the abdominal wall, and it can be congenital or acquired. An indirect inguinal hernia is the most common hernia in young athletes.
8. Signs and symptoms indicating a possible intra-abdominal condition include the following:
   - Shock
   - Severe abdominal pain
   - Nausea or vomiting
   - Distended abdomen
   - Tenderness, rigidity, or muscle spasm
   - Rebound pain
   - Absence of bowel sounds
   - Blood in the urine or stool
9. Individuals diagnosed with mononucleosis or having mono-like symptoms should not participate in collision sports until cleared by a physician.
10. Certain injuries may not develop until hours, days, or weeks later. As such, the presumption of possible intrathoracic or intra-abdominal injuries with any blunt trauma necessitates a complete assessment.
11. Injury assessment for the thorax and visceral region should focus on the vital signs and history of the injury.
12. Observation, palpation, and sites of referred pain can confirm suspicions of an existing internal injury.
13. If, at any time, signs and symptoms indicate an intrathoracic or intra-abdominal injury, EMS should be activated immediately. The ABCs should be monitored regularly to determine whether the individual is improving or deteriorating.
14. If the individual recovers on site, he or she should be informed of any signs and symptoms that might develop later, indicating that the condition is getting worse. If this occurs, the athlete should then seek immediate medical care.

References

1. Cvengros RD, and Lazor JA. 1996. Pneumothorax—a medical emergency. J Ath Train, 31(2):167-168.
2. Moeller JL. 1996. Contraindications to athletic participation: Cardiac, respiratory, and central nervous system conditions. Phys Sportsmed, 24(8):47-58.
3. Van Camp SP, Bloor CM, Mueller FO, et al. 1995. Nontraumatic sports death in high school and college athletes. Med Sci Sports Exerc, 27(5):641-647.
4. Nichols AW. Abdominal and thoracic injuries. In *Athletic injuries and rehabilitation*, edited by JE Zachazewski, DJ Magee, and WS Quillen. Philadelphia: WB Saunders, 1996.

8

Shoulder Conditions

OBJECTIVES

1. List the joints that make up the shoulder girdle.
2. Locate the important bony and soft-tissue structures of the shoulder.
3. Describe the major motions at the shoulder.
4. Explain general flexibility and strengthening exercises used to prevent injuries to the shoulder.
5. List common mechanisms of injury that may lead to instability in the sternoclavicular joint, acromioclavicular joint, and glenohumeral joint.
6. Describe common signs and symptoms associated with joint sprains and overuse injuries in the shoulder region.
7. Describe the signs and symptoms of thoracic outlet syndrome and its management.
8. Locate common fracture sites in the shoulder region and describe their management.
9. Explain a basic assessment of the shoulder region.

The loose structure of the shoulder complex enables extreme mobility but provides little stability. As a result, shoulder injuries are a major concern in activities involving an overhead motion, such as in baseball, swimming, tennis, volleyball, and weightlifting. These activities place significant demands on the shoulder and other joints of the upper extremity, leading to many acute and chronic conditions. This chapter begins with a general anatomy review of the shoulder region, followed by an overview of common injuries to the shoulder complex. Finally, a basic assessment of the region is presented.

ANATOMY OF THE SHOULDER

The shoulder region encompasses five separate articulations—the sternoclavicular (SC) joint, acromioclavicular (AC) joint, coracoclavicular joint, glenohumeral joint, and the scapulothoracic joint **(Fig. 8-1)**. The articulation referred to specifically as the

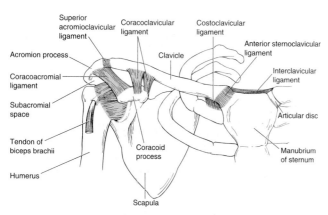

➤ **FIGURE 8-1.** Bony and ligamentous structure of the shoulder girdle.

shoulder joint is the glenohumeral joint, whereas the other articulations are joints of the shoulder girdle. The SC and AC joints enhance motion of the clavicle and scapula that position the glenohumeral joint to provide a greater range of motion for the humerus.

Sternoclavicular Joint

The SC joint consists of the articulation of the superior sternum, or manubrium, with the proximal clavicle. The joint allows motion of the distal clavicle in superior, inferior, anterior, and posterior directions, along with some forward and backward rotation of the clavicle. Thus, rotation occurs at the SC joint during motions such as shrugging the shoulders, reaching above the head, and throwing an object.

Acromioclavicular Joint

The AC joint consists of the articulation of the acromion process of the scapula with the distal end of the clavicle. The AC joint is an irregular, diarthrodial joint; therefore, limited motion is permitted in all three planes.

Coracoclavicular Joint

The coracoclavicular joint is located between the coracoid process of the scapula and the inferior surface of the

clavicle and is joined by the coracoclavicular ligament. This ligament resists independent upward movement of the clavicle, downward movement of the scapula, and anteroposterior movement of the clavicle or scapula. Little movement is allowed at this joint.

Glenohumeral Joint

The glenohumeral joint is the articulation between the glenoid fossa of the scapula and the head of the humerus. Although the joint enables a greater total range of motion than any other joint in the human body, it is lacking in bony stability **(Fig. 8-2)**. This is partially because the hemisphere-shaped head of the humerus has three to four times the amount of surface area of the shallow glenoid fossa. The glenoid fossa is somewhat deepened around its perimeter by the **glenoid labrum**, a narrow rim of fibrocartilage around the edge of the fossa. Because the glenoid fossa is also less curved than the humeral head, the humerus not only rotates, but moves linearly across the surface of the glenoid fossa when humeral motion occurs, thus predisposing the joint to impingement injuries.

The tendons of four muscles, including the supraspinatus, infraspinatus, teres minor, and subscapularis, also join the joint capsule **(Figs. 8-3 and 8-4)**. These muscles are referred to as the SITS muscles, after the first letter of each muscle's name. They are also known as the **rotator cuff** muscles because they all act to rotate the humerus and because their tendons merge to form a collagenous cuff around the joint. Tension in the rotator cuff muscles helps to hold the head of the humerus against the glenoid fossa, further contributing to joint stability.

Scapulothoracic Joint

Because muscles attaching to the scapula permit its motion with respect to the trunk or thorax, this region is sometimes described as the scapulothoracic joint **(Figs. 8-5 and 8-6)**. The scapular muscles perform two functions. The first is stabilization of the shoulder region. For example, when a barbell is lifted from the floor, the lev-

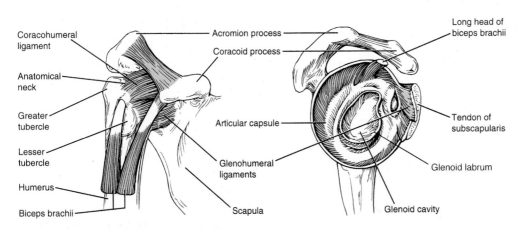

➤ **FIGURE 8-2.** Glenohumeral joint.

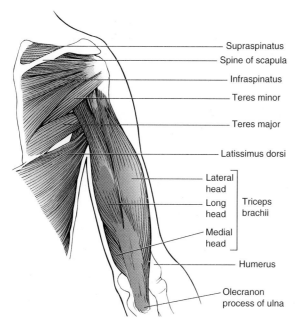

FIGURE 8-3. Deep posterior muscles that move the gleno-humeral joint.

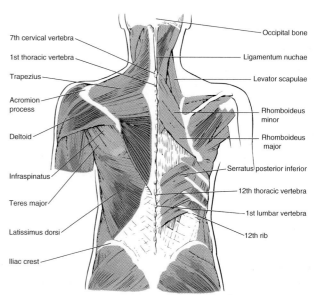

FIGURE 8-5. Superficial and deep posterior muscles of the back.

ator scapula, trapezius, and rhomboids develop tension to support the scapula and, in turn, the entire shoulder through the AC joint. The second function is to facilitate movements of the upper extremity through appropriate positioning of the glenohumeral joint. During an overhand throw, for example, the rhomboids contract to move the entire shoulder posteriorly as the arm and hand move backward during the preparatory phase. As the arm and hand then move forward to execute the throw, tension in the rhomboids is released to permit forward movement of the shoulder, enabling medial rotation of the humerus.

The shoulder is the most freely moveable joint in the body; motion is possible in all three planes **(Fig. 8-7)**. Sagittal plane movements of the humerus at the shoulder include flexion, extension, and hyperextension. Frontal plane movements include abduction and adduction. Transverse plane movements include horizontal abduction and horizontal adduction. The humerus can also rotate medially and laterally.

Bursae

In addition to muscles that move the shoulder joint, the shoulder is surrounded by several bursae. The most important, the subacromial bursa, lies in the subacromial

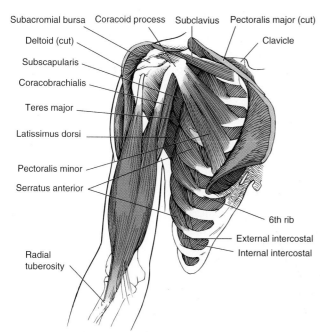

FIGURE 8-4. Deep anterior muscles that move the gleno-humeral joint.

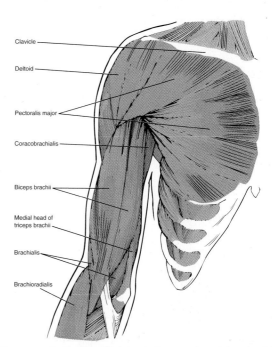

FIGURE 8-6. Superficial anterior muscles of the shoulder.

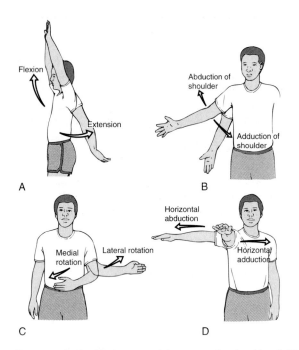

A

B

C

D

➤ **FIGURE 8-7.** Movements of the arm at the shoulder. **A.** Flexion and extension. **B.** Abduction and adduction. **C.** Medial and lateral rotation. **D.** Horizontal abduction and adduction. Combined movements are called circumduction.

space where it is surrounded by the acromion process of the scapula and the coracoacromial ligament above and the glenohumeral joint below **(Fig. 8-4)**. The bursa cushions the rotator cuff muscles, particularly the supraspinatus, from the overlying bony acromion. This bursa can become irritated when repeatedly compressed during overhead arm action.

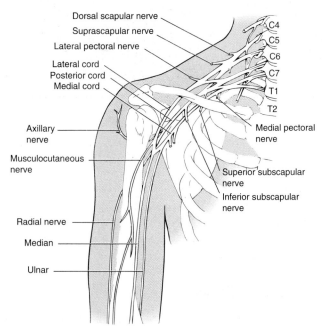

➤ **FIGURE 8-8.** Brachial plexus nerve supply to the shoulder region.

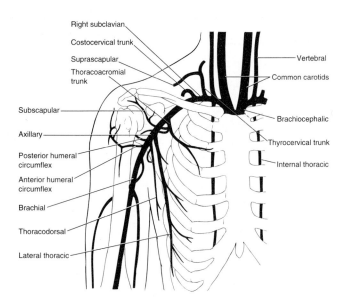

➤ **FIGURE 8-9.** Brachial plexus nerve supply to the shoulder region.

Nerves and Blood Vessels of the Shoulder

Innervation of the upper extremity arises from the **brachial plexus**, a combination of nerves branching primarily from the lower four cervical (C5 to C8) and the first thoracic (T1) spinal nerves **(Fig. 8-8)**. The branches from these nerves extend from the neck anteriorly and laterally, passing between the clavicle and first rib. Injuries to the clavicle in this region can damage the brachial plexus. Also in the area beneath the clavicle is the subclavian artery, which becomes the axillary artery as it passes through the axilla (armpit), providing the major blood supply to the shoulder **(Fig. 8-9)**.

PREVENTION OF INJURIES

Acute and chronic injuries to the shoulder complex are common in sport participation. Many contact and collision sports, such as football, lacrosse, and ice hockey, require shoulder pads to protect exposed bony protuberances. However, in other sports, flexibility and strengthening programs are essential to reduce the incidence of many shoulder injuries.

Shoulder Protection

Shoulder pads should protect the soft and bony tissue structures in the shoulder, upper back, and chest. The external shell is generally made of a lightweight yet hard plastic. The inner lining may be composed of closed-cell or open-cell padding to absorb and disperse the shock. However, use of open-cell padding results in lower peak impact forces compared with closed-cell pads.

Football shoulder pads are either cantilevered or flat. A channel system, incorporated into both types, uses a series of long, thinner pads attached by Velcro® in the

FIELD STRATEGY 8.1 FITTING FOOTBALL SHOULDER PADS

1. Determine the chest girth measurement at the nipple line or measure the distance between shoulder tips. Select pads based on the player's position. Place the pads on the shoulders and tighten all straps and laces. The laces should be pulled together until touching. The straps should have equal tension and be as tight as functionally tolerable to ensure proper force distribution over the pads. Tension on the straps should prevent no more than two fingers from being inserted under the strap. The entire clavicle should be covered and protected by the pads. If the clavicles can be palpated without moving the pads, refit with a smaller pad (**Fig. A**).

2. Anterior view: The laces should be centered over the sternum with no gap between the two halves. There should be full coverage of the acromioclavicular joint, clavicles, and pectoral muscles. Caps should cover the upper portion of the arch and entire deltoid muscle (**Fig. B**).

3. Posterior view: The entire scapula and trapezius should be covered with the lower pad arch extending below the inferior angle of the scapula to adequately protect the latissimus dorsi. The laces should be pulled tight and centered over the spine (**Fig. C**).

4. With the arms abducted, the neck opening should not be uncomfortable or pinch the neck. Finally, inspection should include the shoulder pads with the helmet and jersey in place to ensure that no impingement of the cervical region is present (**Fig. D**).

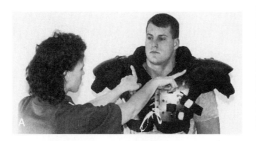
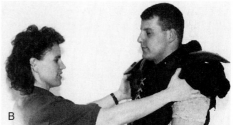
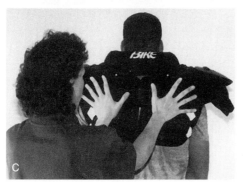
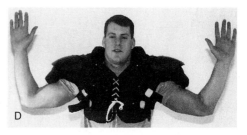

shoulder pads. The pads can be fitted individually to create an air space at the AC joint. The impact forces are placed entirely on the anterior and posterior aspect of the shoulder.

Cantilever pads have a hard plastic bridge over the superior aspect of the shoulder to protect the AC joint. These bridges are lightweight, allow maximal range of motion at the shoulder, and can distribute the impact forces throughout the entire shoulder girdle. Flat shoulder pads are lightweight and provide less protection to the shoulder region, but they allow more glenohumeral joint motion. These pads are often used by quarterbacks or receivers who must raise their arms above the head to throw or catch a pass.

Football shoulder pads should be selected based on the player's position, body type, and medical history. Linemen need protection against constant contact and therefore use larger cantilevers. Quarterbacks, offensive backs, and receivers require smaller shoulder cups and flaps to allow greater range of motion in passing and catching. **Field Strategy 8-1** lists the general steps used in fitting football shoulder pads.

Physical Conditioning

Lack of flexibility can predispose an individual to joint sprains and muscular strains. Warm-up exercises should focus on general joint flexibility and can be performed

FIELD STRATEGY 8.2   FLEXIBILITY EXERCISES FOR THE SHOULDER REGION

A. **Posterior capsular stretch**. Horizontally adduct the arm across the chest while the opposite hand assists the stretch.

B. **Inferior capsular stretch**. Hold the involved arm over the head with the elbow flexed. Use the opposite hand to assist in the stretching. Add a side stretch.

C. **Anterior and posterior capsular stretch**. Hold onto both sides of a doorway with your hands behind you. Let the arms straighten as you lean forward. Repeat with your hands in front of you as you lean backward.

D. **Medial and lateral rotators**. Using a towel, bat, or racquet, pull the arm to be stretched into lateral rotation. Repeat in medial rotation.

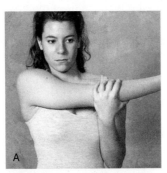

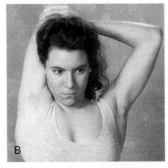

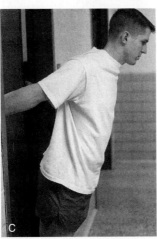

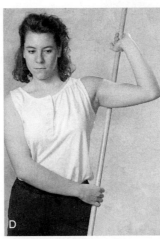

alone or with a partner. Individuals using the throwing motion in their sport should increase range of motion in external rotation, as it has been shown to increase the velocity of the throwing arm and decrease shearing forces on the glenohumeral joint.[1] Several flexibility exercises for the shoulder complex are demonstrated in **Field Strategy 8-2**.

Strengthening programs should focus on muscles acting on both the glenohumeral and scapulothoracic region. Strength in the infraspinatus, teres minor, and posterior shoulder musculature is necessary to begin the cocking phase of throwing. It is also necessary to fix the shoulder girdle during the acceleration phase and provide adequate muscle tension through eccentric contractions for smooth deceleration through the follow-through phase .

In many chronic shoulder problems, particularly among throwers, a weakened supraspinatus is present.

Concentric and eccentric contractions, with light resistance in the first 30° of abduction, can strengthen this muscle. To strengthen the scapular stabilizers, do wide-stance push-ups or move the arm through a resisted diagonal pattern of external rotation and horizontal abduction. Other strengthening exercises are demonstrated in **Field Strategy 8-3**.

Proper Skill Technique

Throwing and related motions can produce a variety of both acute and chronic injuries to the shoulder. Throwing styles vary from individual to individual, even across overarm, sidearm, and underarm styles of throw. Nevertheless, overarm throwing can be described in distinct phases (**Box 8-1**).

In the preparatory or cocking phase, the arm and hand are drawn behind the body through horizontal

FIELD STRATEGY 8.3   STRENGTHENING EXERCISES FOR THE SHOULDER COMPLEX

A. **Shoulder shrugs**. Elevate the shoulders toward the ears and hold. Pull the shoulders back, pinch the shoulder blades together, and hold. Relax and repeat.

B. **Scapular abduction (protraction)**. Thrust the weight directly upward, lifting the posterior shoulder from the table. Relax and repeat.

C. **Scapular adduction (retraction)**. Do bent-over rowing while flexing the elbows. At the end of the motion, pinch the shoulder blades together and hold.

D. **Bench press or incline press**. Use a weight belt and spotter. Place the hands shoulder-width apart and push the barbell directly above the shoulder joint. (Individuals with multidirectional instability of the glenohumeral joint should refrain from this exercise.)

E. **Bent arm lateral flies, supine position**. With the elbows slightly flexed, bring the dumbbells directly over the shoulders. Lower the dumbbells until they are parallel to the floor, then repeat. An alternative method is to move the dumbbells in a diagonal pattern. In the prone position, the exercise strengthens the trapezius (trap flies).

F. **Lat pull-downs**. In a seated position, grasp the handle and pull the bar behind the head, unless there is a predisposing condition, such as a rotator cuff injury. An alternative method is to pull the bar in front of the body.

G. **Surgical tubing**. With the tubing secured, work in diagonal functional patterns similar to those skills experienced in the specific sport.

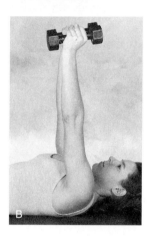
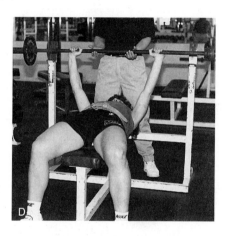
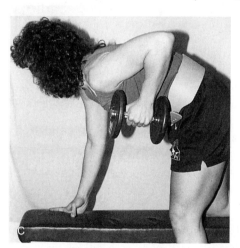
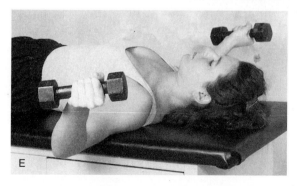
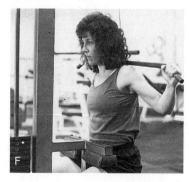
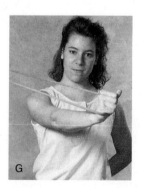

abduction, hyperextension, and maximal external rotation of the humerus **(Fig. 8-10)**. Eccentric loading of the horizontal adductors (pectoralis major) and internal rotators (subscapularis, latissimus dorsi) of the shoulder is high during this action. They function to protect the anterior joint, which is under extreme tension at this time. To facilitate this arm motion, the rhomboids must contract concentrically to pull the scapula and the glenohumeral joint posteriorly, while the serratus anterior provides additional scapular stabilization. As the motion continues, the humeral head tends to sublux, first posteriorly and then anteriorly, against the anterior capsule; consequently, tendinitis of the anterior muscle tendons is quite common.[2] Just before maximal shoulder external rotation, elbow extension begins, immediately followed by the onset of shoulder internal rotation.

➤➤ B O X   8 - 1

Phases of the Throwing Motion

• Wind-up Phase	From first movement until hands separate. Arms begin with downward swing, then are raised overhead (gathered position). Shoulders and hips rotate as arms go overhead, and body shifts from facing target to being perpendicular to the line of throw. Balance is maintained on "stance leg" (right leg) as the lead leg or "stride leg" (left leg) lifts up; hip and knee flex at about chest-high level.
• Stride Phase	From hand separation until the lead foot contacts the ground.
• Cocking Phase	From foot contact until maximum shoulder external rotation.
• Acceleration Phase	From maximum shoulder external rotation until ball release.
• Deceleration and Follow-through Phase	From ball release until maximum shoulder internal rotation and balanced position is achieved.

During the acceleration or delivery phase, the ball is brought forward and released. Humeral horizontal adduction, elbow extension, and rapid internal rotation of the humerus by the pectoralis major, latissimus dorsi, and subscapularis are coupled with relaxation of the rhomboids to enable anterior movement of the glenohumeral joint. If the internal rotators are weak, the reduced ability to provide forceful arm depression can lead to increased external rotation, superior humeral migration, and impaired scapular rotation, which can cause or aggravate an impingement syndrome. At ball release, the elbow is almost fully extended and positioned slightly anterior to the trunk. Because throwing can involve a whiplike action of the arm, large stresses can be placed on the tendons, ligaments, and epiphyses of the throwing arm during delivery.[2]

Arm deceleration occurs after ball release until maximal shoulder internal rotation occurs, and it consists primarily of a snaplike flexion of the wrist and pronation of the forearm. Large eccentric loads at the elbow and shoulder decelerate the arm. The infraspinatus, supraspinatus, teres major and minor, latissimus dorsi, and posterior deltoid play major roles in resisting shoulder distraction and anterior subluxation forces. If the rotator cuff muscles are weak, fatigued, or injured, the humeral head distracts and translates in an anterior

direction, leading to stress on the posterior capsule. The serratus anterior contracts either concentrically or isometrically to decelerate scapular protraction and is assisted by the middle trapezius and rhomboids. Injuries common to the specific phases of throwing are shown in **Box 8-2**.

In addition to proper throwing techniques, participants in contact and collision sports should be taught the shoulder roll method of falling, rather than falling on an outstretched arm. This technique reduces direct compression of the articular joints and disperses the force over a wider area.

SPRAINS TO THE SHOULDER COMPLEX

Ligamentous injuries to the SC joint, AC joint, and glenohumeral joint can result from compression, tension, and shearing forces occurring in a single episode or from repetitive overload **(Fig. 8-11)**. A common method of injury is a fall or direct hit on the lateral aspect of the acromion. The force is first transmitted to the site of impact, then to the AC joint, the clavicle, and, finally, to the SC joint. Failure can occur at any one of these sites. Acute sprains are commonly seen in hockey, rugby, football, soccer, and equestrian sports.

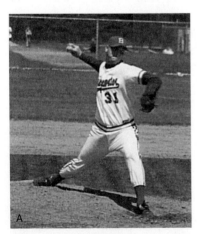 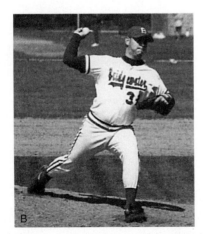 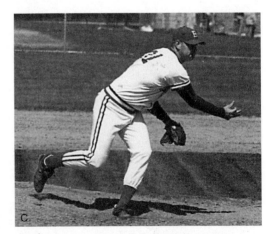

➤ **F I G U R E   8 - 1 0 .** The overarm throwing motion. **A.** Cocking phase. **B.** Acceleration phase. **C.** Deceleration and follow-through phase.

Sternoclavicular Joint Sprain

The SC joint is the main axis for movements of the clavicle and scapula. Nearly all injuries result from compression from a direct blow, as when a supine athlete is landed on by another participant, or more commonly, by indirect forces transmitted from a blow to the shoulder or a fall on an outstretched arm. The disruption typically drives the proximal clavicle superior, medial, and anterior, causing anterior displacement. Posterior displacement, although rare, is more serious because of possible injury to the esophagus, trachea, and subclavian artery.

SIGNS AND SYMPTOMS

First-degree injuries are characterized by point tenderness and mild pain over the SC joint, with no visible deformity. Second-degree injuries cause bruising, swelling, and pain, and the individual is unable to do shoulder elevation without considerable pain. The athlete may hold the arm forward and close to the body, supporting it across the chest, indicating disruption of the stabilizing ligaments. Third-degree sprains involve a prominent displacement of the sternal end of the clavicle and may involve a fracture. Pain is severe when the shoulders are brought together by a lateral force.

MANAGEMENT

Field Strategy 8-4 summarizes the management of anterior sternoclavicular sprains. If a posterior dislocation is suspected and the athlete is having difficulty swallowing or breathing, summon emergency medical services.

Acromioclavicular or Coracoclavicular Joint Sprains

The AC joint is weak and easily injured by a direct blow, a fall on the point of the shoulder (called a shoulder pointer), and, occasionally, by a force transmitted up the long axis of the humerus during a fall on an outstretched arm.

SIGNS AND SYMPTOMS

As with other joint sprains, symptoms parallel the amount of damage done to the supporting ligaments. In a first-degree injury, minimal swelling and pain are present. In a second-degree injury, the AC ligaments are torn, but the coracoclavicular ligament is only mildly sprained and still intact. The distal clavicle rides above the level of the acromion, and a minor step or gap is present at the joint line **(Fig. 8-12)**. Pain increases when the distal clavicle is depressed or moved in an anteroposterior direction and during passive horizontal adduction. In a third-degree injury, the coracoclavicular and AC ligaments tear completely, resulting in obvious swelling and bruising, and a step deformity is present.

MANAGEMENT

Field Strategy 8-5 summarizes management of acromioclavicular sprains.

Glenohumeral Joint Sprain

Damage to the glenohumeral joint can occur when the arm is forcefully abducted (i.e., when making an arm tackle in football), or abducted and externally rotated. In nearly all cases (95%), the anterior capsule is stretched or torn, leading to the humeral head slipping out of the glenoid fossa in an anterior-inferior direction **(Fig. 8-13)**. A direct blow or forceful movement that pushes the humerus posteriorly can also result in damage to the joint capsule.

SIGNS AND SYMPTOMS

In a first-degree injury, the anterior shoulder is particularly painful to palpation and movement, especially when the mechanism of injury is reproduced. A second-degree sprain produces some joint laxity. Pain, swelling, and bruising are usually severe, and range of motion, particularly abduction, is limited. A third-degree injury is considered a dislocation and is discussed in the next section.

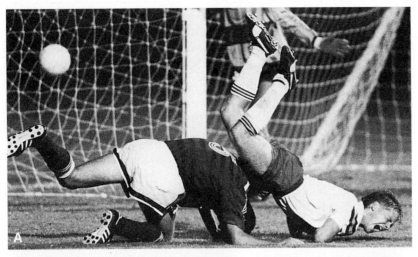

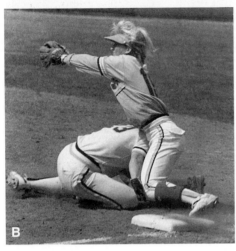

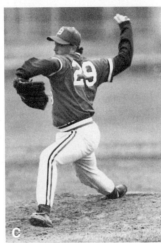

➤ **FIGURE 8-11.** Common mechanisms of injury to the shoulder. **A.** Indirect forces. **B.** Direct forces. **C.** Microtraumatic repetitive forces.

MANAGEMENT

Treatment involves cryotherapy, rest, nonsteroidal anti-inflammatory drugs (NSAIDs), and immobilization with a sling during the initial 12 to 24 hours. If pain persists, encourage this individual to see a physician.

Glenohumeral Dislocations

ANTERIOR DISLOCATIONS

Anterior dislocations are commonly caused by excessive indirect forces that push the arm into abduction, external rotation, and extension. The ligaments are significantly damaged, causing the head of the humerus to lodge under the anterior-inferior portion of the glenoid fossa adjacent to the coracoid process. The labrum may also be damaged or avulsed from the anterior lip of the glenoid as the humerus slides forward (**Bankart lesion**).

SIGNS AND SYMPTOMS

Intense pain occurs with the initial dislocation, although recurrent dislocations may be less painful. Tingling and numbness may extend down the arm into the hand. With a first-time dislocation, the injured arm is often held in slight abduction (20 to 30°) and external rotation, and is stabilized against the body by the opposite hand. Visually, a sharp contour on the affected shoulder, with a prominent acromion process, can be seen when compared to the smooth deltoid outline on the unaffected shoulder **(Fig. 8-14)**. The individual will not allow the arm to be brought across the chest. Assessment of both circulation and nerve integrity is imperative because both structures can be damaged in a dislocation. A pulse may be taken on the medial proximal humerus over the brachial artery, and the axillary nerve can be assessed by stroking the skin on the upper lateral arm. Ask the individual if it feels the same on both arms.

MANAGEMENT

Management of a first-time dislocation requires immediate reduction by a physician because many of these dislocations are associated with a fracture. Treat the injury as a fracture and immobilize the arm in a comfortable position. To prevent unnecessary movement of the humerus, place a rolled towel or thin pillow between the thoracic wall and humerus before applying a sling. Ice is then applied to control hemorrhage and muscle spasm as the individual is transported to the nearest medical facility.

FIELD STRATEGY 8.4 **MANAGEMENT OF A STERNOCLAVICULAR SPRAIN**

Signs and Symptoms	First Degree	Second Degree	Third Degree
Deformity	None	Slight prominence of medial end of the clavicle	Gross prominence of medial end of the clavicle
Swelling	Slight	Moderate	Severe
Palpable pain	Mild	Moderate	Severe
Movement	Usually unlimited, but may have discomfort with movement	Unable to abduct the arm or horizontally adduct the arm across the chest without noticeable pain	Limited as in 2°, but pain more severe
Treatment	Ice, rest; immobilize with sling/swathe	Ice, rest; immobilize with figure-8 or clavicular strap with sling, and refer to a physician	Figure-8 immobilizer with scapulae retracted. Immediately refer to physician. Check pulse, swallowing, or breathing difficulty. If present, activate EMS

EMS—emergency medical services.

POSTERIOR DISLOCATIONS
Occasionally, a posterior dislocation occurs from a fall on, or blow to, the anterior surface of the shoulder, driving the head of the humerus posterior.

SIGNS AND SYMPTOMS
If dislocated, the arm is carried tightly against the chest and across the front of the trunk in rigid adduction and internal rotation. The anterior shoulder appears flat, the coracoid process is prominent, and a corresponding bulge may be seen posteriorly, if not masked by a heavy deltoid musculature.[3] Any attempt to move the arm produces severe pain.

MANAGEMENT
Treatment is the same as with an acute anterior dislocation—ice, immobilization in a sling, and immediate transportation to a physician.

RECURRENT SUBLUXATIONS AND DISLOCATIONS
Recurrent posterior subluxations are common in many activities, such as the follow-through phase of throwing or a racquet swing, ascent phase of push-ups or bench pressing, certain swimming strokes, or during crew sweep strokes. The mechanism of injury is the same as acute dislocations. As the number of occurrences increases, however, the forces needed to produce the injury decrease, as does the associated muscle spasm, pain, and swelling. The individual is aware of the shoulder displacing because the arm gives the sensation of "going dead," referred to as the **dead arm syndrome**. Often it is reduced by the individual or with the help of a teammate.

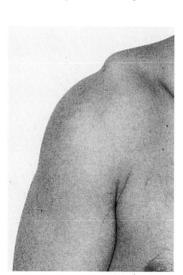
➤ **FIGURE 8-12.** Acromioclavicular sprain. With a moderate acromioclavicular sprain, the distal clavicle is elevated by injury to the acromioclavicular and coracoclavicular ligaments.

SIGNS AND SYMPTOMS
Pain is the major report, followed by crepitation or clicking when the arm shifts into the appropriate position.

FIELD STRATEGY 8.5   MANAGEMENT OF AN ACROMIOCLAVICULAR SPRAIN

Signs and Symptoms	First Degree	Second Degree	Third Degree
Deformity	None, ligaments are still intact	Slight elevation of lateral clavicle; AC ligaments are disrupted, but coracoclavicular is still intact	Prominent elevation of clavicle; AC ligaments and coracoclavicular ligaments are disrupted
Swelling	Slight	Moderate	Severe
Palpable pain	Mild over joint line	Moderate with downward pressure on distal clavicle; palpable gap or minor step present; snapping may be felt on horizontal adduction	Severe on palpation and depression of the acromion process; definite palpable step deformity will be present
Movement	Usually unlimited, but may have some discomfort on abduction over 90°	Unable to abduct the arm or horizontally adduct the arm across the chest without noticeable pain	Limited as in 2°, but pain will be more severe
Stability	No instability	Some instability	Demonstrable instability
Treatment	Ice, NSAIDs, regain full ROM and strength; return to activity as tolerated, with protection	Ice, NSAIDs; immobilize with sling and refer to a physician	Ice, immobilize, and immediately refer to a physician

AC—acromioclavicular; NSAIDs—nonsteroidal anti-inflammatory drugs; ROM—range of motion.

MANAGEMENT

After reduction by a physician, conservative treatment involves resting and immobilization, restoring shoulder motion, and strengthening the rotator cuff muscles. If persistent instability occurs, surgery may be indicated.

OVERUSE INJURIES

During abduction, the strong deltoid muscle pulls the humeral head superiorly, relative to the glenoid fossa. The rotator cuff muscles are critical in counteracting this migration. If the tendons are weak, they are incapable of depressing the humeral head in the glenoid fossa during overhead motions. This can lead to impingement of the supraspinatus tendon and subacromial bursa between the acromion, the coracoacromial ligament, and the greater tubercle of the humerus. This compressive action can lead to a rotator cuff strain, impingement syndrome, bursitis, or bicipital tendinitis, or a combination of these injuries.

Rotator Cuff/Impingement Injuries

Chronic rotator cuff tears result from repetitive microtraumatic episodes that primarily impinge the supraspinatus tendon just proximal to the greater tubercle of the humerus **(Fig. 8-15)**. Partial tears are usually seen in young individuals, with total tears occurring in adults older than 30 years.[4] **Impingement syndrome** implies that, in addition to damage to the supraspinatus tendon, the glenoid labrum, long head of the biceps brachii, and subacromial bursa may also be injured.

SIGNS AND SYMPTOMS

Initially, pain occurs with activity, usually only in the impingement position. As repetitive trauma continues, however, pain becomes progressively worse, particularly between 70 and 120° ("painful arc") of active and resisted abduction. Because forced scapular protraction leads to fur-

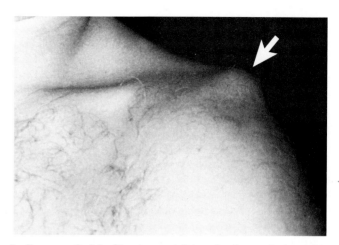

➤ **FIGURE 8-14.** Glenohumeral dislocation. In a typical anterior dislocation, the head of the humerus is forced out of the glenoid fossa and comes to rest adjacent to the coracoid process. As a result, the acromion process becomes prominent (*arrow*), the deltoid musculature appears flat, and the athlete may hold the arm away from the side.

Point tenderness can be elicited on the anterior and lateral edges of the acromion process. A painful arc exists between 70 and 120° of passive abduction.

➤ **FIGURE 8-13.** Glenohumeral sprains. **A.** Normal abduction with some stretching of the fibers. **B.** Forced external rotation and abduction with minimal tears to the joint capsule leading to a moderate or second-degree sprain. **C.** Continuation of the forced movement causes a third-degree sprain or shoulder dislocation.

ther impingement and pain in the structures, the individual may be unable to sleep at night on the involved side.

MANAGEMENT

Treatment involves cryotherapy, NSAIDs, pain-relieving medication, rest, and activity modification. If initial treatment and a reduction in activity do not relieve symptoms, this individual should be referred to a physician. The condition may not improve without a supervised and graduated rehabilitation program. Once the shoulder develops a protective response to the injury, it must be retrained to reestablish the synchronization of all joints in the complex.

Bursitis

The bursa of the shoulder is the first line of defense to protect the rotator cuff musculature, especially the supraspinatus muscle. Therefore, a rotator cuff injury does not occur without bursitis. Because of its location, the subacromial bursa is the most commonly injured bursa in the shoulder region.

SIGNS AND SYMPTOMS

Frequently, sudden shoulder pain is reported during the initiation and acceleration phase of the throwing motion.

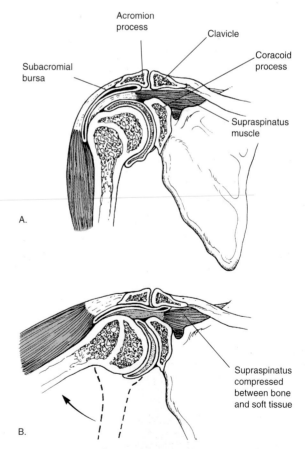

➤ **FIGURE 8-15.** Supraspinatus tendon during abduction. **A.** Normal position. **B.** Abducted position. Repetitive overhead motions can impinge the muscle or tendon between the acromion process and coracoacromial ligament, resulting in a chronic rotator cuff injury.

MANAGEMENT

Treatment is the same as for a rotator cuff strain or impingement syndrome.

Bicipital Tendinitis

Injury to the biceps brachii tendon often occurs from repetitive overuse during rapid overhead movements involving excessive elbow flexion and supination activities, such as in racquet sports players, shot-putters, baseball/softball pitchers, football quarterbacks, swimmers, and javelin throwers. Irritation of the tendon occurs as it passes back and forth in the intertubercular (bicipital) groove of the humerus. The tendon may partially sublux.

SIGNS AND SYMPTOMS

Diffuse pain and tenderness is present over the anterior shoulder. Point tenderness exists directly over the bicipital groove when the tendon is passively stretched, and during resisted supination and elbow flexion.

MANAGEMENT

Treatment involves restriction of rotational activities that exacerbate symptoms; cryotherapy; and NSAIDs to control inflammation. Ice before and after activity can be combined with a gradual program of stretching and strengthening as soon as pain subsides.

Biceps Tendon Rupture

Prolonged tendinitis can make the tendon vulnerable to forceful rupture during repetitive overhead motions, commonly seen in swimmers, or in forceful flexion activities against excessive resistance, commonly seen in weightlifters or gymnasts.

SIGNS AND SYMPTOMS

The individual often hears and feels a snapping sensation and experiences intense pain. Ecchymosis and a visible, palpable defect can be seen in the muscle belly when the individual flexes the biceps.

MANAGEMENT

This individual should be referred immediately to a physician.

Thoracic Outlet Compression Syndrome

Thoracic outlet compression syndrome is a condition in which the lower trunk of the brachial plexus or the subclavian artery and vein become compressed in the proximal neck or the axilla **(Fig. 8-16)**. The condition is often aggravated in activities that require overhead rotational stresses while muscles are loaded, such as in weightlifting and swimming.

SIGNS AND SYMPTOMS

If a nerve is compressed, an aching pain, pins-and-needles sensation, or numbness in the side or back of the neck extends across the shoulder down the medial arm to the ulnar aspect of the hand (ulnar nerve distribution). Weakness in grasp and atrophy of the hand muscles may also be present. If arterial or venous vessels are compressed, signs and symptoms vary depending on the specific structure being obstructed. Blockage of the subclavian vein produces edema, stiffness (especially in the hand), and venous engorgement of the arm with cyanosis. If untreated, this may result in thrombophlebitis. The athlete may present these signs and symptoms several hours after a bout of intense exercise. Occlusion of the subclavian artery results in a rapid onset of coolness, numbness in the entire arm, and fatigue after exertional overhead activity.

MANAGEMENT

Immediate referral to a physician is necessary for more extensive assessment to rule out serious vascular involvement. Conservative treatment involves assessing muscle strength and posture. Noted deficits should lead to an appropriate retraining program to develop strength and muscle balance in the shoulder girdle and facilitate the maintenance of a corrected posture. If the condition was precipitated by a sudden increase in activity, treatment involves anti-inflammatory medication, activity modification, and a reassessment of the training program. Return to full activity can occur after range of motion and strength in the shoulder musculature have been regained.

FRACTURES

Most fractures to the shoulder region result from a fall on the point of the shoulder, rolling over onto the top of the shoulder, or indirectly by falling on an outstretched arm.

Clavicular Fractures

Clavicular fractures are more common than fractures to the scapula and proximal humerus—nearly 80% occur in the midclavicular region **(Fig. 8-17)**. The sternocleidomastoid muscle pulls the proximal bone fragment superiorly, allowing the distal shoulder to droop downward and medially from the force of gravity and pull of the pectoralis major muscle.

SIGNS AND SYMPTOMS

The athlete often tilts the head toward the side of the fracture, supporting the arm next to the body and giving a rounded shoulder appearance. Swelling, ecchymosis,

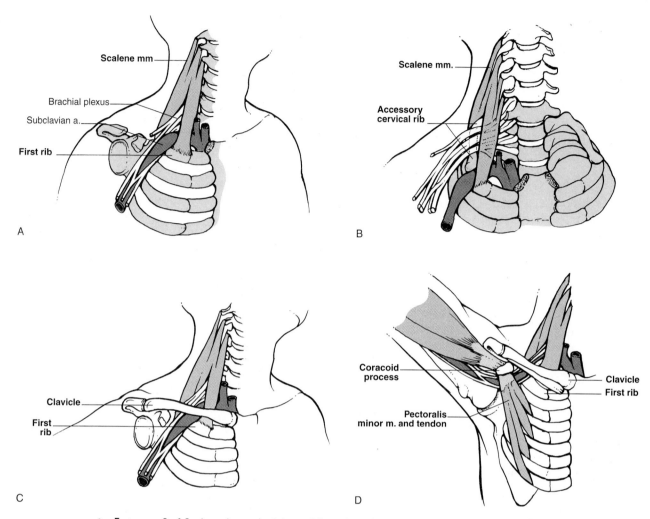

➤ FIGURE 8-16. Location and etiology of thoracic outlet syndrome. **A.** Scalenus anterior syndrome. **B.** Cervical rib syndrome. **C.** Costoclavicular space syndrome. **D.** Hyperabduction syndrome.

and a deformity may be visible and palpable at the fracture site. Greenstick fractures, typically seen in adolescents, also produce a noticeable deformity.

MANAGEMENT

Immediate treatment involves immobilization in a sling and swathe. After the individual is assessed by the physician, a figure-8 brace or strapping is used to pull the shoulders backward and upward for 4 to 6 weeks in young adults and 6 or more weeks in older adults **(Fig. 8-18)** .

Scapular Fractures

Scapular fractures may involve the body, spine and acromion process, coracoid process, or glenohumeral joint.

SIGNS AND SYMPTOMS

Most fractures result in minimal displacement and exhibit localized hemorrhage, pain, and tenderness. The individ-

ual is reluctant to move the injured arm and prefers to maintain it in adduction.

MANAGEMENT

The arm should be immobilized immediately with a sling and swathe, and the individual should be referred to a physician.

Epiphyseal Fractures

Epiphyseal centers around the shoulder region remain unfused for a longer span of time than is typically seen at other epiphyseal sites. For example, the proximal humeral epiphysis does not close until ages 18 to 21 years, thus predisposing an individual to this injury throughout the competitive high school and collegiate years. An epiphyseal fracture at this site, called **little league shoulder**, is often caused by repetitive medial rotation and adduction traction forces placed on the shoulder during pitching **(Fig. 8-19)**. Catchers may also

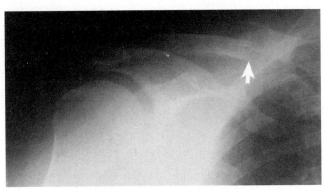

➤ FIGURE 8-17. Midclavicular fracture. *Arrow* indicates the fracture site.

get this fracture because they throw the ball as hard and as often as pitchers, but with less of a wind-up.

SIGNS AND SYMPTOMS

With an epiphyseal fracture, the individual reports acute shoulder pain when attempting to throw hard, which, if ignored, may result in an acute displacement of the weakened physis. Pain may be elicited with deep palpation in the axilla.

MANAGEMENT

The arm should be immobilized in a sling and swathe. Apply ice to control pain and swelling, and refer the athlete immediately to a physician for further care. Radiographs are necessary to see the widened epiphyseal line and demineralization. Treatment is conservative, with symptoms disappearing after 3 to 4 weeks of rest. If activity is resumed too quickly, the condition may recur.

Humeral Fractures

Humeral fractures result from violent compressive forces because of a direct blow, a fall on the upper arm, or a fall on an outstretched hand with the elbow extended. The surgical neck is the most common site for proximal humeral fractures, and may display an appearance similar to a dislocation **(Fig. 8-20)**.

SIGNS AND SYMPTOMS

Pain, swelling, hemorrhage, discoloration, an inability to move the arm, and possible paralysis may be present. The arm is often held splinted against the body.

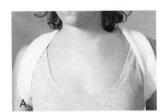
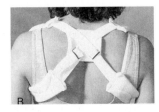

➤ FIGURE 8-18. Figure-8 clavicular straps. **A.** Anterior view. **B.** Posterior view.

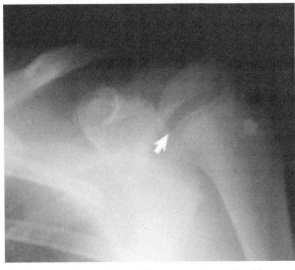

➤ FIGURE 8-19. Epiphyseal fracture to the proximal humeral growth center. *Arrow* indicates the fracture site.

MANAGEMENT

The arm should be immobilized in a sling and swathe. Check the radial pulse to rule out vascular damage. Apply ice to control pain and swelling, and refer the athlete immediately to a physician for further care. Fortunately, these fractures are often impacted, which facilitates closed reduction and allows early movement after 3 to 4 weeks of immobilization.

ASSESSMENT OF THE SHOULDER

The shoulder complex is a complicated region to assess because of the many important structures located in such a small area. At this level of understanding, a basic assessment can be conducted by a coach. However, if pain is

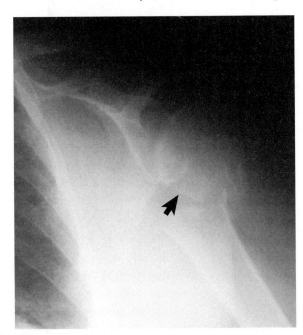

➤ FIGURE 8-20. Fracture to the surgical neck of the humerus. *Arrow* indicates the fracture site.

Signs and Symptoms That Necessitate Immediate Referral to a Physician

- Obvious deformity suggesting a suspected fracture, separation, or dislocation
- Significant loss of motion or weakness in the myotomes
- Joint instability
- Abnormal sensation in the shoulder, arm, or hand
- Absent or weak pulse distal to the injury
- Any significant, unexplained pain

moderate to severe, or if shoulder movement is compromised by the injury, the athlete should be referred to a physician for further assessment and treatment (**Box 8-3**).

History

Questions about a shoulder injury should focus on the current primary complaint, past injuries to the region, and other factors that may have contributed to the current problem (e.g., referred pain, alterations in posture, change in technique, or overuse). Many conditions may be related to improper execution of skills and recent changes in training programs. Keep questions open ended to allow the individual to fully describe the injury. Specific questions related to the shoulder region are shown in **Field Strategy 8-6**.

Observation and Inspection

On-the-field assessment may be somewhat limited because of uniforms and protective equipment that may obstruct the region from observation and inspection. Initially, you may have to slide your hands under the pads to palpate the region to determine the presence of a possible fracture or major ligament damage. If necessary, the pads should be cut and removed gently to expose the area more fully. After the initial examination, the individual may need to be removed from the field and undergo more complete assessment.

Ideally, women should wear a bathing suit or halter top to expose the entire shoulder and arm. Complete a general postural examination as you look for faulty posture or congenital abnormalities that could place additional strain on the anatomic structures. The individual should be viewed from the anterior, lateral, and posterior views. During movement, look for symmetry and fluid scapular motion. Inspect the specific injury site for obvious deformity, swelling, discoloration, symmetry, hypertrophy, muscle atrophy, or previous surgical incisions. Compare the affected limb with the unaffected limb.

Palpation

Bilateral palpation can determine temperature, swelling, point tenderness, crepitus, deformity, muscle spasm, and cutaneous sensation. Increased skin temperature could indicate inflammation or infection. Decreased skin temperature could indicate a reduction in circulation. Vascular pulses can be taken at the radial and ulnar arteries in the wrist, brachial artery on the medial arm, or axillary artery in the armpit. Stand behind the individual to begin bilateral palpation, moving proximal to distal. Leave the most painful area until last. The following areas can be palpated:

- Bony Palpation
  1. Clavicle, acromion process, coracoid process
  2. Greater tubercle of the humerus, bicipital groove, and humeral shaft
  3. Scapula

- Soft-Tissue Palpation
  1. SC joint and sternocleidomastoid muscle
  2. AC joint, subacromial bursa, and coracoacromial ligament
  3. Rotator cuff muscles, pectoralis major, deltoid muscle, and biceps brachii muscle and tendon
  4. Trapezius, rhomboid muscles, latissimus dorsi, and serratus anterior

Fractures can be assessed through palpation of pain at the fracture site, compression of the humeral head against the glenoid fossa, compression along the long axis of the humerus, and with percussion and vibration on a specific bony landmark. If a fracture or dislocation is suspected, immediately assess circulatory and neural integrity distal to the site. Take a pulse at the sites indicated in the previous list, and stroke the palm and dorsum of both hands to see if it feels the same bilaterally. Immobilize the extremity in an appropriate sling or splint, and refer the individual to the nearest medical facility.

Special Tests

Place the athlete in a comfortable position and perform any special tests using gentle stress. The shoulder commonly has painful arcs. Note what range of motion is the most painful. Do not force the limb through any sudden motions, nor cause undue pain. Proceed cautiously through the assessment.

RANGE OF MOTION TESTS

Because pain is frequently referred from the cervical region into the shoulder, perform active range of motion at the neck first. Neck flexion, extension, rotation, and lateral flexion should be assessed for fluid motion and presence of pain. If pain is present at the neck, immediately complete a full neck evaluation. If necessary, immobilize the neck in a cervical collar and refer the individual to a physician.

If no problems are noted during neck movement, continue with the shoulder evaluation. Ask the individual to perform movement patterns at the shoulder. These motions include 1) scapular elevation, depression, pro-

FIELD STRATEGY 8.6   DEVELOPING A HISTORY OF THE INJURY

CURRENT INJURY STATUS

1. Where is the pain (or weakness) located? How would you rate the pain (weakness)? What type of pain is it (dull ache, throbbing, sharp, intermittent, red-hot, burning, or radiating)?

2. Did the pain come on suddenly (acute) or gradually (overuse)? Was the pain greatest when the injury first occurred or did it get worse the second or third day?

3. (If acute, ask:) What were you doing at the time of the injury? Was there a direct blow? Did you fall? How—outstretched arm, rolling over the shoulder or side of the shoulder? (If chronic, ask:) What different activities have you been doing in the last week? (Look for changes in technique, frequency, duration, intensity, or changes in equipment.)

4. Did you hear any sounds during the incident? Any snaps, pops, or cracks? Did you notice any swelling, discoloration, muscle spasms, or numbness with the injury?

5. What actions or motions bring on the pain? Is it worse in the morning, during activity, after activity, or at night? Does it wake you up at night? In what part of the arm motion does it hurt the worst? Does the arm tire easily? When the pain sets in, how long does it last?

6. Are there certain activities you are unable to perform because of the pain? Which ones?

7. What has been done for the condition?

PAST INJURY STATUS

1. Have you ever injured your shoulder before? How did that occur? What was done for the injury? Did you have any difficulty returning to your full functional status?

2. Have you had any medical problems recently? (Look for problems that may refer pain to the area.) Are you on any medication?

traction, and retraction; and 2) glenohumeral flexion, extension, abduction, adduction, internal and external rotation, and horizontal adduction and abduction. Watch the arms from an anterior and posterior view. As you stand behind the individual, make sure the scapula and humerus move together in a freely coordinated motion. Move the unaffected arm first to determine what is normal motion.

After the athlete completes these active motions, each can be resisted to test muscular strength. Begin with the muscle on stretch, and apply resistance throughout the full range of motion. Note any lag, muscle weakness, or painful arc. **Figure 8-21** demonstrates scapular motions to be tested, and **Figure 8-22** demonstrates glenohumeral motions at the shoulder to be tested.

STRESS TESTS

At this point in the assessment, the history, observation, palpation, and range of motion tests should have established a strong suspicion of what structures might be damaged. Perform only those stress tests that are absolutely necessary. If pain increases or function is impaired, immobilize the arm in a sling and refer the individual to a physician.

Drop Arm Test

To test the integrity of the supraspinatus muscle and tendon, the shoulder is abducted to 90° with no humeral rotation. Ask the athlete to slowly lower the arm to the side. If positive, the arm does not lower smoothly, or increased pain occurs during the motion. An alternative test is to abduct the arm again at 90° with no rotation, and ask the individual to hold that position. Apply downward resistance to the distal end of the humerus **(Fig. 8-23A)**. A positive test is indicated if the individual is unable to maintain the arm in the abducted position.

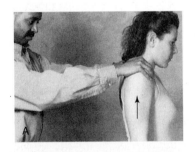
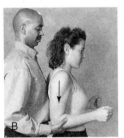
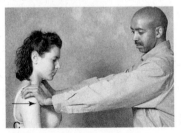
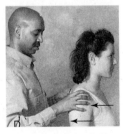

➤ **FIGURE 8-21.** Manual muscle testing for the scapula. **A.** Elevation. **B.** Depression. **C.** Protraction. **D.** Retraction. *Arrows* indicate the direction the athlete moves the scapula against applied resistance.

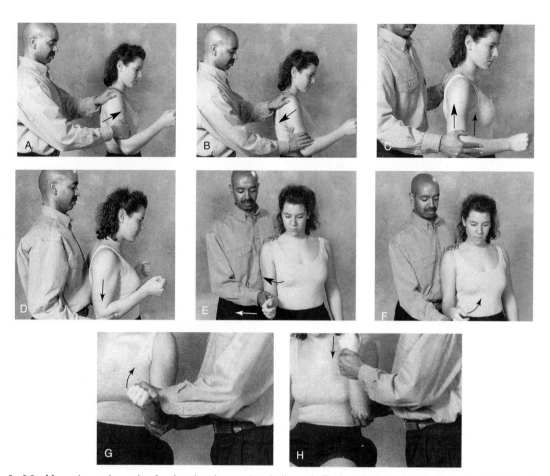

➤ **FIGURE 8-22.** Manual muscle testing for the glenohumeral and elbow. **A.** Flexion. **B.** Extension. **C.** Abduction. **D.** Adduction. **E.** External or lateral rotation. **F.** Internal or medial rotation. **G.** Elbow flexion. **H.** Elbow extension. *Arrows* indicate the direction the athlete moves against applied resistance.

Empty Can Test

Both arms are positioned at 90° of abduction. The arms are then horizontally adducted approximately 30 to 60°, and the humerus is internally rotated with the thumbs pointing downward ("empty can position") **(Fig. 8-23B)**. The coach applies downward pressure proximal to the elbow. Pain or weakness should be assessed. The arms should rebound to the 90° abducted position. A positive test indicates a tear to the supraspinatus muscle or tendon.

Acromioclavicular Distraction/Compression

If the AC joint is unstable, downward traction on the arm leads to downward movement of the acromion process away from the clavicle. Grasp the arm in one hand, and apply steady downward traction while palpating the joint with the other hand **(Fig. 8-24)**. A positive test produces pain or joint movement. Horizontal adduction of the humerus across the chest compresses the AC joint and leads to increased pain if the joint is injured.

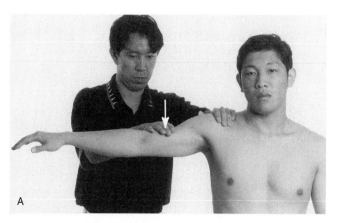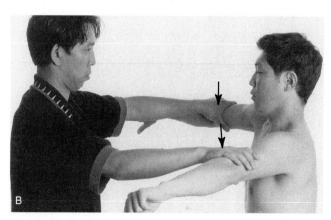

➤ **FIGURE 8-23.** Supraspinatus testing. **A.** Drop-arm test. Abduct the humerus to 90°. Apply mild downward pressure on the distal humerus. **B.** Empty can test. Horizontally adduct the arm approximately 30 to 60° with the humerus internally rotated. Apply mild downward pressure on the distal humerus.

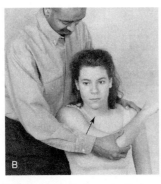

➤ **FIGURE 8-24.** Acromioclavicular testing. **A.** Acromioclavicular traction. **B.** Acromioclavicular compression. *Arrows* indicate the direction the examiner moves the arm.

Apprehension Test for Anterior Shoulder Dislocation

Slowly abduct and externally rotate the individual's humerus **(Fig. 8-25)**. If the individual does not allow passive movement to the extremes of motion, or if apprehension or alarm is shown in the facial expression, the test is positive. This motion should always be done slowly to prevent recurrence of a dislocation.

FUNCTIONAL TESTS

Occasionally, functional movements are the only activities that reproduce the signs and symptoms. Throwing a ball, performing a swimming stroke, or doing an overhead serve or spike may replicate the painful pattern. These movements are also commonly used to determine when the individual can return to sport participation. All functional patterns should be fluid and free of pain.

Summary

1. The shoulder complex does not function in an isolated fashion; rather, a series of joints work together in coordination to allow complicated patterns of motion. Because of this, injury to one structure can affect other structures.
2. A moderate sternoclavicular sprain is characterized by pain and swelling over the joint and an inability to horizontally adduct the arm without increased pain. The arm is typically held forward and close to the body.
3. A moderate acromioclavicular sprain is characterized by an elevated distal clavicle, indicating that the coracoclavicular ligament and the AC ligaments have been torn. The individual typically has a depressed or drooping shoulder.
4. Anterior glenohumeral dislocations are more common than posterior dislocations. The injured arm is often held in slight abduction and external rotation and is stabilized against the body.
5. Impingement syndromes involve an actual abutment of the supraspinatus tendon and subacromial bursa

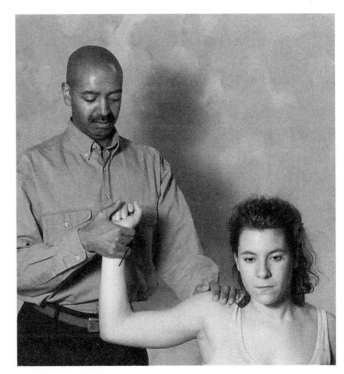

➤ **FIGURE 8-25.** To perform the apprehension test, gently abduct and externally rotate the individual's humerus (indicated by the arrow.

under the coracoacromial ligament and acromion process. The glenoid labrum and long head of the biceps brachii may also be injured.

6. The surgical neck is the most common site for proximal humeral fractures in adults. Adolescents, however, have a high degree of proximal humeral epiphyseal fractures because of repetitive medial rotation and adduction traction forces placed on the shoulder during pitching motions. Adolescents with a suspected epiphyseal fracture should be referred immediately to a physician.
7. If the individual is referred to a physician, remove the individual from activity and immobilize the limb in a sling, swathe, or another commercial product that adequately pads and supports the limb. Apply cryotherapy to reduce inflammation and swelling, and transport the individual appropriately.

References

1. Irrgang JJ, Witney SL, and Harner CD. 1992. Nonoperative treatment of rotator cuff injuries in throwing athletes. J Spt Rehab, 1(3):197-222.
2. Fleisig GS, Escamilla RF, and Andrews JR. Biomechanics of throwing. In *Athletic injuries and rehabilitation*, edited by JE Zachazewski, DJ Magee, and WS Quillen. Philadelphia: WB Saunders, 1996.
3. Magee DJ, and Reid DC. Shoulder injuries. In *Athletic injuries and rehabilitation*, edited by JE Zachazewski, DJ Magee, and WS Quillen. Philadelphia: WB Saunders, 1996.
4. Warren RF. Surgical considerations for rotator cuff tears in athletes. In *Shoulder surgery in the athlete*, edited by DW Jackson. Rockville: Aspen Systems, 1985.

Elbow, Wrist, and Hand Conditions

OBJECTIVES

1. Locate the important bony and soft-tissue structures in the elbow, wrist, and hand.

2. Demonstrate the motions at the elbow, wrist, thumb, and fingers.

3. Describe measures used to prevent injuries to the elbow, wrist, and hand.

4. Recognize and manage joint sprains to the elbow, wrist, and hand.

5. Identify signs and symptoms of medial and lateral epicondylitis.

6. Identify signs and symptoms of carpal tunnel syndrome and ulnar nerve entrapment.

7. Describe tendon injuries to the fingers.

8. Explain how to assess and manage a possible fracture of the elbow, wrist, and hand.

9. Explain how to complete a basic assessment of the elbow, wrist, and hand.

The arms perform lifting and carrying tasks, cushion the body during collisions, and lessen body momentum during falls. Acute injuries to the elbow, wrist, and hand often result from the natural tendency to sustain the force of a fall on the hyperextended wrist, which can sprain or dislocate the wrist or elbow (**Fig. 9-1**). Performance in many sports is also contingent on the ability of the arms to effectively swing a racquet or club, or to position the hands for throwing and catching a ball. This can lead to overuse injuries, such as medial or lateral **epicondylitis**. In addition, sports such as wrestling, football, hockey, and skiing place undue stress on the thumb and fingers, leading to finger sprains and strains.

This chapter begins with a review of the anatomy of the elbow, wrist, and hand. Common signs and symptoms of sprains, strains, overuse injuries, nerve entrapment

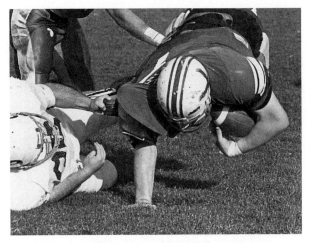

➤ FIGURE 9-1. Mechanism of injury. Falling on an out-stretched arm can lead to serious injury at the elbow, wrist, or hand.

syndromes, and fractures to the region, as well as their management, are then discussed. Finally, a basic assessment of the region is presented.

ANATOMY REVIEW OF THE ELBOW, WRIST, AND HAND

Although the elbow may be generally thought of as a simple hinge joint, the elbow actually encompasses three articulations—the humeroulnar, humeroradial, and proximal radioulnar joints. The bony structure of the elbow and forearm are displayed in **Figure 9-2**.

Elbow Joints

The largest joint at the elbow, the humeroulnar joint, is a hinge joint with motion capabilities of primarily flexion and extension. In some individuals, particularly women, a small amount of overextension (5 to 15°) is allowed. The humeroradial joint is a gliding joint, with motion restricted to the sagittal plane by the adjacent humeroulnar joint. The annular ligament binds the proximal head of the radius to the radial notch of the ulna forming the proximal radioulnar joint. This is a pivot joint with forearm pronation and supination occurring as the radius rolls medially and laterally over the ulna. Several strong ligaments, primarily the ulnar (medial) and radial (lateral) collateral ligaments, bind the three articulations together and a single joint capsule surrounds all three joints **(Fig. 9-3)**. The two collateral ligaments are strong and fan-shaped.

Wrist Articulations

The wrist consists of a series of radiocarpal and intercarpal articulations **(Fig. 9-4)**. Most wrist motion, however, occurs at the radiocarpal joint, a condyloid joint where the radius articulates with the scaphoid, lunate,

and triquetrum. The joint allows sagittal plane motion (flexion, extension, and hyperextension) and frontal plane motion (radial deviation and ulnar deviation), as well as **circumduction (Fig. 9-5)**.

Hand Articulations

In the hand, several joints are required to provide the extensive motion capabilities needed for sports participation. Included are the carpometacarpal (CM), intermetacarpal (IM), metacarpophalangeal (MCP), and interphalangeal (IP) joints. The fingers are numbered digits one through five, with the first digit being the thumb.

CARPOMETACARPAL AND INTERMETACARPAL JOINTS

The CM joint of the thumb is a classic **saddle joint** that allows rotation along its long axis to perform flexion, extension, abduction, adduction, and opposition. The CM joints of the four fingers are essentially gliding joints. The CM and IM joints of the fingers are mutually surrounded by joint capsules that are reinforced by the dorsal, volar, and interosseous CM ligaments.

METACARPOPHALANGEAL JOINTS

The knuckles of the hand are formed by the MCP joints, which are each enclosed in a capsule that is reinforced by strong collateral ligaments. The MCP joints of the fingers allow flexion, extension, abduction, adduction, and circumduction **(Fig. 9-6)**. Among the fingers, abduction is defined as movement away from the middle finger, and adduction is movement toward the middle finger. The MCP joint of the thumb functions more as a hinge joint, and the primary movements are flexion and extension.

INTERPHALANGEAL JOINTS

The proximal interphalangeal (PIP) and distal interphalangeal (DIP) joints of the fingers, and the single IP joint of the thumb, are all hinge joints. An articular capsule joined by volar and collateral ligaments surround each IP joint. The IP joints permit flexion, extension, and, in some individuals, slight hyperextension.

Muscles

A number of muscles cross the elbow, including several that also cross the shoulder or extend down into the hand and fingers. The elbow flexors include those muscles crossing the anterior side of the joint and include the brachialis, biceps brachii, and brachioradialis (see **Fig. 8-6**). The triceps, the major elbow extensor, is assisted by the small anconeus (see **Fig. 8-3**). Pronation and supination of the forearm occur when the radius rotates around the ulna. The pronator quadratus, the primary pronator muscle, is assisted by the pronator teres **(Fig. 9-7)**. As the

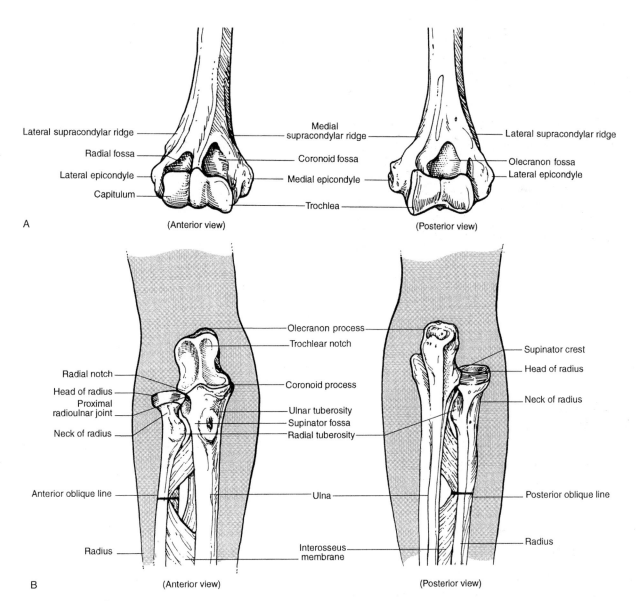

Lateral supracondylar ridge
Radial fossa
Lateral epicondyle
Capitulum

Medial supracondylar ridge
Coronoid fossa
Medial epicondyle
Trochlea

Lateral supracondylar ridge
Olecranon fossa
Lateral epicondyle

A (Anterior view) (Posterior view)

Radial notch
Head of radius
Proximal radioulnar joint
Neck of radius

Olecranon process
Trochlear notch
Coronoid process
Ulnar tuberosity
Supinator fossa
Radial tuberosity

Supinator crest
Head of radius
Neck of radius

Anterior oblique line

Ulna

Posterior oblique line

Radius

Interosseus membrane

Radius

B (Anterior view) (Posterior view)

➤ **FIGURE 9-2.** The bony structure of the right arm and forearm. **A.** Humerus. **B.** Ulna and radius.

name suggests, the supinator is the muscle primarily responsible for supination **(Fig. 9-7)**. During resistance or elbow flexion, the biceps brachii also participates in supination.

Considering the several highly controlled precision movements that the hand and fingers are capable of doing, it is no surprise that a relatively large number of muscles are responsible. The major wrist flexor muscles are the flexor carpi radialis and flexor carpi ulnaris **(Fig. 9-7)**. The palmaris longus, which is often absent in one or both forearms, contributes to flexion when present. Extensor carpi radialis longus, extensor carpi radialis brevis, and extensor carpi ulnaris produce extension and hyperextension at the wrist **(Fig. 9-8)**. The flexor and extensor muscles of the wrist cooperatively develop tension to produce radial and ulnar deviation of the hand at the wrist. The flexor carpi radialis and extensor carpi radialis act to produce radial deviation, and the flexor carpi ulnaris and extensor carpi ulnaris cause ulnar deviation.

Nerves and Blood Vessels to the Elbow, Wrist, and Hand

The major nerves of the elbow region (median, ulnar, and radial) descend from the brachial plexus and extend into the forearm and hand. **(Fig. 9-9A)**. The major arteries of the elbow and forearm region are the brachial, ulnar, and radial arteries **(Fig. 9-9B)**. The brachial artery supplies blood to the elbow joint and the flexor muscles of the arm and can be easily palpated in the anterior elbow. Distal to the elbow, the brachial artery splits into the ulnar and radial arteries to supply the medial forearm and lateral forearm, respectively. Pulses can be taken for both arteries on the anterior aspect of the wrist.

PREVENTION OF INJURIES

The very nature of many contact and collision sports places the wrist and hand in an extremely vulnerable

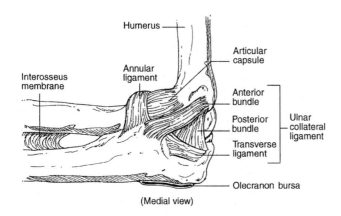

(Medial view)

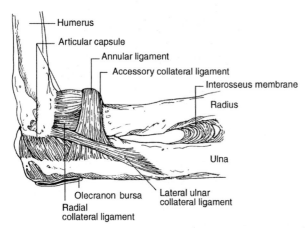

➤ FIGURE 9-3. The major ligaments and olecranon bursa of the left elbow.

position for injury. The elbow, wrist, and hand are often subjected to compressive forces. The hand, in particular, is usually the first point of contact to cushion the body during collisions, to deflect flying objects, or to lessen body impact during a fall. Falling on an outstretched hand is the leading cause of fractures and dislocations at the distal forearm, wrist, and hand.

Protective Equipment

Although hockey and lacrosse do have specific pads to protect the upper arm, elbow, and forearm, most sports do not require any protection for the elbow region. Goalies, baseball and softball catchers, and field players in many sports, such as hockey and lacrosse, are required to wear wrist and hand protection. The padded gloves prevent direct compression from a stick, puck, or ball. Several other gloves have extra padding on high-impact areas, aid in gripping, and protect the hand from abrasions, particularly when playing on artificial turf or on a baseball or softball field.

Physical Conditioning

Many of the muscles that move the elbow also move the shoulder or wrist. Therefore, flexibility and strength exer-

cises must focus on the entire arm. Exercises illustrated in **Field Strategy 9-1** improve general strength at the elbow and wrist and can be combined with strengthening exercises for the shoulder complex (see Chapter 8). Other exercises, such as squeezing a tennis ball or a spring-loaded grip device, can be used to strengthen the finger flexors. Begin with light resistance and progress to a heavier resistance.

Proper Technique

Nearly all overuse injuries at the elbow are directly related to repetitive throwing-type motions that produce microtraumatic tensile forces on the surrounding soft-tissue structures. Children who pitch sidearm motions are three times more likely to develop elbow problems than those who use a more overhand technique.[1] Movement analysis can detect improper technique in the acceleration and follow-through phase that contribute to these excessive tensile forces. Another preventative measure, already discussed in Chapter 8, is teaching sport participants the shoulder roll method of falling to avoid falling on an extended hand or flexed elbow. Failure to roll during falling can lead to excessive compressive forces, which can be transmitted along the long axis of the bones and lead to a fracture or dislocation.

SOFT-TISSUE INJURIES

Direct blows to the arm, forearm, and hand are frequently associated with contact and collision sports. Many are managed with standard acute care protocol.

Contusions

Contusions occur most commonly at the bony prominences. Direct compressive forces are the major mechanism of injury.

SIGNS AND SYMPTOMS

Bruising in the soft tissues can lead to internal hemorrhage, rapid swelling, and hematoma formation that can limit range of motion. Direct impact to the dorsum of the hand can produce a soft, painful, bluish-colored contusion.

MANAGEMENT

Although many are minor, always be cautious of an underlying fracture. Initial treatment for contusions involves ice, compression, elevation, and rest, followed by nonsteroidal anti-inflammatory drugs (NSAIDs) and gentle, pain-free exercise. Aggressive stretching and strengthening exercises should be avoided so as not to further injure muscle tissue. If conservative measures do not alleviate the condition, encourage the individual to see a physician.

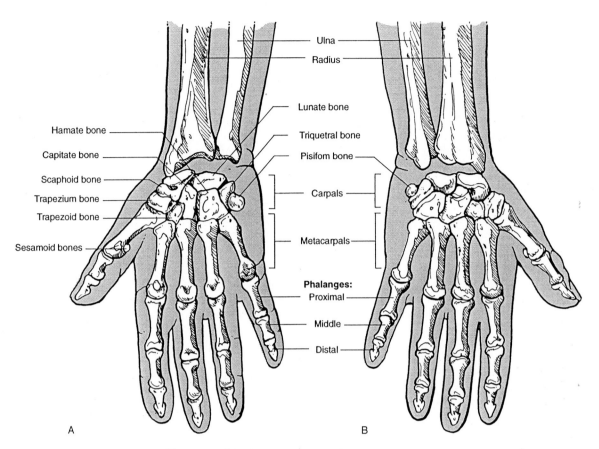

Ulna
Radius
Lunate bone
Hamate bone
Capitate bone
Triquetral bone
Scaphoid bone
Pisifom bone
Trapezium bone
Trapezoid bone
Carpals
Sesamoid bones
Metacarpals
Phalanges:
Proximal
Middle
Distal

A

B

➤ **F I G U R E 9 - 4 .** The bones of the forearm, wrist, and hand. **A.** Anterior view. **B.** Posterior view.

Acute and Chronic Bursitis

A special soft-tissue injury at the elbow is olecranon bursitis. The olecranon bursa is the largest bursa in the elbow region **(Fig. 9-3)**. Injury may occur by falling on a flexed elbow, by constantly leaning on one's elbow ("student's elbow"), by repetitive pressure and friction (as is common in wrestling), or by infections.

SIGNS AND SYMPTOMS

The acutely inflamed bursa presents with rapid swelling, although it may be relatively painless **(Fig. 9-10)**. The swelling may stem from bleeding or seepage of fluid into the bursal sac. Depending on the degree of acute inflammation, heat and redness may occur associated with the swelling.

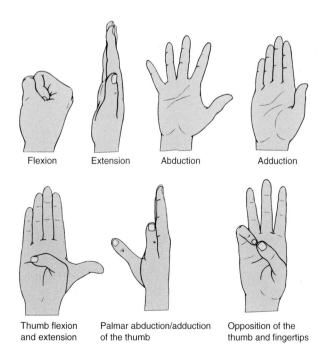

Flexion   Extension   Abduction   Adduction

Thumb flexion   Palmar abduction/adduction   Opposition of the
and extension   of the thumb   thumb and fingertips

➤ **F I G U R E 9 - 6 .** Directional movement capabilities at the fingers and thumb.

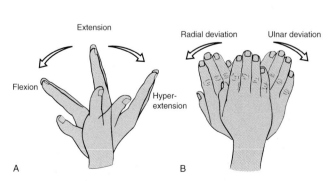

Extension
Radial deviation   Ulnar deviation
Flexion
Hyper-extension

A   B

➤ **F I G U R E 9 - 5 .** Directional movement capabilities at the wrist. **A.** Sagittal plane movements. **B.** Frontal plane movements.

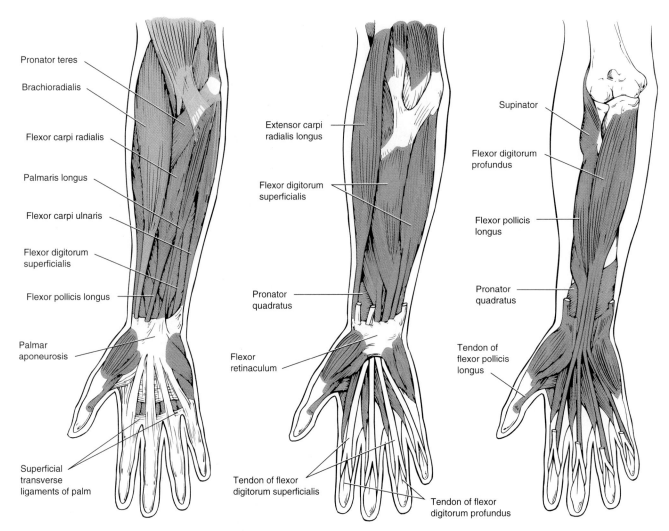

Pronator teres

Brachioradialis

Flexor carpi radialis

Palmaris longus

Flexor carpi ulnaris

Flexor digitorum superficialis

Flexor pollicis longus

Palmar aponeurosis

Superficial transverse ligaments of palm

Extensor carpi radialis longus

Flexor digitorum superficialis

Pronator quadratus

Flexor retinaculum

Tendon of flexor digitorum superficialis

Supinator

Flexor digitorum profundus

Flexor pollicis longus

Pronator quadratus

Tendon of flexor pollicis longus

Tendon of flexor digitorum profundus

➤ **FIGURE 9-7.** The anterior muscles of the forearm, wrist, and hand.

MANAGEMENT

Acute management involves ice, rest, and a compressive wrap applied for the first 24 hours. Significant distention may necessitate aspiration by a physician, followed by a compressive dressing for several days. Chronic bursitis is managed with cryotherapy, NSAIDs, and use of elbow cushions to protect the area from further insult.

Infected Bursitis

Occasionally, the bursa can become infected, regardless of acute trauma to the area. This may result from skin breakdown and a poor blood supply to the area.

SIGNS AND SYMPTOMS

The area is hot to the touch and inflamed. The individual shows traditional signs of infection, including **malaise** (feeling lousy), fever, pain, restricted motion, tenderness, and swelling at the elbow.

MANAGEMENT

An athlete with an infected bursa should be referred to a physician. The physician usually aspirates the bursa and

takes a culture of the fluid to determine the presence of septic bursitis.

Ganglion Cysts

Ganglion cysts are benign tumor masses commonly seen on the dorsal aspect of the wrist. Associated with tissue sheath degeneration, the dorsal cyst contains a jellylike, colorless fluid called mucin and is freely mobile and palpable between the extensor tendons.

SIGNS AND SYMPTOMS

These cysts occur spontaneously. Localized tenderness and maximal aggravation of pain during wrist flexion may occur.

MANAGEMENT

Although these injuries are usually self-limiting, the individual should see a physician if motion is inhibited and painful.

Subungual Hematoma

Direct trauma to the nail bed can result in blood forming under the fingernail—this is called a **subungual hematoma**.

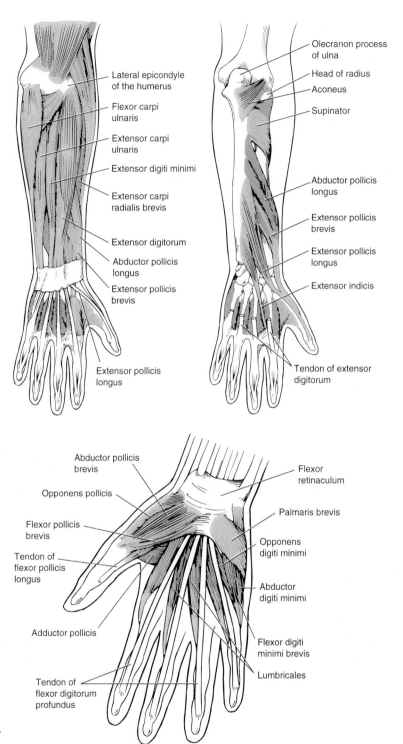

➤ FIGURE 9-8. The posterior muscles of the forearm, wrist, and hand.

SIGNS AND SYMPTOMS
A pocket of blood appears under the fingernail. Increasing pressure from the bleeding can lead to a throbbing, aching pain.

MANAGEMENT
After determining the possibility of an underlying fracture, soak the finger in ice water for 10 to 15 minutes to numb the area and reduce bleeding under the nail bed.

If the discomfort is so great as to prevent the athlete from continuing his or her participation, the individual should immediately see a physician to relieve the pressure under the nail.

SPRAINS AND DISLOCATIONS

Most common ligament tears in the elbow result from repetitive tensile forces that irritate and tear the ligaments, particularly the ulnar collateral ligament. Traumatic elbow

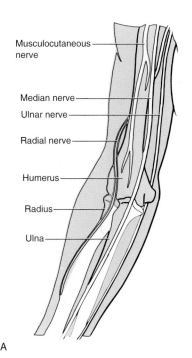

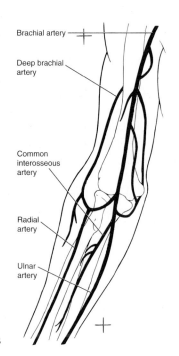

➤ FIGURE 9-9. Nerves and blood vessels of the elbow and forearm. The major nerves at the elbow are the median, ulnar, and radial nerves **A**. The brachial artery crosses the elbow at the cubital fossa and becomes the radial and ulnar arteries at the wrist **B**.

sprains are usually caused by hyperextension or a sudden, violent, unidirectional valgus force that drives the ulna in a posterior or posterolateral direction. In the wrist and hand, hyperextension is also the leading mechanism of injury, although hyperflexion or rotation may also lead to injury. When caused by a single episode, the severity of the injury depends on characteristics of the injury force (its point of application, magnitude, rate, and direction); position of the hand or elbow at impact; and relative strength of the bones and supporting ligaments.

Unfortunately, most individuals do not allow ample time for healing because they need to perform simple daily activities. Consequently, many sprains are neglected, leading to chronic instability.

Elbow Sprain

Repetitive tensile forces irritate and tear the ligaments, particularly the ulnar collateral ligament. When this occurs, pain can be palpated directly over the involved ligament. When forces are excessive, the resulting injury may be an elbow dislocation.

SIGNS AND SYMPTOMS

If the ulnar collateral ligament is injured, a history of pain localized on the medial aspect of the elbow during the late cocking and acceleration phases of throwing is common. Point tenderness can be palpated directly over the ligament and increases with a valgus stress test. If the radial collateral ligament is injured, pain is localized on the lateral aspect of the elbow and increases with a varus stress test.

MANAGEMENT

Ice, compression, NSAIDs, and rest are followed by early, protected range of motion exercises and strengthening exercises.

Elbow Dislocation

The mechanism of injury for an elbow dislocation is usually hyperextension, or a sudden, violent, unidirectional valgus force that drives the ulna posterior or posterolateral.

SIGNS AND SYMPTOMS

Immediately on impact, a snapping or cracking sensation is followed by severe pain, rapid swelling, total loss of function, and an obvious deformity **(Fig. 9-11)**. The ulnar collateral ligament is usually ruptured, and there may be an associated joint fracture. The arm is frequently held in flexion, with the forearm appearing shortened. The olecranon and radial head are palpable posteriorly and a slight indentation in the triceps is visible just proximal to the olecranon. Damage to the ulnar nerve may lead to numbness in the little finger.

MANAGEMENT

Immediate immobilization in a sling or vacuum splint and transportation to the nearest medical facility is warranted because early reduction minimizes muscle spasm. Management of an elbow dislocation is discussed in **Field Strategy 9-2**.

FIELD STRATEGY 9.1   EXERCISES TO PREVENT INJURY TO THE ELBOW REGION

Begin all exercises with light resistance using dumbbells or surgical tubing.

A. **Biceps curl.** Support the involved arm on the leg and fully flex the elbow. This can also be performed bilaterally in a standing position with a barbell.

B. **Triceps curl.** Raise the involved arm over the head. Extend the involved arm at the elbow. This can also be performed bilaterally in a supine or standing position with a barbell.

C. **Wrist flexion.** Support the involved forearm on a table or your leg with the hand off the edge. With the palm facing up, slowly do a full wrist curl and return to the starting position. Repeat.

D. **Wrist extension.** Support the involved forearm on a table or your leg with the hand off the edge. With the palm facing down, slowly do a full reverse wrist curl and return to the starting position. Repeat.

E. **Forearm pronation/supination.** Support the involved forearm on a table or your leg with the hand over the edge. With surgical tubing or a hand dumbbell, roll the forearm into pronation, then return to supination. Adjust the surgical tubing and reverse the exercise, stressing the supinators. Be sure the elbow remains stationary.

F. **Ulnar/radial deviation.** Support the involved forearm on a table or your leg with the hand over the edge. With surgical tubing or a hand dumbbell, perform ulnar deviation. Reverse directions and perform radial deviation. An alternate method is to stand with the arm at the side holding a hammer or weighted bar. Raise the wrist in ulnar deviation. Repeat in radial deviation.

G. **Wrist curl-ups.** To exercise the wrist extensors, grip the bar with both palms facing down. Slowly wind the cord onto the bar until the weight reaches the top, then slowly unwind the cord. Reverse hand position to work the wrist flexors.

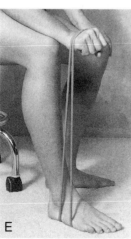
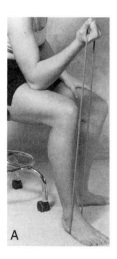
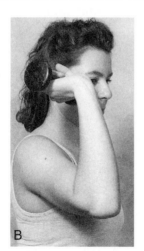
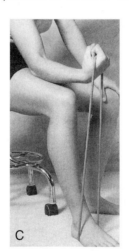
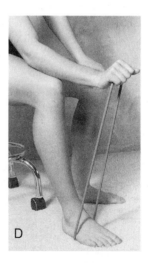
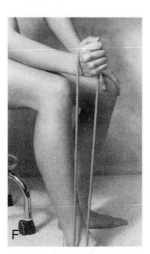
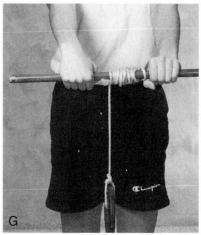

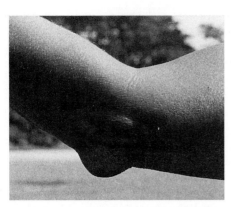

➤ FIGURE 9-10. Olecranon bursitis. When the olecranon bursa ruptures, a discrete, sharply demarcated goose egg is visible directly over the olecranon process.

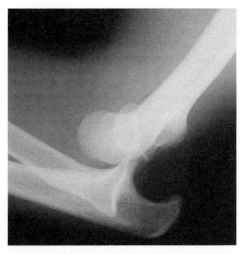

➤ FIGURE 9-11. Elbow dislocation. Posterior dislocations produce a snapping or cracking sensation followed by immediate severe pain, rapid swelling, and total loss of function.

Radial Head Dislocation

In adolescents, subluxation or dislocation of the proximal radial head is often associated with an immature annular ligament. Distraction with rotation, such as when a young child is swung by the arms, can cause the radial head to slip out of the supporting annular ligament.

SIGNS AND SYMPTOMS

Palpation of the radial head causes pain and discomfort that increases with passive pronation and supination of the forearm.

MANAGEMENT

Immobilize the joint, apply ice to reduce any swelling, and refer the individual immediately to a physician.

Wrist Sprain

Axial loading on the proximal palm during a fall on an outstretched hand is the leading cause of wrist sprains (see **Fig. 9-1**). This injury is often neglected, leading to chronic wrist pain.

SIGNS AND SYMPTOMS

Assessment reveals point tenderness on the dorsum of the radiocarpal joint. Pain increases with active or passive extension. Because of the shape of the lunate and its position between the large capitate and lower end of the radius, this carpal bone is particularly prone to dislocation during axial loading **(Fig. 9-12)**. The dorsum of the hand is point tender, and a thickened area on the palm can be palpated just distal to the end of the radius if not obscured by swelling. Passive and active motion may not be painful. If the bone moves into the carpal tunnel, compression of the median nerve leads to pain, numbness, and tingling in the first and second fingers.

MANAGEMENT

Ice, compression, NSAIDs, and rest are followed by early, progressive strengthening exercises for the wrist flexors.

Thumb and Finger Sprains

Sprains of the thumb and fingers are common. The thumb is exposed to more force than the fingers because of its position on the hand. Integrity of the ulnar collateral ligament at the MCP joint is critical for normal hand function because it stabilizes the joint as the thumb is pushed against the index and middle fingers while performing many pinching, grasping, and gripping motions.

GAMEKEEPER'S THUMB

Gamekeeper's thumb occurs when the MCP joint is near full extension and the thumb is forcefully abducted away from the hand, tearing the ulnar collateral ligament at the MCP joint **(Fig. 9-13)**.

SIGNS AND SYMPTOMS

The palmar aspect of the joint is painful, swollen, and may have visible bruising. Instability is detected by replicating the mechanism of injury or by stressing the thumb in flexion.

MANAGEMENT

Initial treatment includes ice, compression, elevation, and referral to a physician for further care. With no instability, treatment involves early range of motion exercises and NSAIDs. Strapping or taping the thumb can prevent reinjury. If joint instability is present, a thumb spica cast may be applied for 3 to 6 weeks. If the ligament has ruptured, however, it may not heal with rest and immobilization and may require surgery to repair the damage.

FIELD STRATEGY 9.2 — MANAGEMENT OF A POSTERIOR ELBOW DISLOCATION

1. This injury should be regarded as an emergency! Activate EMS.

2. Apply ice immediately to reduce swelling and inflammation.

3. To rule out circulatory impairment, assess:
   • Radial pulse
   • Skin color
   • Blanching of the nails

4. To rule out nerve impairment, assess motor and sensory function:
   • Have the athlete (if able) flex, extend, abduct, and adduct the fingers.
   • With the athlete looking away, stroke the palm and dorsum of the hand in several different locations with a blunt and sharp object. Ask the individual to identify where you are touching and whether it is sharp or dull.

5. Immobilize the area with a vacuum splint or other appropriate splint.

6. Take vital signs, recheck pulse and sensory functions, and treat for shock.

7. Transport immediately to the nearest medical facility.

FINGER SPRAINS AND DISLOCATIONS

Excessive varus/valgus stress and hyperextension can damage the collateral ligaments of the fingers. Although many athletes and coaches call this injury a simple "jammed finger," this injury often involves an avulsion fracture from a tendon rupture, which requires immediate surgery to repair the damage. Hyperextension of the proximal phalanx can stretch or rupture the volar plate on the palmar side of the joint. As such, it is critical to refer this individual to a physician to rule out a more extensive injury.

SIGNS AND SYMPTOMS

A swollen, painful finger caused by a ball striking the extended finger is the most frequent initial report. An obvious deformity may not be present unless there is a fracture. The most common dislocation in the body occurs at the PIP joint **(Fig. 9-14)**. Pain is present at the joint line and increases when the mechanism of injury is reproduced. Because digital nerves and vessels run along the sides of the fingers and thumb, dislocations here can be potentially serious.

MANAGEMENT

Because of the probability of entrapping the volar plate in an IP joint, which can lead to permanent dysfunction of the finger, no attempt should be made to reduce a finger dislocation by an untrained individual. Immediate treatment for all dislocations involves immobilization in a finger splint, application of ice to reduce swelling and inflammation, and referral to a physician. The prognosis and rehabilitation program depend on the extent of tissue damage and instability.

STRAINS

Muscular strains commonly result from inadequate warm-up, excessive training past the point of fatigue, and inadequate rehabilitation of previous muscular injuries. Less commonly, they result from a single massive contraction or sudden overstretching.

➤ FIGURE 9-12. Lunate dislocation. The lunate can dislocate during a fall on an outstretched hand when the load from the radius compresses the lunate in a volar direction A. If the bone moves into the carpal tunnel, the median nerve can become compressed, leading to sensory changes in the first and second fingers B.

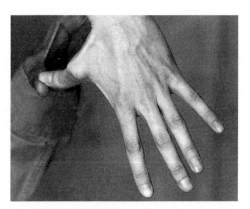

➤ FIGURE 9-13. Clinical appearance of a Gamekeeper's thumb.

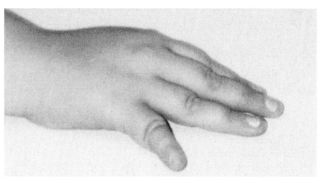

➤ FIGURE 9-14. Dislocation at the proximal interphalangeal joint.

Elbow Strains

SIGNS AND SYMPTOMS

Injury to the elbow flexors (brachialis, biceps brachii, and brachioradialis) will result in point tenderness on the anterior distal arm. Pain increases with resisted elbow flexion. With a triceps strain, resisted elbow extension produces discomfort. Strains to the common wrist flexor group result in pain on resisted wrist flexion, whereas strains to the wrist extensors produce pain with wrist extension.

MANAGEMENT

Most muscle strains are self-limiting, requiring only modified rest, ice, compression, and activity modification. Major tears or ruptures seldom occur. If they do, the athlete will have considerable ecchymosis, a palpable defect, and limited, weak motion.

Wrist and Finger Strains

In the hand, muscle strains involving the finger flexors or extensors tend to be more serious. These injuries may involve avulsing the tendon from the bone.

JERSEY FINGER

A "**jersey finger**" typically occurs when an individual grips an opponent's jersey while the opponent simultaneously twists and turns to get away. This jerking action may force the fingers to rapidly extend, rupturing the flexor digitorum profundus tendon from its attachment on the distal phalanx, hence the name "jersey finger." The ring finger is more commonly involved.

SIGNS AND SYMPTOMS

If avulsed, the tendon can be palpated at the proximal aspect of the involved finger. The individual is unable to flex the DIP joint against resistance.

MANAGEMENT

Treatment involves standard acute care with ice, compression, elevation, and protected rest. If a palpable defect is noted or an avulsion fracture is suspected, immobilization in a finger splint is followed by referral to a physician for possible surgical reattachment.

MALLET FINGER

Mallet finger occurs when an object hits the end of the finger while the extensor tendon is taut, such as when catching a ball. The resulting forceful flexion of the distal phalanx avulses the lateral bands of the extensor mechanism from its distal attachment.

SIGNS AND SYMPTOMS

If the common extensor tendon is avulsed, a characteristic mallet deformity is present **(Fig. 9-15)**, and the athlete is unable to fully extend the DIP joint with the forearm pronated.

MANAGEMENT

Treatment is the same as with a jersey finger.

OVERUSE CONDITIONS

The throwing mechanism can lead to significant overuse injuries at the elbow. During the initial acceleration phase, the body is brought rapidly forward, but the elbow and hand lag behind the upper arm. This results in a tremendous tensile valgus stress placed on the medial aspect of the elbow, particularly the ulnar collateral ligament and adjacent tissues. As acceleration continues, the elbow extensors and wrist flexors contract to add velocity to the throw. This whipping action produces significant valgus stress on the medial elbow and concomitant lateral compressive stress in the radiocapitellar joint **(Fig. 9-16)**. At ball release, the elbow is almost fully extended and is positioned slightly anterior to the trunk. At release, the elbow is flexed approximately 20 to 30°. As these forces

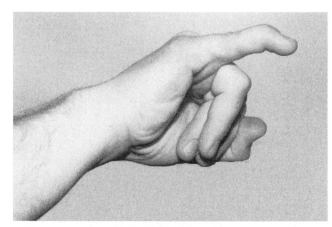

➤ FIGURE 9-15. Mallet finger. Mallet finger is caused when the extensor tendon is avulsed from the attachment on the distal phalanx. The tendon may also avulse a small piece of bone, leading to an avulsion fracture.

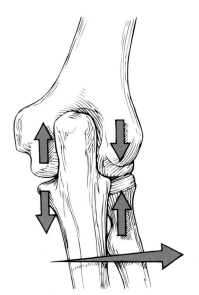

➤ FIGURE 9-16. Forces exerted on the elbow during the throwing motion. An excessive valgus force can lead to both medial tensile stress and lateral compression stress, causing injury to both sides of the joint.

decrease, however, the extreme pronation of the forearm places the lateral ligaments under tension. During deceleration, eccentric contractions of the long head of the biceps brachii, supinator, and extensor muscles decelerate the forearm in pronation. Additional stress occurs on structures around the olecranon as pronation and extension jam the olecranon into the olecranon fossa. Impingement can occur during this jamming.

Medial Epicondylitis

Epicondylitis is a common chronic condition in activities involving pronation and supination, such as tennis, javelin throwing, pitching, volleyball, or golf. Often, the individual reveals a pattern of poor technique, fatigue, and overuse. Medial epicondylitis, common in adolescent athletes, is caused by repeated medial tension/lateral compression (valgus) forces placed on the arm during the acceleration phase of the throwing motion. Valgus forces often produce a combined flexor muscle strain, ulnar collateral ligament sprain, and ulnar neuritis. If the medial humeral growth plate is affected, it may be called "**little league elbow.**" However, this term negates that other individuals, such as golfers, gymnasts, javelin throwers, tennis players, and wrestlers, are also susceptible to the condition. Simultaneously, lateral compressive forces can damage the lateral condyle of the humerus and radial head. Posterior stresses may lead to triceps strain, olecranon impingement, olecranon fractures, or loose bodies.

SIGNS AND SYMPTOMS

Assessment reveals swelling, ecchymosis, and point tenderness directly over the humeroulnar joint, or on the

> ➤ ➤ BOX 9-1
>
> ## Signs and Symptoms of Medial Epicondylitis
> - Swelling, ecchymosis, and point tenderness over the humeroulnar joint
> - Pain over the medial epicondyle, extending distally 1 to 2 cm along the track of the flexor carpi radialis and pronator teres
> - Increased pain with resisted wrist flexion and forearm pronation
> - Increased pain with valgus stress at 30° flexion

medial epicondyle **(Box 9-1)**. Pain is usually severe and aggravated by resisted wrist flexion and pronation and by a valgus stress. If the ulnar nerve is involved, tingling and numbness may radiate into the forearm and hand, particularly the fourth and fifth fingers.

MANAGEMENT

Most conditions are managed with ice, NSAIDs, and immobilization in a wrist splint for 2 to 3 weeks. Activity should not resume until the individual can complete all sport-specific skills without pain. **Field Strategy 9-3** describes the basic management of elbow pain resulting from overuse.

Lateral Epicondylitis

Lateral epicondylitis is the most common overuse injury in the adult elbow. The condition is typically caused by eccentric loading of the extensor muscles, predominantly the extensor carpi radialis brevis, during the deceleration phase of the throwing motion or tennis stroke. Gripping a racquet too tightly, improper grip size, excessive string tension, excessive racquet weight or stiffness, faulty backhand technique, putting top spin on backhand strokes, or hitting the ball off-center all contribute to this condition.

SIGNS AND SYMPTOMS

Pain is anterior or just distal to the lateral epicondyle and may radiate into the forearm extensors during and after activity **(Box 9-2)**. Pain increases with resisted wrist extension or in an action similar to picking up a full cup of coffee ("coffee cup" test).

MANAGEMENT
See **Field Strategy 9-3**.

Tendinitis and Stenosing Tenosynovitis

Individuals involved in strenuous and repetitive training often inflame tendons and tendon sheaths in the wrist and

> FIELD STRATEGY 9.3   MANAGEMENT OF ELBOW PAIN FROM OVERUSE

- Use ice, compression, elevation, NSAIDs, and rest to limit pain and inflammation.
- If an avulsion fracture of the medial epicondyle or apophyseal fracture is suspected in the adolescent, refer the individual to a physician.
- Avoid all activities that lead to pain; immobilization of wrist may be necessary if simple daily activities cause pain.
- Ice massage, contrast baths, and friction massage over the proximal tendons can supplement the treatment plan.
- Maintain range of motion and strength at the wrist and shoulder.
- Stretching exercises should be within pain-free motions, and include wrist flexion/extension, forearm pronation/supination, and radial and ulnar deviation.
- Begin with fast contractions using light resistance. Perform tennis ball squeezes and other strengthening exercises within pain-free ranges. Add surgical tubing as tolerated. Work up to 3 to 5 sets of 10 repetitions per session before moving on to heavier resistance.
- Incorporate early, closed-chain exercises such as press-ups, wall push-ups, or walking on the hands.
- Add strengthening exercises for all shoulder, elbow, and wrist motions.
- Do a biomechanical analysis of the throwing motion to determine proper technique, and make adjustments as necessary.
- After return to protected activity, continue stretching exercises before and after practice, and ice after practice to control any inflammation. Return to full activity as tolerated.

hand. In the wrist, the abductor pollicis longus and extensor pollicis brevis are commonly affected. These two tendons share a single synovial tendon sheath that turns sharply, as much as 105°, to enter the thumb when the wrist is in radial deviation **(Fig. 9-17)**. Friction between the tendons, the **stenosing** sheath, and bony process lead to a condition called "**de Quervain's tenosynovitis**."

SIGNS AND SYMPTOMS

Tendinitis in the wrist flexors or extensors leads to stiffness and an aching pain that is aggravated by activity. It may appear several hours after participation in sports. Pain is usually localized over the involved tendons and is aggravated with passive stretching and resisted motion of the affected tendons.

MANAGEMENT

Treatment involves ice, rest, and NSAIDs as prescribed by a physician.

> ➤ BOX 9-2

Signs and Symptoms of Lateral Epicondylitis

- Pain anterior or just distal to the lateral epicondyle that may radiate into the forearm extensors
- Pain that initially subsides but becomes more severe with repetition
- Pain that increases with resisted wrist extension
- Positive "coffee cup" test and tennis elbow test

NERVE ENTRAPMENT SYNDROMES

Neurovascular syndromes in the elbow, wrist, and hand are seen in several activities, including bowling, cycling, karate, rowing, baseball/softball, field hockey, lacrosse, rugby, weightlifting, and handball, and in wheelchair athletes. The two most common nerve entrapment conditions are carpal tunnel syndrome and ulnar entrapment.

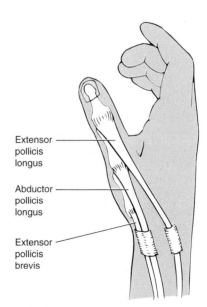

Extensor pollicis longus

Abductor pollicis longus

Extensor pollicis brevis

➤ FIGURE 9-17. Tenosynovitis. The abductor pollicis longus and extensor pollicis brevis share the same synovial sheath. Excessive friction among the tendons, sheath, and bony process lead to tenosynovitis of the tendons.

Carpal Tunnel Syndrome

Carpal tunnel syndrome is caused by direct trauma or repetitive overuse. The condition is three times more common in women and peaks between ages 30 and 50 years. The right hand is more affected than the left.[2] This higher incidence may be largely caused by occupational tasks that demand repetitive digital manipulations, such as typing or computer keyboard work. Sporting activities that predispose athletes to carpal tunnel syndrome include those that involve repetitive or continuous flexion and extension of the wrist, such as in cycling, throwing sports, racquet sports, archery, and gymnastics.

The carpal tunnel runs between the floor of the volar wrist capsule and the transverse retinacular ligament that courses from the hamate and pisiform on the lateral side to the trapezium and scaphoid on the medial side. This unyielding tunnel accommodates the median nerve, the finger flexors in a common sheath, and the flexor pollicis longus in an independent sheath **(Fig. 9-18)**. Therefore, any irritation of the synovial sheath covering these tendons can produce swelling or edema that can put pressure on the median nerve.

SIGNS AND SYMPTOMS

The individual reports that pain wakes him or her in the middle of the night and is often relieved by shaking the hands. Pain and numbness may be felt only in the fingertips on the palmar aspect of the thumb, index, and middle finger. Grip strength and pinch strength may be limited. Symptoms are reproduced when direct compression is applied over the carpal tunnel for about 30 seconds.

MANAGEMENT

Individuals with suspected carpal tunnel syndrome should be referred to a physician for care. Conservative care involves splinting, NSAIDs, and cessation of any activity that contributes to the nerve compression.

Ulnar Neuropathy at the Elbow

In the elbow, the ulnar nerve passes behind the medial epicondyle of the humerus via the ulnar groove, through the cubital tunnel, and underneath the ulnar collateral ligament to enter the forearm **(Fig. 9-19)**. Here the nerve is vulnerable to compression and tensile stress.

SIGNS AND SYMPTOMS

The individual reports sharp pain along the medial aspect of the elbow, radiating as if it was "hitting the crazy bone." Palpation in the ulnar groove generally reproduces symptoms that differentiate this injury from a strain or sprain. Tingling and numbness is typically felt in the ring and little finger. Because the ulnar nerve innervates several **intrinsic muscles** of the hand, grip strength may be weak.

MANAGEMENT

Treatment involves cessation of activities that contribute to the compression; rest; cryotherapy; and NSAIDs to minimize pain and inflammation. If symptoms do not rapidly improve, the individual should be encouraged to

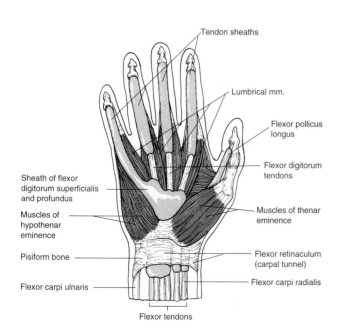

➤ **FIGURE 9-18.** Carpal tunnel. The flexor tendons of the fingers pass through the carpal tunnel in a single synovial sheath.

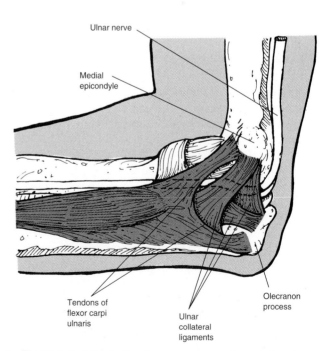

➤ **FIGURE 9-19.** As the ulnar nerve passes through the ulnar groove between the ulnar collateral ligament and the olecranon fossa, it passes under the two heads of the flexor carpi ulnaris. This tendon is slack during extension, but becomes taut during flexion, contributing to ulnar nerve compression.

see a physician because surgical decompression may be necessary to alleviate symptoms.

Ulnar Neuropathy at the Hand

The ulnar nerve can also become entrapped between the hook of the hamate and pisiform, which is frequently seen in cycling, racquet sports, and in baseball or softball catchers who experience repetitive trauma to the palm.

SIGNS AND SYMPTOMS

The individual has numbness in the ulnar nerve distribution, particularly the little finger, and may have a weakened grip strength and atrophy of muscles in the **hypothenar** mass. **Cyclist's palsy** occurs when a biker leans on the handlebar for an extended period, leading to temporary swelling in the hypothenar area that compresses the ulnar nerve. Symptoms mimic the more serious ulnar nerve entrapment syndrome, but they usually disappear rapidly after completion of the ride.

MANAGEMENT

Properly padding the handlebars, wearing padded gloves, varying hand position, and properly fitting the bike to the rider can greatly reduce the incidence of this condition. If symptoms do not rapidly improve, the individual should be encouraged to see a physician because surgical decompression may be necessary to alleviate symptoms.

FRACTURES

Displaced and undisplaced fractures to the humerus, radius, and ulna usually result from violent compressive forces from direct trauma, such as impact with a helmet or implement, axial loading from a fall on a flexed elbow or outstretched hand, with or without a valgus/varus stress, or tensile forces associated with throwing. Likewise, traumatic fractures of the wrist and hand occur during axial loading when falling on an outstretched hand or are caused by compressive forces when the hand or fingers are stepped on or impact a solid object.

Radial and Ulnar Fractures

Although the radius and ulna can be fractured anywhere along their length, two particular fractures to one or both distal bones can lead to serious complications. A **Colles fracture** occurs to the distal radius and ulna within 1½ inches of the wrist joint. The injury often results from falling on an outstretched hand with the wrist extended. The resulting deformity is characterized as a "silver fork" deformity when the distal fragments of the radius and ulna displace in a dorsal and radial direction relative to their proximal shafts **(Fig. 9-20A)**. A reverse of this frac-

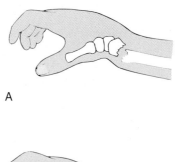

A

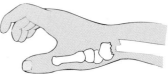

B

➤ **F I G U R E 9 - 2 0 .** Fractures of the forearm. Fractures may result in the wrist and hand angulating in a dorsal direction, called a Colles fracture **(A)**, or in a volar direction, called a Smith fracture **(B)**.

ture is a **Smith's fracture**, where the displacement of the distal radius and ulna moves in a volar direction **(Fig. 9-20B)**. The mechanism of injury is usually a fall onto the back of the hand, causing hyperflexion of the wrist.

SIGNS AND SYMPTOMS

Signs and symptoms of a possible fracture include immediate severe pain, deformity, loss of function, swelling, and ecchymosis. A catastrophic complication from a forearm fracture is a condition called **Volkmann's contracture**. This condition is caused by increased pressure and swelling inside one of the forearm compartments that compromise circulation to the surrounding muscles and nerves. As the pressure builds unabated, **ischemic necrosis** can lead to permanent loss of nerve and muscular function. As a result, the hand is cold, white, and numb. Passive extension of the fingers leads to severe pain. These symptoms indicate a serious problem.

MANAGEMENT

Fractures should be suspected in all forearm injuries, particularly in adolescents. Methods to determine a possible fracture in the forearm were demonstrated in **Figure 4-12**. A suspected fracture should be immobilized in a vacuum splint or other appropriate splint, and the individual should be referred to a physician immediately.

Carpal Fractures

Scaphoid fractures account for 60 to 70% of all carpal bone injuries in the general population and are the most common wrist bone fracture in the athlete.[3] The individual may fall on an extended wrist or have direct contact with the palm of the hand (i.e., during blocking), which

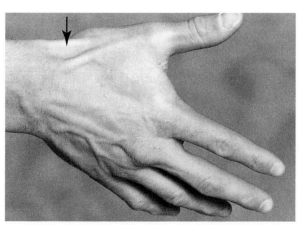

➤ FIGURE 9-21. Anatomic snuff box. The scaphoid forms the floor of the anatomic snuff box. It is bounded by the extensor pollicis brevis medially and the extensor pollicis longus laterally. Increased pain during palpation in this region indicates a possible fracture to the scaphoid bone.

compresses the scaphoid against the radius. Initial radiographs may be normal, and the athlete is discharged with a diagnosis of a wrist sprain without further care. Several months later, however, the individual continues to experience persistent wrist pain. Radiographs at this time may reveal an established nonunion fracture of the scaphoid.

SIGNS AND SYMPTOMS
Because of the high incidence of overlooking this fracture, it is critical to suspect a fracture if any pain is present in the "**anatomic snuff box**" **(Fig. 9-21)**, which lies directly over the scaphoid. Pain may also be present with inward pressure along the long axis of the first metacarpal bone and increases with wrist extension and radial deviation. Because of a poor blood supply to the area, **aseptic necrosis** (death of tissue caused by poor blood supply) is a common complication of this fracture.

MANAGEMENT
Immediately immobilize the wrist in a wrist splint. Apply ice to reduce swelling, and refer the individual to a physician.

Metacarpal and Phalangeal Fractures

Striking an object with a closed fist can lead to excessive axial compressive forces that may fracture the neck, shaft, or base of the metacarpals. Axial compression can also lead to phalangeal fractures when an object impacts the tip of the finger. Fractures may also be caused by having the hand or fingers stepped on, having them impinged between two hard objects, or during hyperextension where the injury may occur in combination with a joint sprain, leading to a fracture-dislocation.

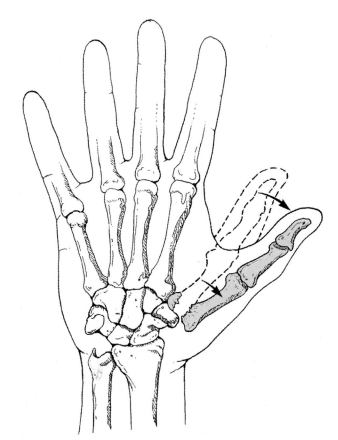

➤ FIGURE 9-22. Bennett's fracture. A Bennett's fracture is usually associated with a dislocation of the metacarpophalangeal joint of the thumb. An avulsion fracture, however, occurs when a segment of the metacarpal is held in place by the deep volar ligament.

SIGNS AND SYMPTOMS
Uncomplicated fractures to the metacarpals result in severe pain, dorsal swelling, and deformity. **Bennett's fracture** is a more serious articular fracture to the proximal end of the first metacarpal. During axial compression, such as when a punch is thrown with a closed fist, the abductor pollicis longus tendon pulls the metacarpal shaft proximally. A small medial fragment, however, is held in place by the deep volar ligament, leading to a fracture-dislocation **(Fig. 9-22)**. Pain and swelling are localized, but deformity may or may not be present. **Field Strategy 9-4** demonstrates how to determine a possible metacarpal fracture. These techniques can also detect possible fractures in the carpals and phalanges.

MANAGEMENT
Acute care of a metacarpal fracture involves ice, compression, and immobilization in a wrist splint with the palm face down and fingers slightly flexed over a gauze roll or a series of gauze pads. This position places the fingers in about 30° of finger flexion, which reduces the pull of the flexor tendons. Phalangeal fractures are immobilized with a finger splint. Apply ice to reduce swelling and pain, and refer the athlete to a physician. Most frac-

FIELD STRATEGY 9.4   DETERMINING A POSSIBLE FRACTURE TO A METACARPAL

1. Observe any deformity or loss of motion (unable to clench the fist or extend fingers).
2. Palpate for pain along the shaft of the bone.
3. Apply compression along the long axis of the bone **(Fig. A)**.
   • Positive sign occurs if pain is felt at the injury site.
4. Apply percussion or vibration at the end of the bone **(Fig. B)**.
   • Positive sign occurs if pain is felt at the injury site.
5. Apply distraction at the end of the bone **(Fig. C)**.
   • Positive sign occurs if pain is decreased. Increased pain may indicate a ligamentous injury.

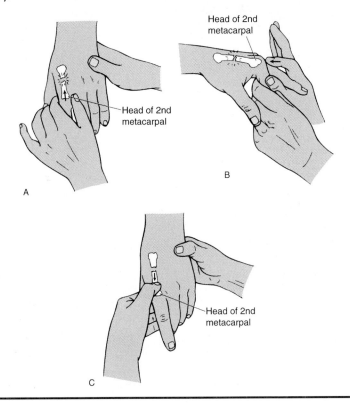

tures are easily managed with proper immobilization, followed by an early exercise program to prevent extension contractures.[3]

ASSESSMENT OF THE ELBOW, WRIST, AND HAND

The elbow's primary role is to position the forearm and hand in the most appropriate position to perform efficient motion. If the individual uses any equipment, such as a bat, racquet, or field hockey or lacrosse stick, check for proper grip size, excessive string tension, and excessive weight or stiffness. Assess skill technique to rule out possible contributing factors. During the evaluation, keep in mind that pain may be referred from the cervical region or shoulder. Although many injuries can be handled on site, any injury that impairs the function of the hand or fingers should be referred immediately to a physician for more extensive evaluation **(Box 9-3)**.

History

To gather information about the primary complaint, ask questions that focus on the individual's perception of pain, weakness, or sensory changes. When was the problem first noticed? Is the injury acute or chronic? Ask specific questions related to equipment, technique, recent changes in training intensity, frequency, or duration. Are there specific actions that aggravate the condition, such as throwing? Is the region subjected to repetitive trauma, such as from constant impact from a ball, racquet, bat, or stick? Is there any noticeable locking, catching, or general muscle weakness? Specific questions to ask during an elbow, wrist, and hand evaluation are listed in **Field Strategy 9-5**.

Observation and Inspection

Both arms should be clearly visible for bilateral comparison. With an acute injury, it is critical early in the assessment to recognize possible fractures and dislocations before moving the wrist or hand. If the individual is in great pain or is unable or unwilling to move the wrist or hand, perform the fracture tests demonstrated in **Figure 4-12** and in **Field Strategy 9-4.** If a fracture is suspected, treat accordingly. Immobilize the wrist and hand in a vacuum splint or wrist splint, apply ice to control pain and inflammation, and transport the individual to a physician.

If a fracture is not suspected but the individual is still in pain or is unable or unwilling to move the elbow, wrist, or hand, complete the assessment in a position most comfortable for the individual. First, observe the position of the arm. Is there a noticeable deformity? How is the individual holding the arm? If swelling is present in a joint, the individual may be unable to fully extend the joint, which results in a slightly flexed position. This resting position allows the joint to have maximal volume to accommodate intra-articular swelling. Inspect the region for symmetry, any abnormal deformity, muscle atrophy

or hypertrophy, and for obvious signs of abrasions, swelling, and discoloration. **Field Strategy 9-6** summarizes observations at the wrist and hand from a dorsal and palmar view.

Palpation

Begin palpation proximal to distal and leave the most painful areas for last. Support the injured arm during palpation and compare bilaterally. At the wrist and hand, begin on the dorsal aspect, then move to the palmar aspect. Bilateral palpation should determine temperature, swelling, point tenderness, crepitus, deformity, muscle spasm, and cutaneous sensation. Vascular pulses can be taken at the radial and ulnar arteries at the wrist (see **Fig. 9-9**). Circulation can also be assessed by blanching the fingernails. Squeeze the nail. Initially the nail should turn white, but color should return immediately upon release of pressure.

- Bony Palpation
  1. Medial and lateral supracondylar ridges and epicondyles of the humerus
  2. Head of the radius and annular ligament facilitated by supination and pronation of the forearm
  3. Olecranon process, olecranon fossa, and ulna (flex the elbow at 45° to relax the triceps)
  4. Radius and ulna
  5. Carpal bones and "anatomic snuffbox"
  6. Metacarpal bones and phalanges
- Soft-Tissue Palpation
  1. Common wrist flexor-pronator tendons and muscles
  2. Ulnar (medial) collateral ligament and ulnar nerve in the ulnar groove
  3. Common wrist extensors and brachioradialis muscle

FIELD STRATEGY 9.5   DEVELOPING A HISTORY OF THE INJURY

CURRENT INJURY STATUS

1. How did the injury occur (mechanism)? Was the region subjected to repetitive impact from a ball, bat, racquet, or stick?

2. Where is the pain (or weakness)? How severe is it? Is it worse in the morning, during activity, after activity, or at night? Does it wake you up at night? What type of pain is it (e.g., sharp, aching, burning, or radiating)?

3. Did the pain come on suddenly (acute) or gradually (overuse)? Was the pain greatest when the injury first occurred or did it get worse the second or third day?

4. Did you hear any sounds during the incident, such as snaps, pops, or cracks? Was there any swelling, discoloration, muscle spasm, or numbness with the injury?

5. Are there certain activities you are unable to perform because of the pain? What action or motions replicate the pain?

PAST INJURY STATUS

1. Have you ever injured this area before? When? How did that occur? What was done for the injury?

2. Have you had any medical problems recently? (You are looking for possible referred pain from the cervical neck or shoulder.)

FIELD STRATEGY 9.6   OBSERVATION AND INSPECTION OF THE WRIST AND HAND

DORSAL VIEW

1. Check bilateral shape and contour of the bony and soft-tissue structures of the forearm, wrist, and hand. Note how the individual moves the hand into the requested positions.

2. Note skin color, presence of ganglions, or muscular wasting. Do the hands appear healthy? Many vascular problems, such as peripheral vascular disorders, Raynaud's disease, or diabetes mellitus, can be indicated by changes in skin color and temperature.

3. Note any localized swelling, effusion, or synovial thickening at the metacarpophalangeal (MCP) or interphalangeal (IP) joints.

4. Observe for any angular deformities of the fingers that may indicate a previous fracture or dislocation.

5. With the forearm in pronation, note whether the distal phalanx fails to remain in an extended position (possible mallet finger).

6. Observe the fingernails for any abnormality or change in color during blanching.

PALMAR VIEW

1. Check the smooth contours of the bony and soft-tissue structures of the forearm, wrist, and hand.

2. Look for muscle wasting in the thenar eminence (median nerve) and hypothenar eminence (ulnar nerve) that may indicate a nerve injury.

3. Have the individual flex the MCP and proximal interphalangeal (PIP) joints, and keep the distal interphalangeal (DIP) joint extended. Note any angular deformity of the fingers that may indicate a previous fracture.

4. Note any localized swelling, effusion, or synovial thickening at the MCP, PIP, and DIP joints. (This may be more visible on the dorsal view.)

5. Check skin color and presence of any abrasions or scars. Scars may decrease the mobility of a joint because of the formation of scar tissue around the tendons and joint.

---

4. Radial (lateral) collateral ligament
5. Biceps brachii, brachialis muscle, and brachial artery in cubital fossa
6. Triceps muscle and olecranon bursa (grasp the skin overlying the olecranon process and note any thickening)
7. Finger and thumb extensors and thumb abductor
8. Carpal tunnel and flexor tendons
9. Palmar fascia and intrinsic muscles within the **thenar** and hypothenar muscle masses

Special Tests

If a fracture or dislocation is suspected, do not attempt any special tests. Immobilize the arm in an appropriate splint and refer the individual to a physician. For other injuries, do only those tests necessary to assess the current injury.

RANGE OF MOTION TESTS

As with previous assessments, bilateral comparison with the uninvolved arm should always be completed. In addition, painful active movements should be performed last to prevent painful symptoms from overflowing into

the next movement. Ask the athlete to perform movement patterns at the elbow, wrist, and hand. These motions include 1) elbow flexion and extension; 2) forearm supination and pronation; 3) wrist flexion and extension; and 4) wrist radial and ulnar deviation. Finger active motion is usually done in a continuous pattern. Ask the individual to 1) make a tight fist (flexion); 2) straighten the fingers (extension); 3) spread the fingers (abduction); 4) bring the fingers together (adduction); and 5) touch the tip of each finger with the tip of the thumb (opposition). Note how fluid each digit moves throughout the range of motion (ROM). If one finger does not move through the full ROM, that finger can be evaluated separately. **Figure 9-23** demonstrates resisted motions at the elbow and wrist that should be tested.

STRESS TESTS

Stress tests are performed when a clear indication exists of what structures may be damaged. Because of the complexity of the wrist and hand and basic level of information in this text, any impairment in motor or sensory function should be referred immediately to a physician for a more complete evaluation. Only basic tests are presented.

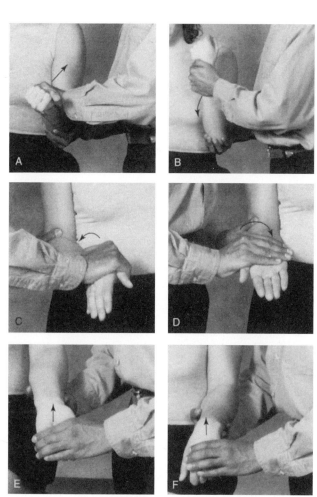

➤ **FIGURE 9-23.** Resisted manual muscle testing. **A.** Forearm supination and pronation. **B.** Wrist flexion and extension. **C.** Ulnar and radial deviation. **D.** Finger flexion and extension. **E.** Finger abduction and adduction. **F.** Thumb flexion and extension. Arrows indicate the direction the athlete moves against resistance.

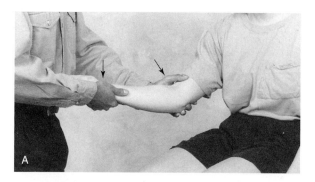

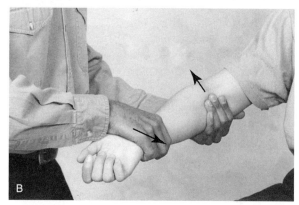

➤ **FIGURE 9-24.** Ligamentous instability tests at the elbow. To stress the ulnar collateral ligament apply a valgus force at multiple angles **A**. To stress the radial collateral ligament, apply a varus force at multiple angles **B**. *Arrows* indicate the direction the athletic trainer applies stress.

Elbow Ligamentous Instability Tests

With the individual seated, stabilize the arm and apply a valgus force to the distal forearm to stress the ulnar collateral ligament **(Fig. 9-24A)**. A varus force is then applied at the forearm to stress the radial collateral ligament **(Fig. 9-24B)**. Perform these tests at full extension, and again at 20 to 30° of flexion, to "unlock" the joint and isolate the ligamentous structures. Note any pain or joint laxity.

Tests for Common Extensor Tendinitis

Stabilize the individual's flexed elbow, and palpate the lateral epicondyle. The athlete should make a fist and pronate the forearm. Ask the athlete to radially deviate and extend the wrist while you resist the motion **(Fig. 9-25A)**. A positive sign is indicated if severe pain is present over the lateral epicondyle of the humerus. The same results can be elicited by stretching the extensor muscles by slowly pronating the forearm, flexing the wrist, and extending the elbow simultaneously **(Fig. 9-25B)**.

Medial Epicondylitis Test

With the flexed elbow stabilized against the body and the forearm supinated, the examiner palpates the medial epicondyle. The examiner then extends the wrist and elbow while the athlete resists this movement. A positive sign is indicated by pain over the medial epicondyle of the humerus.

Finger Ligamentous Instability Test

Stabilize the thumb or finger with one hand proximal to the joint being tested. Apply valgus and varus stresses to the joint to test the integrity of the collateral ligaments **(Fig. 9-26)**. Do bilateral comparison with the uninvolved hand. This test is used to determine gamekeeper's thumb or joint sprains of the fingers.

Carpal Tunnel Compression Test

Exert even pressure with both thumbs directly over the carpal tunnel and hold for at least 30 seconds **(Fig. 9-27A)**. A positive test produces numbness or tingling into the palmar aspect of the thumb, index finger, and middle finger.

Phalen's (Wrist Flexion) Test

Place the dorsum of the hands together to maximally flex the wrists. Hold this position for one minute by gently

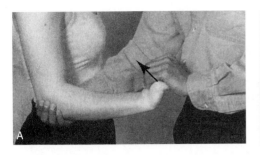

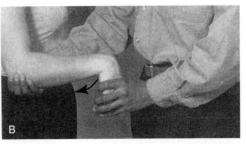

➤ ➤ **FIGURE 9-25.** Tests for common extensor tendinitis. Resisted extension and radial deviation of the wrist **A**. Passive stretching of the wrist extensors **B**. *Arrows* indicate the direction the athlete moves the joint.

pushing the wrists together **(Fig. 9-27B)**. A positive test, indicating either median nerve or ulnar nerve compression, produces numbness or tingling into the fingers.

FUNCTIONAL TESTS

The elbow must function properly to position the hand so that daily activities can be performed smoothly and efficiently. Likewise, the wrist, hand, and fingers should be assessed for manual dexterity and coordination. Activities such as combing the hair, throwing a ball, lifting an object, or pushing an object should be performed pain-free. Ask the individual to perform those skills needed to complete daily living activities and to perform skills specific to the sport. Each movement should be pain-free and fluid. Before returning to sport, the individual should be able to perform these functional skills, have bilateral range of motion and strength in the elbow, wrist, and fingers, and be cleared to participate by the supervising physician.

Summary

1. The elbow encompasses three articulations—the humeroulnar, humeroradial, and proximal radioulnar joints.
2. The medial collateral ligament is the most important ligament for stability of the elbow joint.

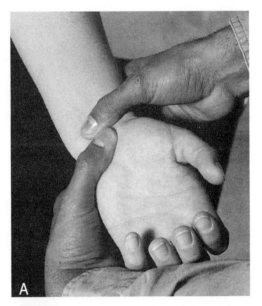

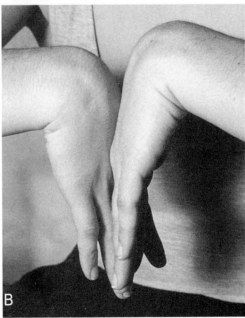

FIGURE 9-27. Nerve compression tests. Carpal tunnel compression test: Compression over the carpal tunnel may lead to tingling into the palmar aspect of the thumb, index finger, and middle finger, and indicates a carpal tunnel syndrome **A**. Phalen's test: Phalen's (wrist flexion) test indicates that the median or ulnar nerve is compressed if it produces numbness or tingling into the specific nerve distribution pattern **B**.

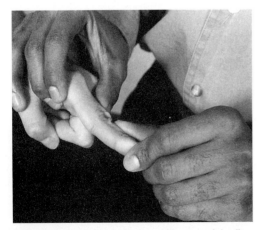

➤ ➤ **FIGURE 9-26.** Ligament instability test of the fingers. To stress the ligamentous structures around the joints, apply varus and valgus forces at the specific joint.

3. The subcutaneous olecranon bursa is the largest bursa in the elbow region. Bursitis may be acute or chronic. If the skin is warm to the touch, the individual should be referred to a physician.

4. Most ulnar dislocations occur in individuals younger than 20 years, with a peak incidence in early adolescence. The mechanism is usually hyperextension, or a sudden, violent unidirectional valgus force that drives the ulna posterior or posterolateral. Because 60% of all elbow dislocations have an associated fracture, the limb should be immobilized in a splint and the athlete transported immediately to the nearest medical facility.

5. Chronic injuries result from inadequate warm-up, excessive training past the point of fatigue, inadequate rehabilitation of previous injuries, or neglect of seemingly minor conditions that progress to major complications.

6. Repetitive throwing motions place a tremendous tensile stress on the medial joint structures (medial collateral ligament, ulnar nerve, and common flexor tendons) and concomitant lateral compressive stress in the radiocapitellar joint.

7. Medial epicondylitis produces severe pain on resisted wrist flexion and pronation, and with a valgus stress.

8. Common extensor tendinitis produces severe pain on resisted wrist extension and supination, and with a varus stress.

9. Most injuries to the wrist are caused by axial loading on the proximal palm during a fall on an outstretched hand.

10. Excessive varus/valgus stress and hyperextension can damage the collateral ligaments of the fingers. Ligament failure usually occurs at its attachment to the proximal phalanx or, less frequently, in the midportion.

11. The most common dislocation in the body occurs at the PIP joint. Because digital nerves and vessels run along the sides of the fingers and thumb, dislocation can be serious if it is reduced by an untrained individual.

12. Muscular strains occur from excessive overload against resistance or from stretching the tendon beyond its normal range. Ruptures of a muscle tendon may cause the tendon to retract, necessitating surgical reattachment of the tendon in its proper position.

13. Carpal tunnel syndrome is the most common compression syndrome of the wrist and hand. It is characterized by pain and numbness that wakes the individual in the middle of the night, and it is often relieved by shaking the hands.

14. Compression of the ulnar nerve leads to weakness in grip strength, atrophy of the hypothenar mass, and loss of sensation over the little finger.

15. If pain is present during palpation of the anatomic snuff box, suspect a fracture of the scaphoid and refer the athlete immediately to a physician..

16. In a serious elbow injury, immobilize the limb by wrapping the arm to the body, or use a sling and swathe, posterior splint, vacuum splint, or a commercial product that can pad and protect the area. With a wrist or hand injury, immobilize the limb in a wrist or finger splint, apply ice to control hemorrhage and swelling, and transport the individual to the nearest medical facility.

References

1. Stanitski CL. 1993. Combating overuse injuries: a focus on children and adolescents. Phys Sportsmed, 21(1):87-106.

2. Halikis MN, and Taleisnik J. Soft-tissue injuries of the wrist. In *Clinics in sports medicine*, edited by KD Plancher, vol. 15, no. 2. Philadelphia: WB Saunders, 1996.

3. Griggs SM, and Weiss AC. 1997. Bony injuries of the wrist, forearm, and elbow. Clin Sports Med, 15(2):373-400.

CHAPTER 10

Pelvis, Hip, and Thigh Conditions

KEY TERMS:

Hip pointer

Hypovolemic shock

Innominate

Legg-Calvé-Perthes disease

Lumbar plexus

Myositis ossificans

Osteitis pubis

Osteochondrosis

Q-angle

Sacral plexus

Snapping hip syndrome

OBJECTIVES

1. Locate the important bony and soft tissue structures of the pelvis, hip, and thigh.

2. Describe the motions of the hip and identify the primary muscles that produce them.

3. Describe flexibility and strengthening exercises that can prevent injury to this region.

4. Identify common sites for contusions to this region, and explain their management.

5. Explain the signs, symptoms, and management of a hip pointer.

6. List risk factors that can predispose an athlete to myositis ossificans of the quadriceps.

7. Describe the management of trochanteric bursitis.

8. Describe signs and symptoms of a hip dislocation and how to manage the situation.

9. List risk factors that increase the probability of sustaining a hamstring strain.

10. Describe how to manage a hamstring or groin strain.

11. Explain the signs and symptoms of pelvic and femoral fractures, and describe their management.

12. Describe a basic assessment of the pelvis, hip, and thigh region.

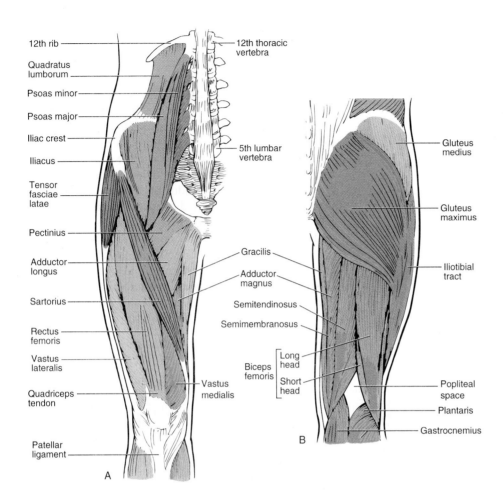

12th rib

Quadratus
lumborum

Psoas minor

Psoas major

Iliac crest

Iliacus

Tensor
fasciae
latae

Pectinius

Adductor
longus

Sartorius

Rectus
femoris

Vastus
lateralis

Quadriceps
tendon

Patellar
ligament

A

12th thoracic
vertebra

5th lumbar
vertebra

Gracilis

Adductor
magnus

Semitendinosus

Semimembranosus

Biceps
femoris [Long
head

Short
head]

Vastus
medialis

Gluteus
medius

Gluteus
maximus

Iliotibial
tract

Popliteal
space

Plantaris

Gastrocnemius

B

➤ **FIGURE 10-4.** The superficial muscles of the hip and thigh. **A.** Anterior view. **B.** Posterior view.

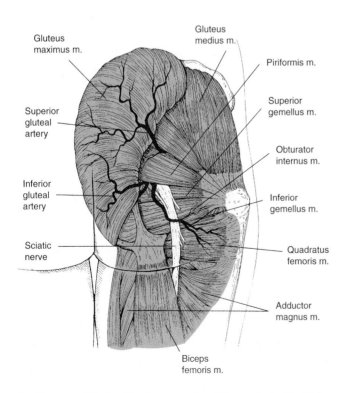

Gluteus
maximus m.

Superior
gluteal
artery

Inferior
gluteal
artery

Sciatic
nerve

Gluteus
medius m.

Piriformis m.

Superior
gemellus m.

Obturator
internus m.

Inferior
gemellus m.

Quadratus
femoris m.

Adductor
magnus m.

Biceps
femoris m.

➤ **FIGURE 10-5.** The deep muscles of the posterior hip. Note that the sciatic nerve passes inferior to the piriformis muscle to enter the posterior thigh.

protective equipment, wearing shoes with adequate cushion and support, and participating in an extensive physical conditioning program, can reduce the incidence of many injuries to the region.

Protective Equipment

Several collision and contact sports require special pads to protect vulnerable areas such as the iliac crests, sacrum and coccyx, and genital region. A girdle with special pockets can hold the pads in place. The male genital region is best protected by a protective cup placed in the athletic supporter. Special commercial thigh pads can also be used to prevent contusions to the anterior thigh, and neoprene sleeves can provide uniform compression, therapeutic warmth, and support for a quadriceps or hamstrings strain.

In addition to wearing appropriate protective equipment, the athlete should also wear proper footwear to prevent microtraumatic forces from being transmitted up the leg to the hip region. Sport activities take place on a variety of terrains and floor surfaces. Shoes should adequately cushion impact forces, and they should support and guide the foot during the stance and final pushoff phases of running, regardless of the terrain or surface. Inadequate cushioning in the heel region can transmit

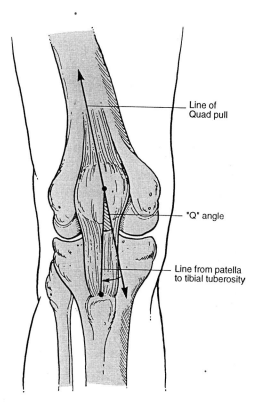

➤ **FIGURE 10-6.** Q-Angle. The Q-angle is formed between the line of quadriceps pull and the imaginary line connecting the center of the patella to the center of the tibial tubercle. An increased Q-angle can lead to a higher risk of trochanteric bursitis and patellofemoral injuries.

forces up the leg, leading to inflammation of the hip joint or stress fractures of the femoral neck or pubis. Therefore, it is important to purchase shoes that provide an adequate heel cushion and a thermoplastic heel counter, which can maintain its shape and firmness even in adverse weather conditions. The soles should be designed for the specific type of surface that the athlete is playing on to avoid slipping or sliding. Information on the proper fitting of shoes is presented in Chapter 12.

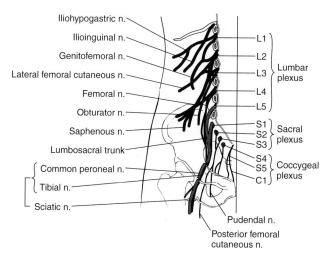

➤ **FIGURE 10-7.** The lumbar plexus and sacral plexus.

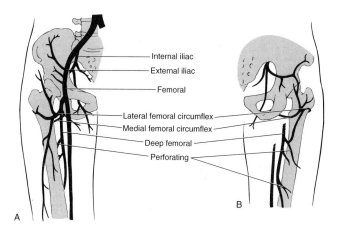

➤ **FIGURE 10-8.** The arterial supply to the hip and thigh region. **A.** Anterior view. **B.** Posterior view.

Physical Conditioning

Exercises to prevent injury to the pelvis, hip, and thigh are primarily concerned with flexibility and strengthening muscles in the area. **Field Strategy 10-1** illustrates several exercises for the hip flexors, extensors, adductors, abductors, and medial and lateral rotators. Because many of the muscles that move the hip also move the knee, flexibility and strengthening exercises of the quadriceps, hamstrings, and tensor fascia latae are illustrated in Chapter 11.

CONTUSIONS

Direct impact to soft tissue, such as a kick to the thigh or a fall onto a hard surface, causes a compressive force to crush soft tissue. The condition may be mild and resolve itself in a matter of days, or the bleeding and swelling may be more extensive, resulting in a large, deep hematoma that takes months to resolve. Contusions can occur anywhere in the hip region but are typically seen on the crest of the ilium (i.e., a hip pointer) or in the quadriceps muscle group. This type of contusion is called a charley horse.

Hip Pointers

Hip pointers are contusions to an unprotected iliac crest. Because so many trunk and abdominal muscles attach to the iliac crest, any movement of the trunk, including coughing, laughing, and even breathing, can be painful.

SIGNS AND SYMPTOMS

Immediate pain, discoloration, spasm, and loss of function prevent the individual from rotating the trunk or laterally flexing the trunk toward the injured side. In a severe injury, the individual may be unable to walk or bear weight, even with crutches, because of the intense pain caused by muscular tension pulling on the injury site.

FIELD STRATEGY 10.1   EXERCISES TO PREVENT INJURY AT THE THIGH, HIP, AND PELVIS

The following exercises can be performed for motions at the hip. Exercises for the hamstrings, quadriceps, and iliotibial band, which cross the knee joint, are described in Chapter 11.

A. **Hip flexor stretch (lunge)**. Place the leg to be stretched in front of you. Bend the contralateral knee as you move the hips forward. Keep the back straight. Alternative method: Place the foot on a chair or table and lean forward until a stretch is felt.

B. **Lateral rotator stretch, seated position**. Cross one leg over the thigh and place the elbow on the outside of the knee. Gently stretch the buttock muscles by pushing the bent knee across the body while keeping the pelvis on the floor.

C. **Adductor stretch, standing position**. Place the leg to be stretched out to the side. Slowly bend the contralateral knee. Keep the hips in a neutral or extended position.

D. **TheraBand®** or tubing exercises. Secure TheraBand (KAS Enterprises, Covington, LA) or surgical tubing to a table. Perform hip flexion, extension, abduction, adduction, and medial and lateral rotation in a single plane or in multidirectional patterns.

E. **Half squats**. A weight belt should be worn during this exercise. Place the feet at shoulder width or wider. Keep the back straight by keeping the chest out and the head up at all times. Flex the knees and hips to no greater than 90°. Begin the upward motion by extending the hips first.

F. **Hip extension**. With the trunk stabilized and the back flat, extend the hip while keeping the knee flexed. Alternate legs.

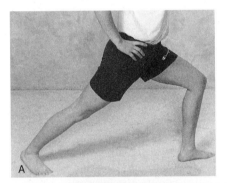

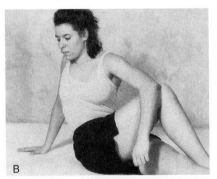

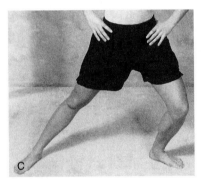

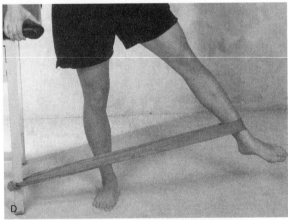

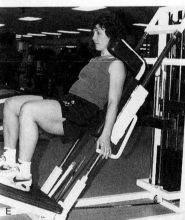

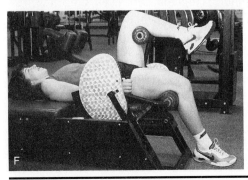

MANAGEMENT

Treatment involves ice, compression, and total inactivity during the first 2 to 3 days after injury. If intense pain was palpated directly over the iliac crest, the athlete should be referred to a physician to rule out a possible fracture of the iliac crest because the same mechanism of injury may cause both injuries. With an uncomplicated hip pointer, the athlete can return to activity in 3 to 7 days; however, the area should be protected with a pad to prevent reinjury.

Quadriceps Contusion

The most common site for a quadriceps contusion is the anterolateral thigh. If the contusion is severe enough, it can damage muscle tissue.

SIGNS AND SYMPTOMS

Pain and swelling may be extensive immediately after impact. In a mild contusion, the individual has mild pain and swelling and is able to walk without a limp. In a moderate contusion, the individual can flex the knee only between 45 and 90° and will walk with a noticeable limp. If the contusion is severe, the individual is unable to bear weight or fully flex the knee. Within 24 hours, there may be a palpable firm hematoma, resulting in an inability to contract the quadriceps or do a straight-leg raise.

MANAGEMENT

Treatment involves ice application and a compressive wrap for the first 24 to 48 hours, applied with the knee in maximal flexion **(Fig. 10-9)**. This position preserves the needed flexion and limits intramuscular bleeding and spasm. Continued swelling despite proper acute care protocol necessitates immediate referral to a physician.

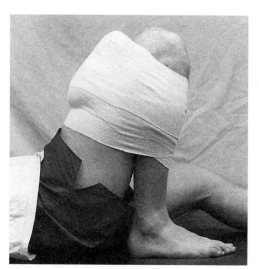

➤ **FIGURE 10-9.** Ice a quadriceps contusion with the knee in maximal flexion to place the muscles on stretch.

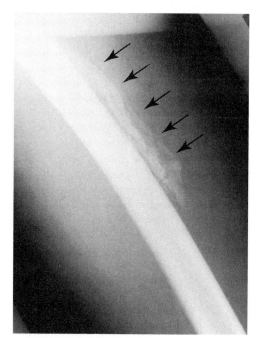

➤ **FIGURE 10-10.** Myositis ossificans. With myositis ossificans, full resorption of the calcification may not occur, leaving a visible cortical-type bony lesion.

Myositis Ossificans

An athlete who receives a severe blow to the quadriceps muscle group, such as from an opponent's knee, can develop significant bleeding and damage within the muscle tissue itself. If the initial contusion is not properly cared for or if further insult occurs, the internal hemorrhaging increases and over a period of time, abnormal bone growth or calcification within the muscle occurs **(Fig. 10-10)**. **Myositis ossificans** is an abnormal ossification involving bone deposition within muscle tissue. Several risk factors following a quadriceps contusion can predispose an athlete to this condition **(Box 10-1)**. Common sites are the anterior and lateral thigh, but it may also occur on the hip, groin, leg, and lateral aspect of the mid humerus.

SIGNS AND SYMPTOMS

Examination reveals a warm, firm, swollen thigh nearly 2 to 4 cm larger than the unaffected side. A palpable, painful mass may limit passive knee flexion to 20 to 30°.

➤ ➤ **BOX 10-1**

Risk Factors for Developing Myositis Ossificans

- Innate predisposition to ectopic bone formation
- Continuing to play after injury
- Early massage, hydrotherapy, or thermotherapy during acute stage
- Passive, forceful stretching
- Too rapid a progression in rehabilitation program
- Premature return to play
- Re-injury of same area

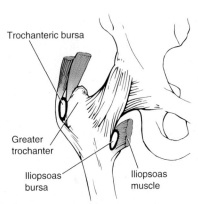

▶ FIGURE 10-11. Bursa of the hip. Bursitis at the hip may involve the trochanteric bursa, iliopsoas bursa, or ischial bursa.

Active quadriceps contractions and straight-leg raises may be impossible.

MANAGEMENT

Apply ice and compression immediately, and refer this individual to a physician. Periodic radiographs usually are taken until the abnormal ossification matures, which typically occurs within 6 to 12 months. If the mass fails to reabsorb completely, many individuals return safely to participation, with adequate protection from subsequent blows. Surgery is indicated only in cases where activity is limited by pain, weakness, and decreased range of motion. Excision before the mass matures may result in reformation, sometimes larger than the original mass.

BURSITIS

Bursitis is common in runners and joggers. It typically affects the greater trochanteric bursa, iliopsoas bursa, and ischial bursa **(Fig. 10-11)**. The trochanteric bursa lies between the greater trochanter and the gluteus maximus and tensor fascia latae (iliotibial tract). Bursitis occurs commonly in female runners because of the wider pelvis and larger Q angle **(Fig. 10-6)**; it is also seen in cross-country skiers and ballet dancers. Because streets are crowned to allow for run off, the condition usually affects the down leg, referring to the leg closest to the gutter.

Acute Bursitis

SIGNS AND SYMPTOMS

Trochanteric bursitis is characterized by a burning or aching pain over or just posterior to the greater trochanter that intensifies with walking or exercise. The condition is aggravated by contracting the hip abductors against resistance. The iliopsoas bursa can be irritated when the iliopsoas muscle repeatedly compresses the bursa against either the joint capsule of the hip or the lesser trochanter of the femur. Pain is felt medial and anterior to the joint and cannot be palpated easily. Passive rotary motions at the hip, as well as resisted hip flexion, abduction, and external rotation, may reproduce symptoms. Direct bruising from a fall can con-

tuse the ischial bursa. However, there is often a history of prolonged sitting on a hard surface ("benchwarmer's bursitis") or of prolonged sitting with the legs crossed.

MANAGEMENT

Treatment for bursitis involves cryotherapy, protected rest, nonsteroidal anti-inflammatory drugs (NSAIDs), and a stretching program for the involved muscle or muscles. Wearing different shoes, using orthotics, or altering the running technique may correct the problem and avoid recurrence. If the condition does not rapidly improve, a bone scan should be conducted to rule out possible femoral neck stress fractures.

Snapping Hip Syndrome

Chronic bursitis can lead to **snapping hip syndrome,** a condition prevalent in dancers, runners, and cheerleaders. It can develop secondary to a variety of other causes.

SIGNS AND SYMPTOMS

The condition is characterized by a snapping sensation, rather than pain, either heard or felt during certain motions at the hip. It usually occurs when an individual laterally rotates and flexes the hip joint while balancing on one leg.

MANAGEMENT

The condition is usually handled with anti-inflammatories and a stretching program. If this syndrome is associated with pain or a sense of hip joint instability, however, the individual should be referred to a physician.

SPRAINS AND DISLOCATIONS

Hip joint sprains are rare because of the many movements allowed at the ball and socket joint because of the level of protection provided by layers of muscles that add to the hip joint's stability. Injury can occur in violent twisting actions or in catastrophic trauma when the knee is driven into a stationary object, such as in an automobile accident when the knee is driven into the dashboard.

SIGNS AND SYMPTOMS

Symptoms of a mild or moderate hip sprain involve pain on hip rotation. Severe hip sprains and dislocations result in immediate, intense pain and an inability to walk or even move the hip. The hip remains in a characteristic flexed and internally rotated position, which indicates a posterior, superior dislocation **(Fig. 10-12)**.

MANAGEMENT

Treatment for mild and moderate sprains is symptomatic and includes cryotherapy, rest, and protected weightbear-

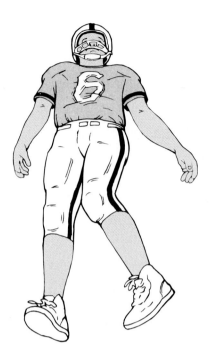

➤ FIGURE 10-12. Hip dislocation. Most hip dislocations drive the head of the femur posterior and superior, leaving the leg in a characteristically flexed and internally rotated position.

ing on crutches until walking is pain-free. Emergency medical services (EMS) should be activated if a hip dislocation occurs. Because the sciatic nerve may be damaged, nerve function must be assessed. This can be done by running the fingers down both lower legs and asking the athlete where you are touching the leg and what it feels like. Ask the athlete whether there is full or partial sensation. It is imperative not to move the individual until the ambulance arrives because of a possible fracture to the acetabulum or head of the femur. The vital signs should be monitored frequently and the individual treated for shock.

STRAINS

Muscular strains to the hip and thigh muscles are frequently seen not only in sport, but also in many occupations involving repetitive motions. Strains range from mild to severe, and the severity of symptoms parallels the amount of disruption to the muscle fibers. General signs and symptoms include a sharp pain in the involved muscle, localized swelling and inflammation, weakness and an inability of the muscle to contract against resistance, and, in severe cases, a visible defect. Although any muscle group can be involved, most of the strains involve the hamstrings or adductor muscles.

Hamstring Strain

The hamstrings are the most frequently strained muscles in the body. This type of strain is typically caused by a rapid contraction of the muscle during a ballistic action or by a violent stretch. Several factors can increase the risk of injury **(Box 10-2)**. A hamstring strain can be both

➤ ➤ BOX 10-2

Risk Factors for Hamstring Strains
- Poor flexibility
- Poor posture
- Muscle imbalance
- Improper warm-up
- Muscle fatigue
- Lack of neuromuscular control
- Previous injury
- Overuse
- Improper technique

chronic and recurring. Most sport participants are fully aware of limited motion after a strain, and they concentrate on regaining flexibility through an aggressive stretching program. However, these individuals fail to restrengthen the hamstrings adequately, setting up a muscle imbalance with the quadriceps.

SIGNS AND SYMPTOMS

In mild strains, the individual reports tightness and tension in the muscle. In second- and third-degree strains, the individual may report a tearing sensation or feeling a "pop," leading to immediate pain and weakness in knee flexion. In more severe cases, a sharp pain is present in the posterior thigh and may occur during mid-stride. The individual limps and is unable to do heelstrike or fully extend the knee. Pain and muscle weakness are elicited during active knee flexion.

MANAGEMENT

Treatment for muscle strains involves immediate ice, compression, elevation, protected rest, and NSAIDs for the first 7 to 10 days. Whenever possible, the injured muscle should be iced in a stretched position, and crutches should be used if the individual walks with a limp. In severe strains, a compression wrap may be indicated from the toe to groin to prevent venous thrombosis or distal edema. If the condition does not improve within 2 to 5 days, refer the individual to a physician to rule out other underlying conditions.

Adductor Strain

Adductor strains, or groin strains, are common in activities that require quick changes of direction and explosive propulsion and acceleration. A strength imbalance between the hip abductors and adductors may be a predisposing factor in many of these injuries.

SIGNS AND SYMPTOMS

The individual often experiences a previous "twinge" or "pull" of the groin muscles, and he or she may be unable

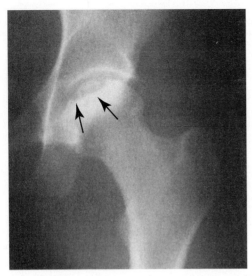

➤ FIGURE 10-13. Osteochondrosis of the left femoral head (Legg-Calvé-Perthes disease). Note the destruction of the articular cartilage. In mild cases, no restriction of activity is indicated.

to walk because of the intense, sharp pain. As the condition worsens, increased pain, stiffness, and weakness in hip adduction and flexion become apparent. Running straight ahead or backwards may be tolerable, but any side-to-side movement leads to more discomfort and pain. Increased pain is present during passive stretching with the hip extended, abducted, and externally rotated, and with resisted hip adduction.

MANAGEMENT
Treatment is the same as for a strain of the hamstrings.

LEGG-CALVÉ-PERTHES DISEASE

Legg-Calvé-Perthes disease, or avascular necrosis of the proximal femoral epiphysis, is a noninflammatory, self-limiting disorder of the hip seen in young children, especially males, between the ages of 3 and 12 years. It is considered an **osteochondrosis** condition of the femoral head, caused by diminished blood supply to the capital region of the femur. The result is a progressive necrosis of the bone and marrow of the epiphysis of the femoral head **(Fig. 10-13)**.

SIGNS AND SYMPTOMS
The most common complaint is a gradual onset of a limp and mild hip or knee pain that lasts for several months. The pain is most often referred to the groin region, but some patients report knee pain as the primary symptom. Pain is generally activity-related, which often contributes to delayed recognition. Examination reveals a decreased range of motion in hip abduction, extension, and external rotation caused by muscle spasm in the hip flexors and adductors.

MANAGEMENT
This condition should be suspected in 3- to 12-year olds when pain in the groin, anterior thigh, or knee region cannot be explained. If pain persists for more than 1 week after initial acute care, or if the individual continues to limp after activity, immediate referral to a physician is needed to rule out nontraumatic causes of the pain that have similar signs and symptoms. Possibilities include a slipped capital femoral epiphysis (discussed later in the chapter), septic arthritis, transient synovitis, juvenile rheumatoid arthritis, or a bone tumor. Confirmation of the condition is made through radiographs, bone scans, or magnetic resonance imaging (MRI).

HIP FRACTURES

Major fractures of the pelvic girdle and hip often result from severe direct trauma, as occurs when an individual is thrown from a horse onto hard ground, a hockey player collides with the side boards, or a football or rugby player falls on top of a downed player. In sports where this trauma is most likely to occur (e.g., football and hockey), the pelvic region is usually protected by padding to prevent such injuries. Fractures that occur in this region include avulsion and apophyseal fractures, epiphyseal fractures, and stress fractures.

Avulsion Fractures

Individuals who perform rapid, sudden acceleration and deceleration moves are at risk for avulsion fractures to

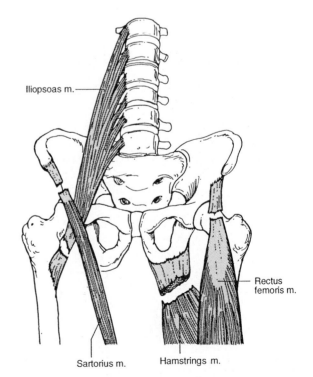

Iliopsoas m.

Rectus femoris m.

Sartorius m.   Hamstrings m.

➤ FIGURE 10-14. Avulsion fractures. Several major muscles attach to the pelvis that can be avulsed from their bony attachments during muscular action.

the ASIS with displacement of the sartorius; anterior inferior iliac spine (AIIS) with displacement of the rectus femoris; ischial tuberosity with displacement of the hamstrings; and the lesser trochanter with displacement of the iliopsoas **(Fig. 10-14)**.

SIGNS AND SYMPTOMS

The individual usually reports sudden, acute, localized pain that may radiate down the muscle. Examination reveals severe pain, swelling, and discoloration directly over the tendinous attachment on the bony landmark. In a complete displaced avulsion fracture, a gap may be palpated between the tendon's attachment and bone. Pain increases with passive stretching of the involved muscle and during active and resisted motion.

MANAGEMENT

Depending on the fracture site, immobilization from an elastic compression spica wrap may limit motion and decrease pain. After the individual is fitted with crutches, he or she should be referred to a physician for radiographic examination.

Slipped Capital Femoral Epiphysis

Slipped capital femoral epiphysis is an epiphyseal fracture seen in adolescent boys ages 12 to 15 years. It occurs across the capital femoral epiphysis, the growth plate at the femoral head **(Fig. 10-15)**. The condition is seen primarily in an obese adolescent with underdeveloped sexual characteristics and occasionally in rapidly growing slender boys.

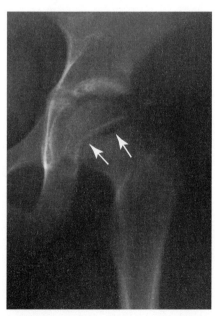

➤ **FIGURE 10-15.** Slipped capital femoral epiphysis. An epiphyseal fracture, seen in adolescents aged 12 to 15 years, occurs through the growth plate at the femoral head. With this fracture, the patient is unable to internally rotate the femur.

SIGNS AND SYMPTOMS

As the proximal femoral growth plate deteriorates, the individual begins to develop a painful limp with groin pain. Pain may also be referred to the anterior thigh or knee region. Early signs and symptoms may go undetected. Frequently, the only complaint is diffuse knee pain. The individual is unable to internally rotate the femur or stand on one leg.

MANAGEMENT

Immediate referral to a physician is indicated because surgery is mandatory in nearly all cases.

Stress Fractures

Stress fractures to the pubis, femoral neck (most common), and proximal third of the femur occur in individuals who do extensive jogging or aerobic dance activities to the point at which muscle fatigue occurs. Other risk factors predispose an athlete to stress fracture of the femur **(Box 10-3)**.

SIGNS AND SYMPTOMS

Signs and symptoms involve a diffuse or localized aching pain in the anterior groin or thigh region during weight-bearing activity that is relieved with rest. Night pain is a frequent complaint.

MANAGEMENT

Bone scans or MRIs are frequently used for early diagnosis to prevent delayed treatment. Biking and swimming can maintain cardiovascular fitness; however, the whip kick and scissors kick should be avoided.

Osteitis Pubis

Osteitis pubis is an inflammatory process that involves continued stress on the symphysis pubis from repeated overload of the adductor muscles or from repetitive running activities.

SIGNS AND SYMPTOMS

The most common complaint is a gradual onset of pain in the adductor musculature, which is aggravated by kicking,

---

➤ ➤ **Box 10-3**

Risk Factors for Stress Fractures of the Femur

- Sudden increase in training (mileage, intensity, or frequency)
- Change in running surface or terrain
- Improper footwear
- Biomechanical abnormalities
- Nutritional and hormonal factors (anorexia, amenorrhea, osteopenia)

running, and pivoting on one leg. Pain over the symphysis pubis and lower abdominal muscles increase with sit-ups and abdominal muscle-strengthening exercises.

MANAGEMENT

Treatment is symptomatic with ice, protected rest, and NSAIDs until the condition is resolved; however, prolonged rest is usually required to alleviate symptoms.

Pelvic Fractures

Major fractures to the pelvis seldom occur in sport participation except in activities such as equestrian sports, hockey, rugby, skiing, or football. Three main mechanisms are involved in traumatic pelvic fractures:

- Avulsion or traction injury of the bony origin or attachment of muscle (see Avulsion Fractures earlier in this chapter)
- Direct compression, with disruption of the pelvic osseous ring
- Direct blow to the pelvis itself

Because the pelvis is a closed ring, an injury to one location in the pelvis causes a countercoup fracture or sprain on the other side of the pelvic ring. For example, if the superior and inferior pubic rami are fractured on the right side, sacroiliac disruption on the left side often results.

SIGNS AND SYMPTOMS

This crushing injury produces severe pain, total loss of function, and in many cases, severe loss of blood leading to **hypovolemic shock**. The extent of blood loss is unknown because hemorrhage within the pelvic cavity is not visible. A possible pelvic fracture can be determined with slight compression to the sides of the ilium and the ASIS. Fractures to the acetabulum can be detected by gently placing upward pressure on the femur against the acetabulum.

MANAGEMENT

If a fracture is suspected, initiate the emergency care plan and activate EMS. Cover the individual with a blanket to maintain body temperature. Monitor vital signs frequently, and watch for signs of internal hemorrhage and shock.

Femoral Fractures

Fractures to the femoral shaft can be serious because of potential damage to the neurovascular structures from bony fragments.

SIGNS AND SYMPTOMS

Severe pain and swelling can occur in the soft tissues of the thigh **(Box 10-4)**. These traumatic fractures tend to

> ➤ ➤ **BOX 10-4**

Signs and Symptoms of Femoral Fractures

- Displaced fracture
- Shortened limb deformity
- Severe angulation with the thigh externally rotated
- Swelling into the soft tissues
- Severe pain
- Total loss of function
- Loss of or change in distal neurovascular functions
- Nondisplaced fractures
- Extreme pain on palpation
- Crepitation
- Muscle weakness
- Muscle spasm
- Swelling into the soft tissues

angulate and displace posteriorly. The adductor muscles contract to rotate and shorten the femoral shaft, giving a characteristic posture **(Fig. 10-16)**. There may be total loss of neurovascular function distal to the fracture site.

MANAGEMENT

Femoral fractures can be life-threatening if the neurovascular structures are damaged by bony fragments and lead to excessive blood loss and hypovolemic shock, similar to that seen in pelvic fractures. Immediately activate EMS, cover the individual with a blanket to maintain body temperature, and monitor vital signs until the ambulance arrives.

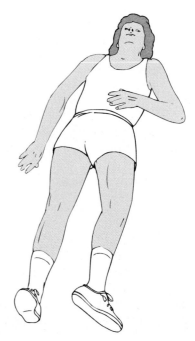

> ➤ **FIGURE 10-16.** Femoral fracture. In a fractured femur, the adductor muscles contract, leading to internal rotation of the proximal femur with external rotation of the tibia. If the fractured bones override each other, the leg will have a shortened appearance.

INJURIES AND CONDITIONS OF THE GENITALIA

The male genitalia are more susceptible to injury than female genitalia because several structures are external to the body, thus exposed to direct trauma. Protective cups can protect the penis and scrotum from injury; these cups are required for baseball catchers and hockey goalies. Direct trauma can damage the penis, urethra, and scrotum, which holds the testes. In addition, congenital variations in testicular suspension make certain individuals susceptible to torsion of the testicle.

Male Genital Injuries

Direct trauma to the groin from a knee, implement, or straddle-like injury, such as falling on a bar, can cause severe pain and dysfunction to the testes and penis. Superficial wounds to the penis or urethra may involve a contusion, abrasion, laceration, avulsion, or penetrating wound. Most injuries resolve without specific treatment. Superficial bleeding can be controlled by applying a sterile dressing, and a cold compress with mild compression can control swelling. Referral to a physician is necessary only if hemorrhage persists or swelling impairs function of the urethra.

SCROTAL INJURIES

Blunt scrotal trauma can cause a contusion, hematoma, torsion, dislocation, or rupture of the testicle.

SIGNS AND SYMPTOMS

A knee, foot, or elbow to the groin commonly compresses the testicle against the pelvis, leading to a nauseating, painful condition. Immediate internal hemorrhage, effusion, and muscle spasm occur.

MANAGEMENT

Testicular spasm can be relieved by placing the individual on his back and flexing the knees toward the chest to relax the muscle spasm **(Fig. 10-17)**. After pain subsides, a cold compress should be placed on the scrotum to reduce swelling and hemorrhage.

TESTICULAR CANCER

A scrotal mass can be indicative of testicular cancer, the most common malignancy in 15- to 35-year-old men. Men who have an undescended or partially descended testicle are at a higher risk of developing testicular cancer than others. Prevention is critical and involves monthly testicular self-examinations **(Box 10-5)**.

SIGNS AND SYMPTOMS

The first sign is a slightly enlarged testicle and a change in its consistency. A dull ache or sensation of dragging

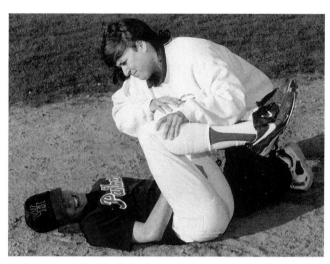

➤ **FIGURE 10-17.** Relieving testicular spasm. To relieve testicular spasm, place the individual on his or her back and flex the knees toward the chest. After pain has diminished, apply ice to control swelling and hemorrhage.

and heaviness is often present in the lower abdomen or groin. Other early warning signs include the following:

- A lump in either testicle
- Dull ache in the lower abdomen or the groin
- Sudden collection of fluid in the scrotum
- Pain or discomfort in a testicle or in the scrotum
- Enlargement or tenderness in the breasts

➤ ➤ **BOX 10-5**

Performing a Testicular Self-examination

Starting at age 15 years, men should perform a monthly testicular self-examination. By doing this, men become familiar with this area of the body and can detect any changes early. The best time to conduct the examination is after a warm bath or shower because the heat makes the scrotum relax. The process takes only a few minutes.

1. Stand in front of a mirror. Look for any swelling on the skin of the scrotum.
2. Examine each testicle with both hands. Place the index and middle fingers under the testicle with the thumbs placed on top. Gently roll the testicle between the thumbs and fingers. Do not be alarmed if one testicle seems slightly larger than the other; this is normal.
3. Find the epididymis—the soft, tubelike structure behind the testicle that collects and carries sperm. If you are familiar with this structure, you will not mistake it for a suspicious lump. Most lumps are found on the sides of the testicle, but some appear on the front.
4. If a lump is detected, contact your physician immediately. Remember: testicular cancer is highly curable, especially when treated promptly.

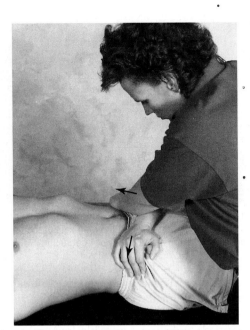

➤ FIGURE 10-19. Gapping test (sacroiliac compression and distraction test). Apply a cross-arm pressure down and outward to the anterior superior iliac spine with your thumbs. Repeat with pressure applied down through the anterior portion of the ilium spreading the superior iliac joint. Unilateral pain or posterior leg pain may indicate a sprain to the anterior sacroiliac ligaments. Sharp pain elsewhere may indicate a pelvic fracture.

5. Hip extension with the knee flexed
6. Knee flexion

STRESS TESTS

Always be alert to possible congenital defects and epiphyseal injuries when dealing with adolescents. As you progress through the assessment process, perform only those tests you believe to be necessary.

Thomas Test for Hip Flexion Contractures

With the patient in a supine, fully extended position, observe any noticeable lumbar lordosis. If contractures are present, you may be able to slip your hand under the low back. Ask the individual to flex the uninvolved leg to the chest and hold it in that position. This should flatten the lumbar region. If the test is negative, the straight leg remains in contact with the table. If the test is positive, however, the straight leg (involved leg) rises off the table **(Fig. 10-21)**. Both legs are tested and compared.

Kendall Test for Rectus Femoris Contracture

The athlete lies supine on the table with both knees flexed at 90° over the edge of the table. The individual flexes the unaffected knee to the chest and holds it in that position. The other knee should remain flexed at 90°. If the knee slightly extends, a contracture in the rectus femoris may be present on that leg **(Fig. 10-22)**. If the results are positive, palpate the muscle for tightness to confirm the contracture.

Hamstrings Contracture Test

In a seated position on a table, flex the hip, bringing one leg against the chest to stabilize the pelvic region. Ask the individual to touch the toes of the extended leg **(Fig. 10-23)**. Inability to do so indicates tight hamstrings on the extended leg. Test both legs and compare.

Straight Leg Raising Test

Although this test is typically used to stretch the dura mater of the spinal cord to assess possible intervertebral disc lesions, it is also used to rule out tight hamstrings. With the patient in a supine position, passively flex the individual's hip while keeping the knee extended until the individual reports tightness or pain **(Fig. 10-24)**. Slowly lower the leg until the pain or tightness disappears. Then, dorsiflex the foot, have the individual flex the neck, or do both actions simultaneously. Pain that increases with dorsiflexion, neck flexion, or both indicates stretching of the dura mater of the spinal cord. Pain that does not increase with dorsiflexion or neck flexion usually indicates tight hamstrings.

FUNCTIONAL TESTS

Functional tests should be performed before clearing any individual for re-entry into sports participation. The individual should be able to perform activity pain free and with no limp or antalgic gait. Examples of functional activities include walking, going up and down stairs, jogging, squatting, jumping, running straight ahead, running sideways, and changing directions while running. Whenever possible, use protective equipment or padding to prevent reinjury.

Summary

1. The hip joint is the most stable joint in the body. It is protected by a deep, bony socket called the acetabulum and is stabilized by several strong ligaments, including the iliofemoral, pubofemoral, and ischiofemoral ligaments.
2. Contusions are typically seen on the crest of the ilium (hip pointer) or in the quadriceps muscle group (charley horse). Severe quadriceps contusions can lead to myositis ossificans or an acute compartment syndrome.
3. Bursitis can result from inflammation secondary to excessive compression between a muscle and a bony prominence. The greater trochanteric bursa is the most commonly injured.
4. Snapping hip syndrome is characterized by a snapping sensation either heard or felt during certain motions at the rip rather than by pain.
5. Testicular spasm can be relieved by placing the individual on his or her back and flexing the knees toward the chest to relax the muscle spasm.

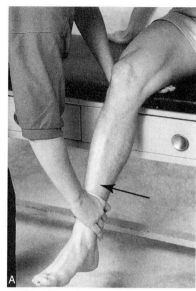

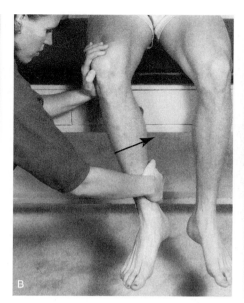

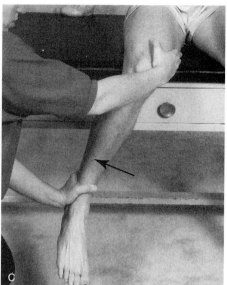

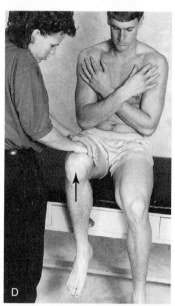

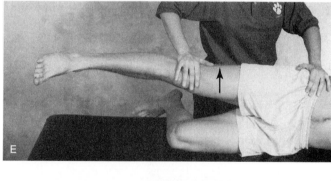

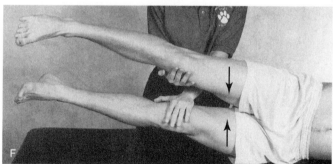

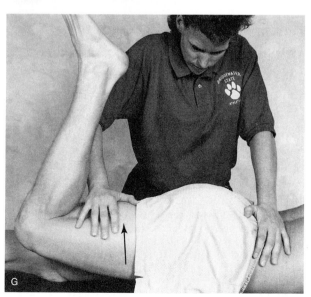

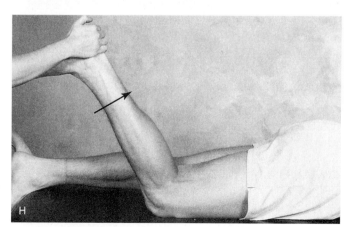

➤ FIGURE 10-20. Resisted manual muscle testing. **A.** Knee extension. **B.** Lateral hip rotation. **C.** Medial hip rotation. **D.** Hip flexion. **E.** Hip abduction. **F.** Hip adduction. **G.** Knee flexion. **H.** Hip extension.

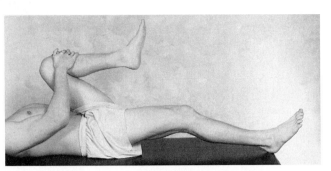

➤ **FIGURE 10-21.** Thomas test. To perform a Thomas test for flexion contractures, ask the individual to flex the uninvolved leg to the chest and hold it. A positive test occurs when the extended leg moves up off the table indicating hip flexion contractures.

6. Hip dislocations result in immediate, intense pain and an inability to walk or even move the hip. The hip remains in a characteristic flexed and internally rotated position, indicating a posterior, superior dislocation.

7. The hamstrings are the most frequently strained muscle group in the body. Injuries are typically caused by a rapid contraction of the muscle during a ballistic action or by a violent stretch.

8. Adductor strains are common in activities that require quick changes of direction, explosive propulsion, and acceleration.

9. Avulsion fractures may occur in individuals who perform rapid, sudden acceleration and deceleration moves. The following sites are the most affected:
   • ASIS—Proximal sartorius muscle or tensor fascia latae
   • AIIS—Proximal rectus femoris muscles
   • Ischial tuberosity—Proximal hamstrings attachment
   • Lesser trochanter—Distal iliopsoas attachment

10. Stress fractures to the pubis, femoral neck (most common), and proximal third of the femur occur in individuals who do extensive jogging or aerobic

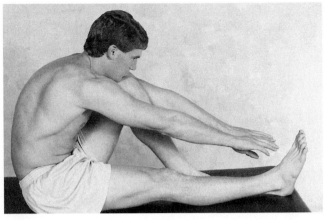

➤ **FIGURE 10-23.** Hamstring contractures. The athlete flexes one hip against the chest to stabilize the pelvic region. The test is positive if the individual cannot touch the toes of the extended leg.

dance activities to the point at which muscle fatigue occurs.

11. Osteitis pubis is an inflammatory process involving continued stress on the symphysis pubis from repeated overload of the adductor muscles or from repetitive running activities. The most common report is a gradual onset of pain in the adductor musculature, aggravated by kicking, running, and pivoting on one leg.

12. Major fractures to the pelvis and femur produce severe pain, total loss of function, and, in many cases, severe loss of blood, which leads to hypovolemic shock.

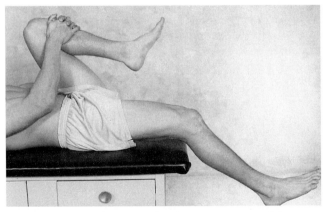

➤ **FIGURE 10-24.** Straight leg raising test. Passively flex the individual's hip while keeping the knee extended until pain or tension occurs in the hamstrings. Slowly lower the leg until the pain or tension disappears. Next, dorsiflex the foot, have the individual flex the neck, or do both simultaneously. If pain does not increase with dorsiflexion of the ankle or flexion of the neck, tight hamstrings are indicated.

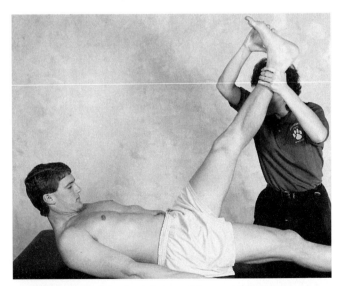

➤ **FIGURE 10-22.** Kendall test. The Kendall test is similar to the Thomas test, except the individual lies supine with both knees flexed over the edge of the table. The uninvolved leg is flexed to the chest and held. A positive test occurs when the leg flexed over the end of the table extends.

11

Knee Conditions

Objectives

1. Locate the important bony and soft tissue structures at the knee.
2. Name the main supporting ligaments of the knee joint, and describe what directional forces they attempt to withstand.
3. Describe the motions of the knee, and identify the primary muscles that produce them.
4. Identify basic principles of preventing knee injuries.
5. Recognize common soft tissue injuries at the knee and describe their management.
6. Identify common soft tissue injuries associated with the patellofemoral joint and describe their management.
7. List factors that increase the risk for iliotibial band friction syndrome.
8. Describe how to manage a traumatic fracture of the patella and tibia.
9. Describe a basic assessment of the knee region.

D uring walking and running, the knee moves through a considerable range of motion while bearing loads equivalent to three to four times body weight. The knee is also positioned between the two longest bones in the body, the femur and tibia, creating the potential for large, injurious torques at the joint. These factors, coupled with minimal bony stability, make the knee susceptible to injury, particularly during participation in field or contact sports. This chapter begins with a review of the anatomy of the knee and major muscle actions at the knee. General principles to prevent injuries are then discussed, followed by a review of common injuries to the knee complex and their management. Finally, a basic assessment protocol for the knee region is introduced.

ANATOMY REVIEW OF THE KNEE

The proximal bone of the knee joint is the femur. The prominent posterior ridge of the femur, the linea aspera, serves as an attachment for many of the muscles that move the hip and knee. As it reaches its distal end, the shaft of the femur broadens to form the medial and lateral epicondyles. Running between the epicondyles on the anterior sur-

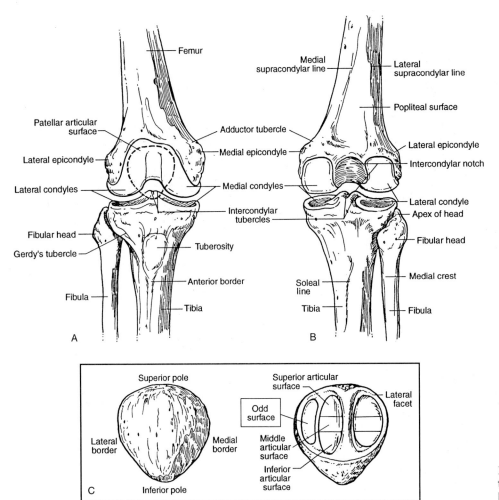

face of the femur is the femoral trochlea, through which the patella glides as the knee moves into flexion and extension **(Fig. 11-1)**. Corresponding to the femoral condyles are the medial and lateral tibial plateaus. The medial tibial plateau (condyle) is 50% larger than the lateral tibial plateau to accommodate the longer medial femoral condyle. On the anterior aspect of the tibia is the prominent tibial tubercle, which serves as the distal attachment of the infrapatellar ligament.

The Knee Joint

The knee is a large synovial joint consisting of three articulations within the joint capsule **(Fig. 11-2)**. The weight-bearing joints are the two condylar articulations of the tibiofemoral joint, with the third articulation being the patellofemoral joint. The soft tissue connections of the proximal tibiofibular joint also exert a minor influence on knee motion.

TIBIOFEMORAL JOINT
The **tibiofemoral joint** functions primarily as a modified hinge joint because of the restricting ligaments, with some lateral and rotational motions allowed. Because the

medial and lateral condyles of the femur differ in size, shape, and orientation, the tibia rotates laterally on the femur during the last few degrees of extension to produce "locking" of the knee. This phenomenon is known as the **"screwing-home" mechanism**.

THE PATELLOFEMORAL JOINT
The patella is a triangular-shaped bone commonly known as the kneecap. It articulates with the patellofemoral groove between the femoral condyles to form the **patellofemoral joint**. In the sagittal plane, the patella serves to increase the angle of pull of the patellar tendon on the tibia, thereby improving the mechanical advantage of the quadriceps muscles for producing knee extension. The patella also provides some protection for the anterior aspect of the knee.

Menisci

The **menisci** are discs of fibrocartilage firmly attached to the superior tibia that deepen the concavities of the tibial plateaus **(Fig. 11-2D)**. They serve several functions, such as absorption and dissipation of force, lubrication and nourishment of the joint structures, and congruency of the

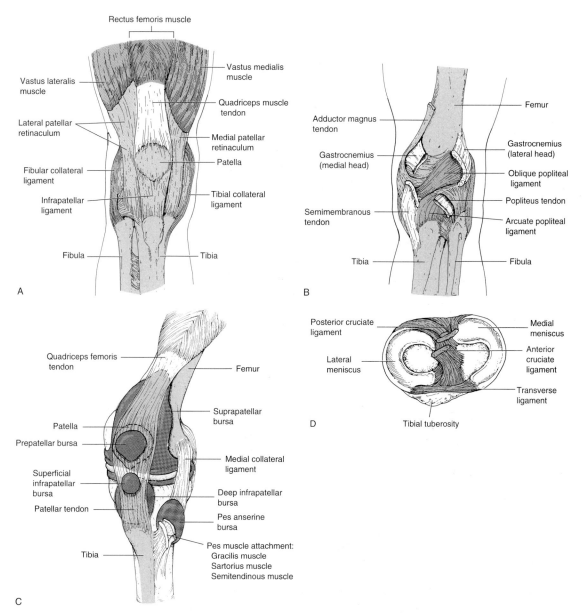

➤ FIGURE 11-2. The knee. **A.** Ligaments of the knee (anterior view). **B.** Ligaments of the knee (posterior view-superficial and deep structures). **C.** Bursae of the knee. **D.** Superior surface of tibia with menisci and associated structures.

joint surfaces to improve weight distribution. The medial meniscus is more frequently injured than the lateral meniscus, partly because the medial meniscus is more securely attached to the tibia and, therefore, less mobile.

Ligaments

Because the shallow articular surfaces of the tibiofemoral joint contribute little to knee stability, the stabilizing role of the ligaments crossing the knee is significant. Two major ligaments of the knee are the anterior and posterior **cruciate ligaments**. The name *cruciate* reflects the fact that these ligaments cross each other, and *anterior* and *posterior* refer to their respective tibial attachments. These ligaments restrict the anterior and posterior sliding of the femur on the tibial plateaus during knee flexion and extension, and they also limit knee hyperextension.

The anterior cruciate (ACL) is considered to be the weaker of the two ligaments and is frequently subject to deceleration injuries.

The medial and lateral **collateral ligaments** are referred to, respectively, as the tibial and fibular collateral ligaments after their distal attachments. The medial collateral ligament resists medially directed shear (valgus) and rotational forces acting on the knee. The lateral collateral ligament resists laterally directed shear (varus) forces and contributes to lateral stability of the knee.

Joint Capsule and Bursa

The joint capsule at the knee is large and lax, encompassing both the tibiofemoral and patellofemoral joints. Anteriorly, it extends above the patella to attach along the edges of the superior patellar surface. The deep bursa formed by this capsule above the patella, the suprapatellar bursa, is the largest bursa in the body **(Fig. 11-2C)**. It lies between the femur and quadriceps femoris tendon and it reduces friction between the two structures. Posteriorly, the subpopliteal bursa lies between the lateral condyle of the femur and popliteal muscle, and the semimembranosus bursa lies between the medial head of the gastrocnemius and semimembranosus tendons.

Three other key bursae associated with the knee, but not contained in the joint capsule, are the prepatellar, superficial infrapatellar, and deep infrapatellar bursae. The prepatellar bursa is located between the skin and anterior surface of the patella, allowing free movement of the skin over the patella during flexion and extension. The superficial infrapatellar bursa is located between the skin and patellar tendon. Inflammation of this bursa caused by excessive kneeling is sometimes referred to as "housemaid's knee." The deep infrapatellar bursa is located between the tibial tubercle and the infrapatellar tendon and is separated from the joint cavity by the infrapatellar fat pad. This bursa reduces friction between the ligament and the bony tubercle.

Muscles

The muscles of the knee develop tension to produce motion at the knee and also contribute to the knee's stability. The primary motions permitted at the tibiofemoral joint are flexion and extension **(Fig. 11-3)**. Knee flexion is primarily carried out by the hamstrings, also assisted by the popliteus, gastrocnemius, gracilis, and sartorius. In addition, the flexor musculature has a secondary responsibility of rotating the tibia. The flexors attaching on the tibia's medial side (e.g., semitendinosus, semimembranosus, gracilis, and sartorius) internally rotate the tibia, while those attaching on the lateral side (e.g., biceps femoris) externally rotate the tibia. Knee extension is carried out by the quadriceps femoris muscle group. Refer to **Figure 10-4** to view the primary muscles that move the knee.

During flexion/extension movements, the patella glides superiorly and inferiorly against the distal end of the femur in a primarily vertical direction with an excursion of as much as 8 cm. The patella also undergoes medial and lateral displacement as the tibia is rotated laterally and medially, respectively. Tracking of the patella against the femur depends on the direction of the net force produced by the attached quadriceps. The vastus lateralis tends to pull the patella laterally in the direction of the muscle's action line, parallel to the femoral shaft. The iliotibial band and lateral extensor retinaculum also exert a lateral force on the patella. Although considerable debate exists over the role of the vastus medialis oblique (VMO), it seems to oppose the lateral pull of the vastus lateralis, thereby keeping the patella centered in the patellofemoral groove. If the magnitude of the force produced by the vastus lateralis exceeds that produced by the VMO, the patella is pulled laterally out of its groove during tracking. Mistracking of the patella during knee movement can lead to pain and dysfunction.

Nerves and Blood Vessels of the Knee

The tibial nerve is the largest and most medial branch of the sciatic nerve. It innervates all of the muscles in the hamstring group, except the short head of the biceps femoris, and then continues to supply all of the remaining posterior muscles in the lower leg **(Fig. 11-4)**. The common peroneal nerve is the lateral branch of the sciatic nerve. It innervates the short head of the biceps femoris, then passes through the popliteal fossa, winds around the head of the fibula, and divides into the superficial and deep peroneal nerves, with an articular branch to the knee. The femoral nerve courses down the anterior aspect of the thigh to supply the quadriceps group and the sartorius.

Just proximal to the knee, the main branch of the femoral artery becomes the popliteal artery. The popliteal artery then courses through the popliteal fossa and branches to form the medial and lateral superior genicular, the middle genicular, and the medial and lateral inferior genicular arteries to supply the knee **(Fig. 11-5)**.

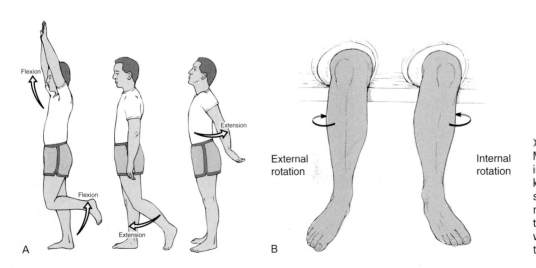

➤ **FIGURE 11-3.** Motions at the knee. **A.** Flexion and extension of the knee. **B.** Supination of the subtalar joint in the foot results in external rotation of the tibia. Pronation is linked with internal rotation of the tibia.

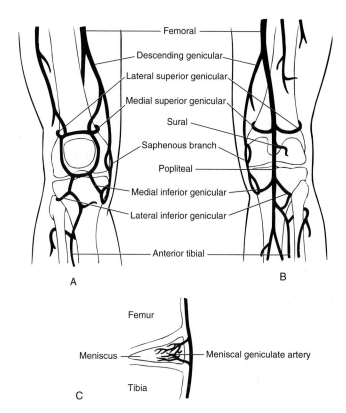

➤ **FIGURE 11-4.** The innervation of the knee. **A.** Anterior view. **B.** Posterior view.

➤ **FIGURE 11-5.** Collateral circulation around the knee. **A.** Anterior view. **B.** Posterior view. **C.** Circulation to meniscus.

PREVENTION OF INJURIES

Prevention of knee injuries must focus on a well-rounded physical conditioning program because many of the muscles that move the knee also move the hip. Although much debate continues as to the effectiveness of prophylactic knee braces, recent rule changes and improved shoe design have contributed significantly to a reduction in knee injuries.

Protective Equipment

Knee braces fall into three broad functional categories: prophylactic, functional, and rehabilitative **(Fig. 11-6)**. Prophylactic knee braces (PKBs) are designed to protect the medial collateral ligament (MCL) by redirecting a lateral valgus force away from the joint itself to points more distal on the tibia and femur. This is done via a single or bilateral bar design. Functional knee braces are widely used to protect moderate anterior cruciate ligament (ACL) injuries and in postsurgical ACL ligament repair or reconstruction cases. Rehabilitative braces provide absolute immobilization at a selected angle after surgery, permit controlled range of motion through predetermined arcs, and prevent accidental loading in non–weight-bearing patients.

The routine use of PKBs has not been proven effec-

tive in reducing the number or severity of knee injuries. In some instances, PKBs may have been a contributing factor to the injury. Functional braces, commonly called derotation braces, may be prescribed by a physician for individuals who have a mild to moderate degree of instability and who participate in activities with low or moderate load potential. Functional knee braces do not guarantee increased stability in sports that require cutting, pivoting, or other quick changes in direction.[1]

Patella braces are designed to dissipate force, maintain patellar alignment, and improve patellar tracking. A horseshoe-type silicone or felt pad is sewn into an elastic or neoprene sleeve to relieve tension in recurring patellofemoral subluxation or dislocations **(Fig. 11-7A)**. An alternative brace for treating patellar pain is a strap worn over the infrapatellar ligament **(Fig. 11-7B)**.

Proper shoe design can also prevent injury. In field sports, shoes may have a flat sole, long cleat, short cleat, or a multicleated design (see **Fig. 12-14**). The cleats should be positioned properly under the major weight-bearing joints of the foot and should not be felt through the sole of the shoe. Research has shown that shoes with the longer irregular cleats placed at the peripheral margin of the sole with a number of smaller pointed cleats in the middle produce higher torsional resistance and are associated with a significantly higher ACL injury rate compared with shoe models that have flat cleats and screw-in cleats or pivot disk models.[2] In football, a cleated shoe with a higher number of shorter, broader cleats can prevent the

FIELD STRATEGY 11.1   EXERCISES TO PREVENT INJURY AT THE KNEE

A. **Hamstrings stretch, seated position.** Place the leg to be stretched straight out with the opposite foot tucked toward the groin. Reach toward the toes until a stretch is felt.

B. **Quadriceps stretch, prone position.** Push the heel toward the buttocks, then raise the knee off the floor until tension is felt.

C. **Iliotibial band stretch, supine position.** With the trunk stabilized, adduct the leg to be stretched over the other leg, and allow gravity to passively stretch the iliotibial band.

D. **Iliotibial band stretch, standing position.** Cross the limb to be stretched behind the other, extending and adducting the hip as far as possible.

E. **Closed-chain exercises:**

   1. Step ups, step downs, and lateral step ups

   2. Squats (Never below 85–90°)

   3. Leg press

   4. Lunges

F. **Open-chain exercises:**

   1. Knee extension (quadriceps)

   2. Knee flexion (hamstrings)

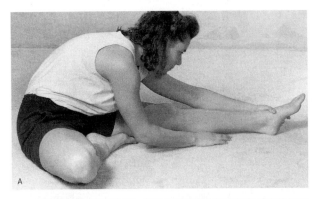

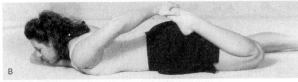

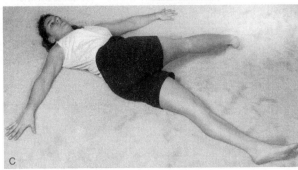

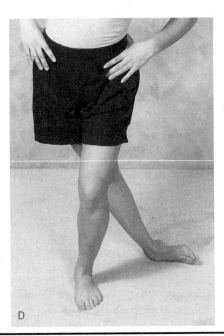

foot from becoming fixed to the ground, yet it still allows for good traction on running and cutting maneuvers. Refer to **Box 12-1** for guidelines in fitting shoes.

Physical Conditioning

The development of a well-rounded physical conditioning program is the key to injury prevention. Exercises should work toward flexibility and muscular strength, endurance, and power, as well as speed, agility, balance, and cardiovascular fitness. Stretching exercises should focus on the quadriceps, hamstrings, gastrocnemius, iliotibial (IT) band, and adductors. Because many of these muscles contribute to knee stability, strengthening programs should also focus on these muscle groups. Specific exercises to prevent injury are provided in **Field Strategy 11-1**. Additional exercises for muscles that cross the hip region were demonstrated in Field Strategy 10-1.

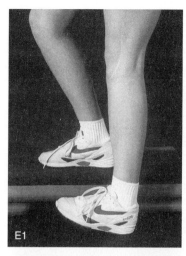

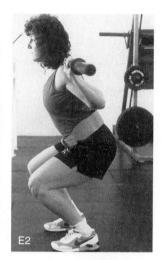

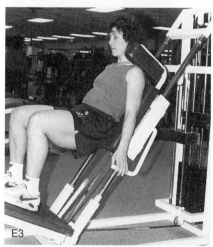

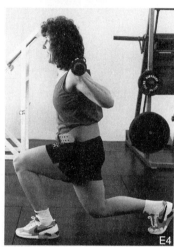

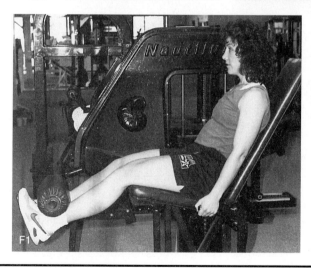

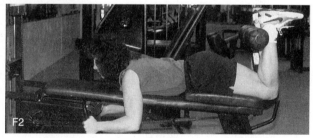

SUPERFICIAL WOUNDS

Because of the very nature of many contact and collision sports, superficial wounds at the knee are common. In most cases, the injuries can be handled on site by following standard acute-care protocol. If, however, the condition does not improve within 48 hours, the athlete should be referred to a physician for further care.

Contusions

Contusions resulting from compressive forces (i.e., a kick, getting hit with a ball, or falling on the knee) are common injuries at the knee.

SIGNS AND SYMPTOMS

General signs and symptoms include localized tenderness, pain, swelling, and ecchymosis. If swelling is exten-

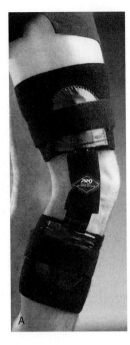
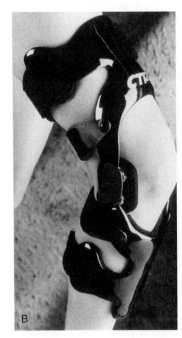
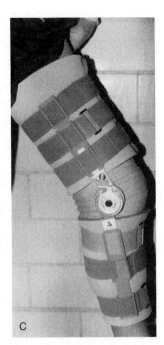

➤ FIGURE 11-6. Knee braces. **A.** Prophylactic knee braces may be a single or bilateral bar design and are used to protect the medial (tibial) collateral ligament. **B.** Functional knee braces control tibial translation and rotational stress relative to the femur, and can provide extension limitations to protect the ACL. **C.** Rehabilitative braces provide absolute or relative immobilization following surgery.

sive, other injuries may be obscured. For example, being kicked on the proximal tibia or fibula may appear as a contusion, when in fact the impact may have caused an avulsion fracture of one of the collateral ligaments or resulted in an epiphyseal injury in an adolescent.

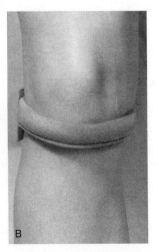

➤ FIGURE 11-7. Patellofemoral braces. **A.** A horseshoe-type silicone or felt pad sewn into a sleeve can relieve chronic patella pain. **B.** A strap worn over the infrapatellar ligament may also relieve patellar pain.

MANAGEMENT

Follow standard acute protocol with ice, compression, elevation, and relative rest. Extreme point tenderness and positive findings on fracture tests often indicate a more serious injury, and referral to a physician is indicated.

Bursitits

Bursitis may be caused by direct trauma, infections, or metabolic disorders. The most commonly injured bursa is the prepatellar bursa because of its location on the anterior surface of the patella.

SIGNS AND SYMPTOMS

Swelling may occur immediately or over a 24-hour period, obscuring the visible outline of the patella **(Fig. 11-8)**. Direct pressure over the bursa and passive flexion of the knee lead to considerable pain. In contrast to inflammations of the prepatellar bursa, inflammations of the deep infrapatellar bursa and pes anserinus bursa (see **Fig. 11-2**) are usually caused by overuse and subsequent friction when local tendons are compressed against the underlying bone.

MANAGEMENT

Treatment consists of cryotherapy, a compressive wrap, nonsteroidal anti-inflammatory medication (NSAIDs), avoidance of activities that irritate the condition, or total rest until acute symptoms subside. A protective foam pad may protect the area from further insult. If signs of infection become

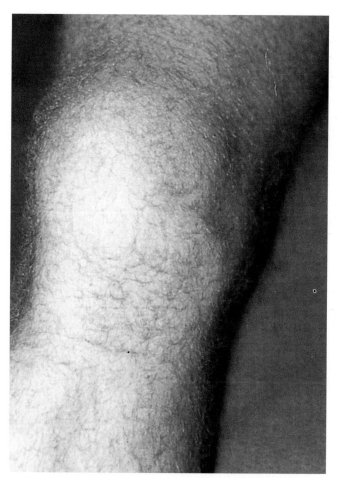

➤ FIGURE 11-8. Prepatellar bursitis. The prepatellar bursa is commonly injured by compression from a direct blow, or during a fall on a flexed knee. When injured, the bursa appears grossly distended and swollen.

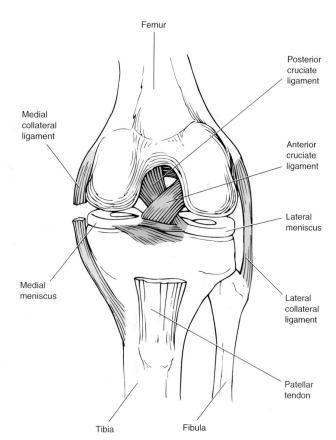

➤ FIGURE 11-9. Valgus instability. When a valgus force is applied to the knee, the tibial collateral ligament and medial capsular ligaments are damaged, leading to valgus laxity.

apparent, or if the joint appears grossly distended and warm to the touch, refer the individual to a physician.

LIGAMENTOUS INJURIES

Knee joint stability depends primarily on a static system of support from its ligaments and capsular structures rather than from the surrounding muscles. Bones and menisci provide some additional stability via their shape and inherent stability. The knee position at impact and the direction in which the tibia displaces or rotates after impact denote what structures are damaged. At this level of understanding, ligamentous injuries are described based on unidirectional or straight laxity.

Unidirectional Instabilities

In straight medial laxity, or **valgus laxity**, lateral forces cause tension on the medial aspect of the knee, potentially damaging the medial (tibial) collateral ligament (MCL), posterior oblique ligament, and posteromedial capsular ligaments **(Fig. 11-9)**.

Straight lateral laxity, or **varus laxity**, results from medial forces that produce tension on the lateral aspect of the knee, damaging the lateral (fibular) collateral ligament, lateral capsular ligaments, and joint structures **(Fig. 11-10)**.

With straight anterior laxity, the anterior cruciate ligament (ACL) is damaged **(Fig. 11-11)**. Isolated anterior laxity is rare. Instead, an anteromedial or anterolateral laxity usually occurs. Damage to the ACL commonly occurs during a cutting or turning maneuver, landing, or sudden deceleration. The rate of ACL injuries is higher in women, particularly those in jumping and pivoting sports. This higher rate may be caused by extrinsic factors, such as skill level, level of experience, muscular strength imbalances, shoe-surface interface, and use of ankle prophylactic braces; or it may be the result of intrinsic factors, such as ligament size, joint laxity, limb alignment, notch dimensions, and estrogen.[3]

In straight posterior laxity, the tibia is displaced posteriorly, damaging the posterior cruciate ligament (PCL) **(Fig. 11-12)**. Hyperextension is the most common mechanism, although the ligament can also be damaged when the knee is flexed and the upper tibia is driven posteriorly, such as when a hockey player collides with the boards.

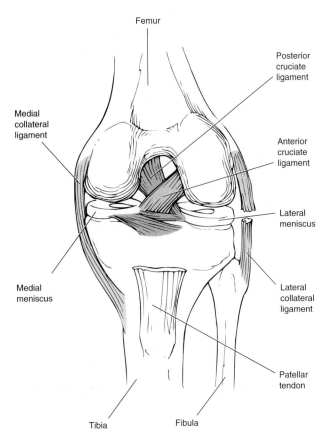

➤ **FIGURE 11-10.** Varus instability. An isolated varus force can damage the fibular collateral ligament leading to varus laxity.

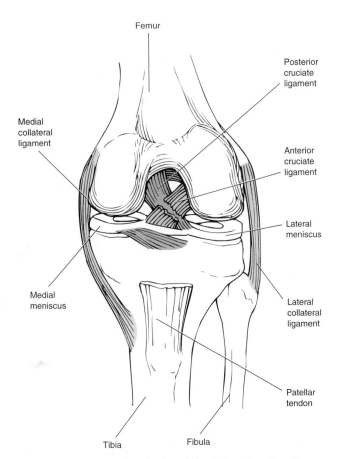

➤ **FIGURE 11-11.** Anterior instability. When changing directions during deceleration, as occurs in basketball, the anterior cruciate ligament can be damaged.

SIGNS AND SYMPTOMS

If the medial collateral ligament is injured, pain and swelling are localized on the medial joint line. If the lateral collateral ligament is injured, swelling and pain are limited to the lateral knee. However, if pain is detected on the head of the fibula, an avulsion fracture should be suspected. With an anterior cruciate injury, pain is often described as being deep in the knee, but it is more often felt anteriorly on either side of the patellar tendon. Joint effusion is typically mixed with blood and may not become evident until 24 hours postinjury, even if standard acute care is followed. With a posterior cruciate injury, intense pain and a sense of stretching are felt in the posterior aspect of the knee. Effusion and **hemarthrosis** occur rapidly, and knee extension is limited because of the effusion and stretching of the posterior capsule and gastrocnemius. **Box 11-1** explains the signs and symptoms seen in various stages of ligament failure.

MANAGEMENT

Injuries involving minimal ligament failure are managed conservatively with ice application, compression, elevation, and protected rest until acute symptoms subside. A compression wrap, consisting of an inverted horseshoe around the patella secured by an elastic wrap, can be used with a knee immobilizer to reduce swelling. How-

ever, the knee immobilizer should be removed while the patient is sleeping. In a moderate injury with partial ligament failure, ice, compression, elevation, and protected rest should be continued for 24 to 72 hours. Crutches are used until the individual can walk without a limp. Progression to partial weight bearing with heel-to-toe gait can begin as tolerated. In ligament injuries in which complete ligament failure has occurred or in which more than one major ligament is involved, referral to an orthopedist is warranted for possible surgical repair.

KNEE DISLOCATION

Knee dislocations and less severe multiple-ligament injuries make up about 20% of all grade III knee ligament injuries. To dislocate the knee, at least three ligaments must be torn. Most often, this involves the ACL, PCL, and one collateral ligament. Although dislocations can occur in any direction, the most common is in an anterior or posterior direction. As with any dislocation, additional damage can occur to other joint structures, including the ligaments, capsular structures, menisci, articular surfaces, tendons, and neurovascular structures. Associated injuries include vascular damage in 20 to 40% and nerve damage in 20 to 30% of all knee dislocations. Posterior

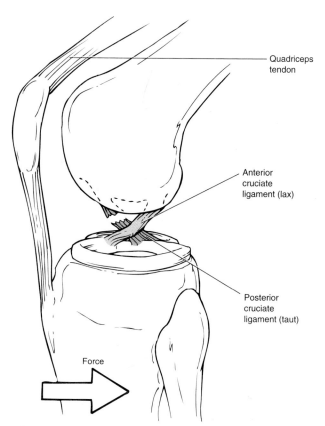

➤ FIGURE 11-12. Posterior instability. During hyperextension of the knee or when the knee is flexed and the tibia is driven posteriorly, the posterior cruciate ligament can be damaged.

➤ ➤ BOX 11-1

Signs and Symptoms of Ligament Failure

MINIMAL LIGAMENT FAILURE (< 5 MM DISTRACTION)
- Less than one third of the fibers are torn
- Mild swelling and pain are localized over the injury site (with the MCL, pain is in the proximal 1 to 2 inches)
- Range of motion is normal, but muscular strength may be slightly decreased

PARTIAL LIGAMENT FAILURE (5–10 MM DISTRACTION)
- One third to two thirds of the ligament has been damaged, with microtears present
- Localized swelling and joint effusion may be caused by deep capsular tears, meniscal damage, or cruciate ligament damage
- Pain is sharp and can be either transient or lasting
- Individual may report instability and an inability to walk with the heel on the ground
- Range of motion is decreased initially by pain and hamstring muscle spasm, then later by soft tissue swelling or effusion
- Individual is unable to fully extend the knee actively

COMPLETE LIGAMENT FAILURE (< 10 MM DISTRACTION)
- More than two thirds of the ligament has been ruptured
- Swelling is diffuse, indicating severe capsular tear and damage to intracapsular structures
- Pain is initially sharp and often disappears within a minute
- Individual is aware of the feeling of instability or the knee giving way
- Significant loss of range of motion

knee dislocations are associated with the highest incidence of damage to the popliteal artery.

SIGNS AND SYMPTOMS

An athlete may describe feeling a severe injury to the knee and hearing a loud pop. Deformity of the knee may be present if the knee dislocated and remained unreduced. Unfortunately, knee dislocations often reduce spontaneously, making identification difficult. Swelling occurs within the first few hours, but the swelling may not be large due to an associated capsular injury and extravasation of the hemarthrosis.

MANAGEMENT

This injury is considered a medical emergency. Emergency medical services (EMS) should be initiated immediately. Do not move the athlete. Check the distal circulation at the posterior tibial artery and dorsalis pedis artery at the foot. Stroke the anterior and posterior lower leg and foot to make sure the athlete has normal sensation. Cover the athlete to maintain body temperature, treat for shock, and wait for the ambulance to arrive. If a vascular injury is present and left untreated or not repaired within 8 hours after injury, there is an 86%

amputation rate. If surgery is completed within 6 to 8 hours, the amputation rate drops to 11%. Associated nerve injury has a poor prognosis, regardless of the treatment.

MENISCAL INJURIES

Menisci, which become stiffer and less resilient with age, are injured similar to ligamentous structures. In addition to compression and tensile forces, shearing forces caused when the femur rotates on a fixed tibia trap the posterior horns of both menisci, leading to some tearing. Peak incidence of injuries occurs in men between the ages of 21 and 40 years and in girls and women between the ages of 11 and 20 years and between 61 and 70 years.[4] Medial meniscus damage is more common than lateral meniscus damage.

SIGNS AND SYMPTOMS

Meniscal injuries are difficult to assess because of the limited sensory nerve supply, and only the outer 10 to 33% is supplied by blood.[5] Localized pain and joint-line tenderness near the collateral ligament are probably the most common findings. The athlete may experience a popping, grinding, or clicking sensation that can lead to the knee buckling or giving way, causing the athlete to stumble or fall. In addition, the individual has difficulty doing a deep squat or a duck walk.

MANAGEMENT

Mild cases of pain and swelling can be managed with standard acute care ice, compression, elevation, protected rest, and crutches as needed. If joint effusion is extensive, aspiration of the fluid by a physician may be necessary. Occasionally, the meniscal tear may lodge in the knee joint, causing the knee to lock in place. When the knee cannot be spontaneously reduced, surgical intervention is necessary.

PATELLA AND RELATED INJURIES

The patellofemoral joint is the region most commonly associated with anterior knee pain. Patellar tracking disorders and instability within the joint, along with overweight, direct trauma, and repetitive motions, contribute to a variety of injuries. The quadriceps mechanism, more accurately called the **extensor mechanism**, places the femur and patella in specific positions to provide stability and function at the knee **(Fig. 11-13)**. The VMO is the dynamic medial stabilizer that resists lateral displacement of the patella. Atrophy of this muscle is nearly always evident in patellofemoral dysfunction. Another factor that can contribute to patellofemoral pain is an increased Q-angle, as discussed in Chapter 10. A Q-angle less than 13° or greater than 18° is considered abnormal and can predispose the sport participant to patellar injuries or degeneration.

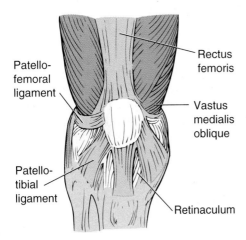

➤ FIGURE 11-13. The extensor mechanism. The extensor mechanism is composed of dynamic and static stabilizers. Working together, they combine rolling and gliding motions to place the femur and patella in specific positions to effect the deceleration mechanism of the patellofemoral articulation to provide stability and function at the knee.

Patellofemoral ligament

Rectus femoris

Vastus medialis oblique

Patello-tibial ligament

Retinaculum

Patellofemoral Stress Syndrome

Patellofemoral stress syndrome occurs when either the VMO is weak or the lateral retinaculum that holds the patella firmly to the femoral condyle is excessively tight. In either case, the end result is lateral excursion of the patella. The condition is found more commonly in women because of their higher Q-angle.

SIGNS AND SYMPTOMS

Pain often results when a tense lateral retinaculum passes over the trochlear groove. The individual may report a dull, aching pain in the anterior knee made worse by squatting, sitting in a tight space with the knee flexed, or descending stairs or slopes. Point tenderness can be located over the lateral edge of the patella. Intense pain and crepitus is elicited when the patella is manually compressed into the patellofemoral groove.

MANAGEMENT

Treatment involves standard acute care and NSAIDs. Performing strengthening exercises for the VMO, normalizing patella mobility, and increasing flexibility and muscle control of the entire lower extremity are essential for full recovery. Patellofemoral support devices may be used to prevent lateral displacement of the patella **(Fig. 11-7)**.

Chondromalacia Patellae

Chondromalacia patellae is a true degenerative change in the articular cartilage of the patella. This condition occurs when compressive forces exceed the normal range or when alterations in patellar excursion produce abnormal shear forces that damage the articular surface. Because articular cartilage does not contain nerve endings, chondromalacia should not be considered the true source of anterior knee pain. (Chrondromalcia is a surgical finding that represents areas of hyaline cartilage trauma or aberrant loading, but it is not the cause of pain.)

SIGNS AND SYMPTOMS

Generalized anterior knee pain and crepitus are present in activities such as walking up and down stairs or doing deep knee bends. Localized pain and tenderness can be palpated on the medial and lateral patellar borders. Pain and crepitus increase with active and resisted knee extension.

MANAGEMENT

Asymptomatic chondromalacia does not require treatment. If it is symptomatic, standard acute-care protocol and mild NSAIDs, medial quadriceps strengthening, and a hamstrings flexibility program may be implemented. Exercises such as crouches or deep-knee bends should be avoided because these positions can aggravate the condition. A knee sleeve with a patellar cutout may help some individuals.

Acute Patellar Subluxation and Dislocation

A subluxation or dislocation of the patella commonly occurs during deceleration with a cutting maneuver. During this action, the patella moves laterally and may tear the medial muscular and retinaculum attachments from the medial aspect of the patella.

SIGNS AND SYMPTOMS

There is an immediate audible pop and violent collapse of the knee. In addition to soft tissue damage, the lateral femoral condyle and medial patellar bone may be bruised. The patella can remain dislocated or can spontaneously reduce, leaving a painful, swollen, tender knee.

MANAGEMENT

The individual resists any attempt to displace the patella laterally (positive patellar apprehension test). Immediate treatment includes ice, elevation, immobilization, and immediate referral to a physician.

Patellar Tendinitis (Jumper's Knee)

The patellar tendon frequently becomes inflamed and tender from repetitive or eccentric knee extension activities, such as in running and jumping, hence the name "jumper's knee."

SIGNS AND SYMPTOMS

Initially, pain after activity is concentrated on the inferior pole of the patella, but it also occurs at the insertion of the patellar tendon into the tibial tubercle (**Fig. 11-14**).

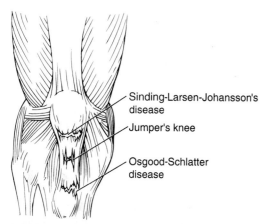

Sinding-Larsen-Johansson's disease

Jumper's knee

Osgood-Schlatter disease

▶ FIGURE 11-14. Patellar tendon conditions. Patellar tendon conditions may involve Sinding-Larsen-Johansson disease, patellar tendinitis, or Osgood-Schlatter disease. The location of pain typically defines which problem is present.

> ▶ ▶ BOX 11-2
>
> ### Signs and Symptoms of Patellar Tendinitis
> - Initially, pain after activity is concentrated on the inferior pole of the patella or the distal attachment of the patellar tendon on the tibial tubercle
> - As the condition progresses, pain is present at the start of activity, subsides with warm-up, then reappears after activity
> - Pain is present while ascending and descending stairs
> - Pain occurs on passive knee flexion beyond 120° and during resisted knee extension

As the condition progresses, pain is present at the beginning of activity, subsides during warm-up, then reappears after activity. Examination reveals point tenderness at the inferior pole of the patella, and less commonly over the body of the patellar tendon (**Box 11-2**).

MANAGEMENT

Immediate treatment includes standard acute care and NSAIDs. Aquatic therapy is useful in early stages to reduce gravitational forces. Eccentric quadriceps strengthening and a stretching program for the quadriceps, hamstrings, plantar flexors, hip flexors, and extensors help absorb some of the strain.

Osgood-Schlatter Disease

Osgood-Schlatter disease (OSD) is a traction-type injury to the tibial apophysis where the patellar tendon attaches onto the tibial tuberosity. OSD typically develops in girls between the ages of 8 and 13 years, and in boys between the ages of 10 and 15 years (at the beginning of their growth spurt).[6]

SIGNS AND SYMPTOMS

The individual points to the tibial tubercle as the source of pain, and the tubercle appears enlarged and prominent. Pain generally occurs during activity and is relieved with rest. Point tenderness can be elicited directly over the tubercle, but range of motion is usually not affected. Pain is present at the extremes of knee extension and forced flexion.

MANAGEMENT

Treatment is symptomatic and self-limiting, but it may take 12 to 24 months to run its course. Shock-absorbent insoles in sports shoes may decrease peak stress on the tendon and tubercle. Icing the knee for 20 minutes after activity may also be beneficial, as is hamstrings and quadriceps stretching. Wrestling gel pads, basketball knee pads, or an Osgood-Sclatter pad may protect the tibial tubercle when kneeling and may prevent repeated contusions to the sensitive area. In most cases, activity is not restricted unless pain is disabling. The condition rectifies itself with closure of the apophysis. A similar condition, Sinding-Larsen-Johansson disease, occurs at the inferior pole of the patella. Treatment is similar to Osgood-Schlatter disease.

ILIOTIBIAL BAND FRICTION SYNDROME

The IT band continues the line of pull from the tensor fascia latae and gluteus maximus muscle to Gerdy's tubercle on the lateral proximal tibia. The band drops posteriorly behind the lateral femoral epicondyle with knee flexion, then snaps forward over the epicondyle during extension **(Fig. 11-15)**. Excessive compression and friction forces over the greater trochanter and lateral femoral condyle can be caused by a large Q-angle, genu valgus, excessive foot pronation, or constantly running on the same side of the street. Most streets are crowned for water runoff; therefore, one leg is always lower than the other, placing considerable strain on lateral joint structures.

SIGNS AND SYMPTOMS
Symptoms are progressive **(Box 11-3)**.

MANAGEMENT
Immediate treatment involves standard acute care and NSAIDs. A flexibility program for the hip abductors, flexors, and lateral thigh muscles should be started immediately.

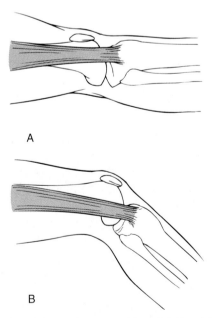

➤ **FIGURE 11-15.** Iliotibial band. The iliotibial band drops posteriorly behind the lateral femoral epicondyle during knee flexion, then snaps forward over the epicondyle during extension. Malalignment problems or constant irritation can inflame the iliotibial band, or lead to bursitis.

> ➤ ➤ **BOX 11-3**
>
> ### Signs and Symptoms of Iliotibial Band Syndrome
> - Initially, pain does not restrict distance or speed
> - As the condition worsens, pain restricts distance and speed, especially during weight-bearing flexion and extension, such as walking down stairs
> - Eventually, pain restricts all running and becomes continuous during activities of daily living
> - Extreme point tenderness is palpated 2 to 3 cm proximal to the lateral joint line over the lateral femoral epicondyle with the leg flexed at 30°
> - Flexion and extension of the knee may produce a creaking sound

FRACTURES

Traumatic fractures around the knee area are rare in sports, unless high-velocity sports such as motorcycling and auto racing are included.

Patella Fractures

SIGNS AND SYMPTOMS
A patella fracture produces diffuse extra-articular swelling on and around the knee. A defect may be palpated and a straight-leg raise is therefore impossible to perform.

MANAGEMENT
Apply ice, elevate, and splint the region with a knee immobilizer. Refer the individual to a physician.

Avulsion Fractures

Avulsion fractures can be caused by compressive forces from direct trauma or by excessive tensile forces.

SIGNS AND SYMPTOMS
The individual has localized pain and tenderness over the bony site, and a fragment may be palpated. If a musculotendinous unit is involved, muscle function is limited. The tibial tuberosity is a common site for apophyseal fractures in boys and may occur because of Osgood-Schlatter disease, which has already been discussed. These injuries are commonly seen in jumping activities like basketball, long jump, high jump, and hurdling. The individual has pain, swelling, and tenderness directly over the tuberosity. When a small fragment of the tuberosity avulses, knee extension is painful and weak.

MANAGEMENT

Treatment involves standard acute care and application of a knee immobilizer. The athlete should be immediately referred to a physician for further care. If necessary, the athlete should be fitted for crutches and instructed to use a non–weight-bearing gait en route to the physician.

Stress Fractures

Stress fractures result from repetitive overload of the bone caused by sudden changes in training intensity, duration, frequency, running surface, or poorly worn shoes.

SIGNS AND SYMPTOMS

The individual reports localized pain, both before and after activity, that is relieved with rest and lack of weight bearing. As the condition progresses, pain becomes more persistent.

MANAGEMENT

Once identified as a stress fracture, treatment involves rest, crutches, or casting. Early bone scans are highly recommended.

Chondral and Osteochondral Fractures

A **chondral fracture** is a fracture involving the articular cartilage at a joint. An **osteochondral fracture** involves the articular cartilage and underlying bone. These fractures occur when compression from a direct blow to the knee causes shearing or forceful rotation. **Osteochondritis dissecans** occurs when a fragment of bone adjacent to the articular surface of a joint is deprived of its blood supply, leading to avascular necrosis. Although found in several joints, it is typically associated with the knee, particularly in males aged 10 to 20 years **(Fig. 11-16).**

SIGNS AND SYMPTOMS

The most common symptom is an aching, diffuse pain or swelling with activity. If the bony fragment has displaced and is free floating within the joint, the knee may momentarily lock.

MANAGEMENT

After standard acute care and immobilization in a splint, the athlete should be referred immediately to a physician for further care. A positive diagnosis is made with a radiograph.

ASSESSMENT OF THE KNEE

The lower extremity works as a unit to provide motion. Several biomechanical problems at the foot directly impact strain on the knee. In addition, the knee plays a

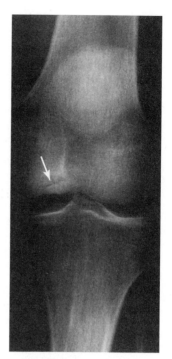

➤ **FIGURE 11-16.** Osteochondritis dissecans. Osteochondritis dissecans occurs when a fragment of bone adjacent to the articular surface of a joint is deprived of its blood supply, leading to avascular necrosis. In this patient, a portion of the medial epicondyle of the femur is damaged.

major role in supporting the body during dynamic and static activities. Furthermore, referred pain from the hip and lumbar spine may also be involved. As such, assessment of the knee complex must encompass an overview of the entire lower extremity. **Box 11-4** identifies conditions that warrant immediate referral to a physician.

History

Many conditions at the knee are related to family history, age, congenital deformities, mechanical dysfunction, and recent changes in training programs, surfaces, or foot attire. Specific questions related to the knee are listed in **Field Strategy 11-2**.

➤ ➤ **BOX 11-4**

Conditions That Necessitate Immediate Referral to a Physician

- Obvious deformity suggesting a dislocation or fracture
- Significant loss of motion or locking of the knee
- Excessive joint swelling
- Gross joint instability
- Reported sounds, such as popping, snapping, or clicking, or giving way of the knee
- Possible epiphyseal injuries
- Abnormal sensations in the leg or foot
- Any unexplained or chronic pain that disrupts an individual's play or performance

FIELD STRATEGY 11.2   DEVELOPING A HISTORY OF THE INJURY

CURRENT INJURY STATUS

1. Where is the pain (or weakness) located? How severe is the pain (weakness)? What type of pain is it? (Dull ache [degenerative problem], stabbing or sharp [mechanical problem], or pain in the morning [arthritic condition]?)

2. Did the pain come on suddenly (acute) or gradually (overuse)? Was the pain greatest when the injury first occurred, or did it get worse the second or third day?

3. (If acute, ask): What position was the knee in when the injury occurred? From what direction, if any, did the traumatic force come from? Was the foot fixed during impact? (If chronic, ask): What different activities have you been doing in the last week? (Look for changes in technique, frequency, duration, intensity, or changes in shoes, equipment, or running surface.)

4. Did you hear any sounds during the incident? Any snaps, pops, or cracks (ligament rupture, patellar dislocation, or osteochondral fracture)? Can you bear weight on the leg or balance on the leg?

5. How soon did the swelling set in? Are there certain activities you are unable to perform because of the pain or swelling?

6. What have you done for the injury?

PAST INJURY STATUS

1. Have you ever injured your knee before? When? How did that occur? What was done at the time of injury?

2. Have you had any medical problems recently? (Look for possible referred pain from the lumbar spine, hip, or ankle). Are you on any medication? Do you have any musculoskeletal problems elsewhere in the body? What shoes do you wear?

Observation and Inspection

Both legs should be clearly visible to denote symmetry, any congenital deformity, swelling, discoloration, hypertrophy, or muscle atrophy. Ask the athlete to bring the shoes he or she normally wears when pain is present. Inspect the sole, heel box, and general condition of the shoe for unusual wear, indicating a biomechanical abnormality that may be affecting the knee.

In an ambulatory patient, observe overall body symmetry. Note any abnormalities in gait (favoring one limb), unusual swelling, or discoloration. Ask the individual to do a deep-knee squat and to step up and down on a low stool or cement block. With the individual sitting on a table, place the injured knee on a folded towel or pillow at 30° flexion to relieve any strain on the joint structures. Inspect the injury site for obvious deformities, discoloration, swelling, and scars that might indicate previous surgery, and note the general condition of the skin. Compare the affected limb with the unaffected limb.

Palpation

Bilateral palpation can determine temperature, swelling, point tenderness, crepitus, deformity, muscle spasm, and cutaneous sensation. Vascular pulses can be taken at the popliteal artery in the posterior knee, or at the ankle (see Chapter 12). Proceed proximal to distal, leaving the most painful area to last. The following structures can be palpated:

- Bony Palpation
  1. Patella
  2. Medial and lateral femoral condyles and epicondyles
  3. Joint line, medial and lateral tibial plateaus, tibial tuberosity, and head of the fibula
- Soft Tissue Palpation
  1. Quadriceps muscles and adductor muscles
  2. Patellar tendon, and medial and lateral collateral ligaments
  3. Posterior joint capsule, popliteus, hamstring muscles, and gastrocnemius

Palpation of bony structures and compression, distraction, and percussion may detect a possible fracture. For example, compression at the distal tibia and fibula causes distraction at the proximal tibiofibular joint. Percussion or tapping on the malleoli and epicondyles of the femur may produce positive fracture signs. If you suspect a fracture, immobilize the joint in a knee immobilizer, or summon EMS if a traction splint is necessary. Assess circulatory and neural integrity distal to the fracture site, and treat for shock until the ambulance arrives.

Special Tests

Perform special tests with the individual in a comfortable position, preferably supine. Pain and muscle spasm can restrict motion and give inaccurate results. Do not force the limb through any sudden motions. It may be necessary to place a rolled towel under the knee to relieve strain on the joint structures.

RANGE OF MOTION TESTS

Active and resisted movements are best with the individual on a table. Stabilize the hip and provide resistance throughout the full range of motion with the individual in a seated position for all motions except knee flexion, which is done in the prone position. As the quadriceps extend the knee, observe any abnormal tibial movement or excessive pain from patellar compression. As always, perform the most painful movements last to prevent painful symptoms from overflowing into the next movement. Perform knee extension and flexion, as well as ankle plantar flexion and dorsiflexion **(Fig. 11-17)**.

Stress Tests

From information gathered during the history, observation, inspection, and palpation, determine which tests most effectively assess the condition. Perform only those tests you believe to be absolutely necessary.

ANTERIOR AND POSTERIOR DRAWER TEST

The anterior cruciate ligament and posterior cruciate ligament should be assessed first before any joint swelling obscures the extent of injury. Have the patient seated while he or she reclines against the room wall. Flex the knee at approximately 90°, and stabilize the foot by placing it under your thigh to prevent any tibial rotation. An alternative position is to have the patient seated at the edge of the table with the foot stabilized between your legs. Place both thumbs on either side of the patella tendon, extending the fingers into the popliteal fossa. Apply alternating anterior and posterior displacement force on the proximal tibia **(Fig. 11-18A)**. Stability can be visualized from a lateral view or palpated with the thumb at the joint line. The test is positive for an anterior cruciate injury if the tibia shifts abnormally anteriorly, and it is positive for a posterior cruciate injury if the tibia shifts abnormally posteriorly.

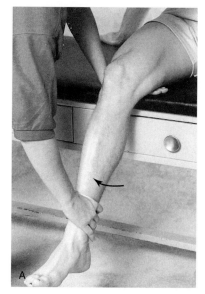

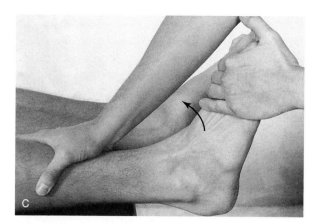

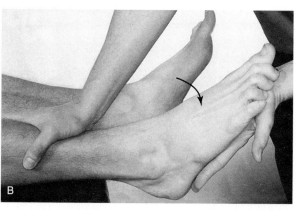

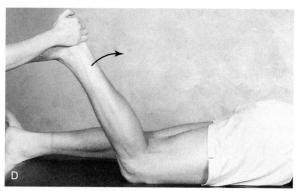

➤ **FIGURE 11-17.** Resisted manual muscle testing. **A.** Knee extension. **B.** Ankle plantar flexion. **C.** Ankle dorsiflexion. **D.** Knee flexion.

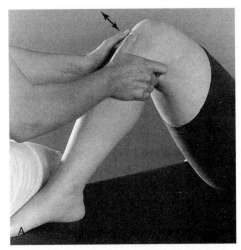

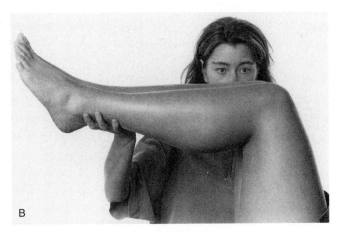

➤ FIGURE 11-18. Cruciate ligament tests. A. Anterior and posterior drawer tests. With the knee flexed, apply an anterior and posterior displacement force on the proximal tibia. B. Posterior sag (gravity) test. Flex both hip and knees. Look from the side and compare the anterior contours of both legs. If one leg sags back and the prominence of the tibial tubercle is lost, the posterior cruciate may be damaged.

GRAVITY DRAWER TEST (POSTERIOR "SAG" SIGN)

One-plane posterior instability can also be tested by flexing the hip and knee at 90°. In this position, the tibia sags back on the femur if the posterior cruciate ligament is torn **(Fig. 11-18B)**. It is important to note the sag because it may produce a false-positive anterior drawer test if the sag goes unnoticed.

VALGUS STRESS TEST

With the individual supine and leg extended, place the heel of one hand on the lateral joint line. The other hand stabilizes the distal lower leg. Apply a lateral or valgus stress at the joint line with the lower leg fully extended, and again at 30° flexion **(Fig. 11-19A)**. If positive (i.e., the tibia abducts), primary damage is to the medial collateral ligament and posteromedial joint structures.

VARUS STRESS TEST

The knee is placed in a similar position as the valgus test; however, a medial or varus stress is applied at the

knee joint **(Fig. 11-19B)**. Laxity in full extension indicates major instability. When testing at 20 to 30° of flexion, the true test for one-plane lateral instability, a positive test indicates damage to the lateral collateral ligament.

MENISCAL TEST

At this level of experience, meniscal injuries are difficult to assess; suspicion is your best tool. Ask the individual to show the maneuver that last reproduced the symptoms. Can they do a deep knee squat? Can they bear weight on the affected limb and cross the opposite foot in front of, and behind, that limb (cross-over test)? You are attempting to trap the torn meniscus in the joint, producing pain and an audible click.

PATELLA APPREHENSION TEST

With the knee in a relaxed position, push the patella laterally **(Fig. 11-20)**. If the individual voluntarily or involuntarily shows apprehension, it is a positive test for subluxating patella.

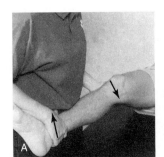
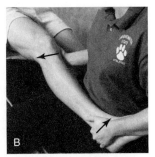

➤ FIGURE 11-19. Valgus and varus stress tests. A. Valgus stress test. With the knee flexed at 30°, apply a gentle valgus stress at the knee joint while moving the lower leg laterally. Repeat the test with the knee fully extended. B. Varus stress test. With the knee flexed at 30°, apply a varus stress at the knee joint while moving the lower leg medially. Repeat the test with the knee fully extended.

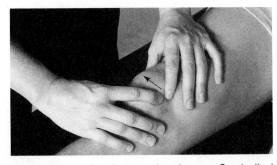

➤ FIGURE 11-20. Patellar apprehension test. Gently displace the patella laterally. The test is a positive sign for subluxating patella if the individual shows apprehension.

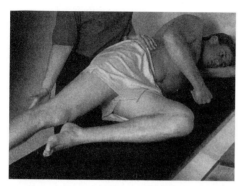

➤ **FIGURE 11-21.** Ober's test for iliotibial band friction syndrome. Passively abduct and slightly extend the hip. Slowly lower the extended leg. If the iliotibial band is tight, the leg remains in the abducted position.

OBER'S TEST FOR ILIOTIBIAL TRACT CONTRACTURE

The individual lies on his or her side with the lower leg slightly flexed at the hip and knee for stability. Stabilize the pelvis with one hand to prevent the pelvis from shifting posteriorly during the test. Passively abduct and slightly extend the hip so the iliotibial tract passes over the greater trochanter **(Fig. 11-21)**. Slowly lower the upper leg. If the iliotibial band is tight, the leg remains in the abducted position.

Functional Tests

Functional tests should be performed pain-free, and the individual should walk without a limp or antalgic gait before returning to participation. Examples of functional tests include forward running, crossover stepping, running figure eights or V-cuts, side-step running, and karioca running. When appropriate, use functional braces or protective supportive devices to prevent reinjury.

Summary

1. The knee (tibiofemoral joint) functions primarily as a modified hinge joint with some lateral and rotational motions allowed.
2. The cruciate ligaments prevent anterior and posterior translation of the tibia on the femur. The ACL is frequently subject to deceleration injuries. The shorter and stronger PCL is considered the primary stabilizer of the knee.
3. The collateral ligaments prevent valgus (medial) and varus (lateral) stress at the knee.

4. The menisci help provide lubrication and nutrition of the joint, reduce friction during movement, provide shock absorption by dissipating stress over the articular cartilage, improve weight distribution, and help the capsule and ligaments prevent hyperextension.
5. Because of its location, the prepatellar bursa is the bursa most commonly injured by compressive forces. The deep infrapatellar bursa, however, is often inflamed by overuse, and subsequent friction results between the infrapatellar tendon and structures behind it (fat pad and tibia).
6. Isolated anterior instability is rare. Instead, an anteromedial or anterolateral laxity usually occurs. The rate of ACL injuries is higher in women, due partially to muscle strength imbalance and to intrinsic and extrinsic factors.
7. Menisci become stiffer and less resilient with age. Because the menisci are not innervated by nerve endings, synovial inflammation and joint effusion may not develop for more than 12 hours after the initial injury.
8. Patellofemoral stress syndrome often occurs when either the VMO is weak or the lateral retinaculum that holds the patella firmly to the femoral condyle is excessively tight. This condition is much more common than chondromalacia patellae, which is a true degeneration in the articular cartilage of the patella.
9. Adolescents are particularly prone to Osgood-Schlatter disease and Sinding-Larsen-Johansson disease.

References

1. Wichman S, and Martin DR. 1996. Bracing for activity. Phys Sportsmed, 24(9):88-94.
2. Moul JL. 1998. Differences in selected predictors of anterior cruciate ligament tears between male and female NCAA Division I collegiate basketball players. J Ath Train, 33(2):118-121.
3. Moeller JL, and Lamb MM. 1997. Anterior cruciate ligament injuries in female athletes: Why are women more susceptible? Phys Sportsmed, 25(4):31-48.
4. Cooper DE, Arnoczky SP, and Warren RF. Arthroscopic meniscal repair. In *Clinics in sports medicine*, edited by KM Singer. Vol. 9, no. 3. Philadelphia: WB Saunders, 1990.
5. Irrgang JJ, Safran MR, and Fu FH. The knee: Ligamentous and meniscal injuries. In *Athletic injuries and rehabilitation*, edited by JE Zachazewski, DJ Magee, and WS Quillen. Philadelphia: WB Saunders, 1996.
6. Wall EJ. 1998. Osgood-Schlatter disease: Practical treatment for a self-limiting condition. Phys Sportsmed, 26(3):29-34.

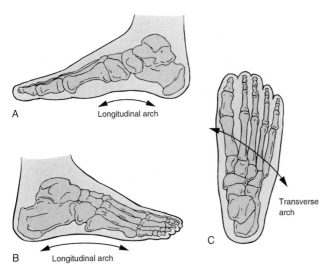

➤ FIGURE 12-10. The arches of the foot. A. Medial view. B. Lateral view. C. Dorsal view.

Protective Equipment

Shin pads made of a high-density foam pad can protect the highly vulnerable anterior tibia. Many styles incorporate padding or plastic shells over the ankle malleoli, which is also subject to repeated contusions. Commercial ankle protectors used to stabilize the ankle joint postinjury may also help reduce chronic ankle sprains (Fig. 12-13). Lace-up braces have been shown to limit all ankle motions, whereas a semirigid orthosis or an air bladder style brace limit only inversion and eversion. Although strapping the ankle with adhesive tape may restrict inver-

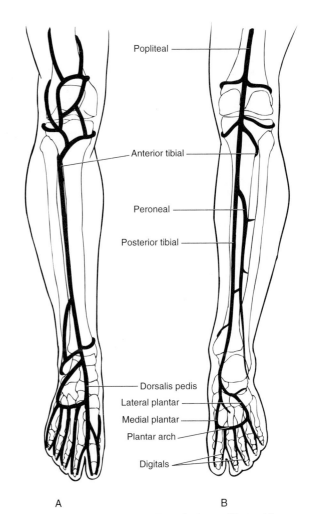

➤ FIGURE 12-12. Blood supply to the leg, ankle, and foot region. A. The dorsalis pedis artery is easily palpated in the midfoot region between the second and third tendons of the extensor digitorum longus. B. The posterior tibial artery can be palpated just posterior to the medial malleolus.

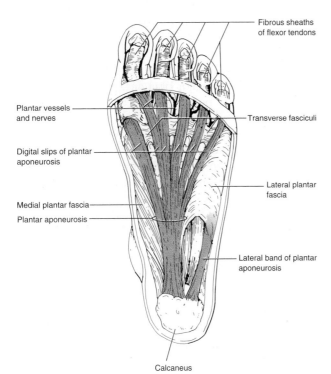

➤ FIGURE 12-11. Plantar fascia. The plantar fascia stores mechanical energy each time the foot deforms during the weight-bearing phase of the gait cycle.

sion and eversion, tape tends to lose maximal protection after 20 minutes or more of exercise. Therefore, ankle braces are more effective in reducing ankle injuries, are easier for the wearer to apply independently, do not produce some of the skin irritation problems associated with adhesive tape, provide better comfort and fit, do not adversely affect performance, and may be more cost effective.

Style, selection, and fit of shoes may also affect injuries to the lower extremity. In field sports, shoes may have a flat sole, long cleat, short cleat, or a multicleated design (Fig. 12-14). The cleats should be positioned properly under the major weight-bearing joints of the foot and should not be felt through the sole of the shoe. Shoes with the longer irregular cleats placed at the peripheral margin of the sole with smaller pointed cleats positioned in the middle of the sole produce significantly higher torsional resistance and are associated with a significantly higher anterior cruciate ligament injury rate compared with shoe models with flat cleats, screw-in cleats, or pivot

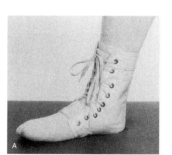
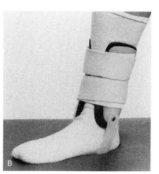
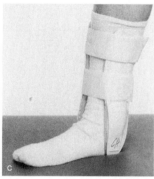

➤ **FIGURE 12-13.** Ankle protectors. Commercial designs include the lace-up brace **(A)**, semirigid orthosis **(B)**, and an air bladder brace **(C)**.

disk models.[1] When increased temperatures are a factor, such as when playing on turf, only the flat-soled basketball-style turf shoe had low-release coefficients at varying elevated temperatures.[2] In individuals with arch problems, the shoe should include adequate forefoot, arch, and heel support. **Box 12-1** lists several important points to remember when purchasing athletic shoes.

Physical Conditioning

In addition to external protection and properly fitted shoes, a flexibility and strengthening program should be initiated before any sport participation. A tight Achilles

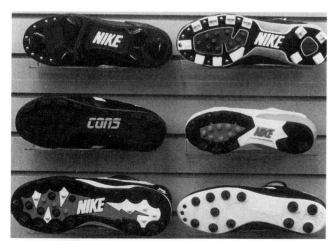

➤ **FIGURE 12-14.** Cleated shoes. Athletic shoes have long cleats, short cleats, or a multicleated design. Selection depends on the surface and weather conditions.

➤ ➤ **BOX 12-1**

Factors in the Selection and Fit of Athletic Shoes

- Fit shoes toward late afternoon or evening, preferably after a workout, and wear socks typically worn during sport participation.
- Fit shoes to the longest toe of the largest foot, providing one thumb's width to the end of the toe box.
- The widest part of the shoe should coincide with the widest part of the foot. Eyelets should be at least 1 inch apart with normal lacing. Women with big or wider feet should consider purchasing boy's or men's shoes.
- The sole of the shoe should provide moderate support but should not be too rigid. Sole tread typically comes in a horizontal bar (commonly used on asphalt or concrete) or waffle design (used on off-road terrain).
- The midsole should be composed of ethylene vinyl acetate (EVA), polyurethane, or preferably, a combination of the two. EVA provides good cushioning but breaks down over time. Polyurethane has minimal compressibility and provides good durability and stability.
- A thermoplastic heel counter maintains its shape and firmness even in adverse weather conditions.
- Running shoes should position the heel at least 1/2 inch above the outsole to minimize stretch on the Achilles tendon.
- While wearing the shoes, approximate athletic skills (walking, running, jumping, and changing directions).
- Individuals with specific conditions need special shoes, such as:
  - Runners with normal feet—more forefoot and toe flexibility
  - Overpronation—greater control on the medial side
  - Achilles tendinitis—at least a 15-mm heel wedge
  - Court sports—added side-to-side stability
  - High, rigid arches—soft midsoles, curved lasts, and low or moderate hindfoot stability
  - Normal arches—firm midsole, semicurved lasts, and moderate hindfoot stability
  - Flexible low arch—very firm midsole, straight last, and strong hindfoot stability
- After purchasing the shoes, walk in the shoes for 2 to 3 days to allow them to adapt to the feet. Then begin running or practicing in the shoes for about 25 to 30% of the workout. To prevent blisters, gradually extend the length of time the shoes are worn.
- Avid runners should replace shoes every 3 months; recreational runners, every 6 months.

tendon increases the risk of plantar fasciitis, Achilles tendinitis, and lateral ankle sprains. To build strength in the foot, for example, pick up marbles or dice with the toes and place them in a container close to the foot. Place a tennis ball between the soles of the feet and roll the ball back and forth from the heel to the forefoot. To increase strength in the lower leg muscles, secure elastic tubing

FIELD STRATEGY 12.1   EXERCISES TO PREVENT INJURY TO THE LOWER LEG

A. Foot Intrinsic Muscle Exercises
1. **Plantar fascia stretch**. Place a towel around the toes and slowly overextend the toes. To stretch the Achilles tendon, dorsiflex the ankle.
2. **Towel crunches**. Place a towel between the plantar surfaces of the toes and feet. Push the toes and feet together, crunching the towel between the toes.
3. **Toe curls**. With the foot resting on a towel, slowly curl the toes under, bunching the towel beneath the foot. Variation: use two feet, a book, or a small weight on the towel for added resistance.
4. **Picking up objects**. Pick up small objects such as marbles or dice with the toes and place in a nearby container, or use therapeutic putty to work the toe flexors.
5. **Shin curls**. Slide the plantar surface of the foot up the opposite shin, moving distal to proximal.
6. **Unilateral balance activities**. Stand on uneven surfaces with the eyes first open, then closed.
7. **BAPS board**. Seated position: roll the board slowly clockwise, then counterclockwise 20 times.

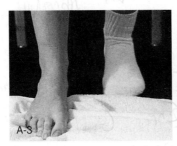

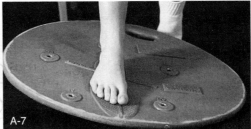

(Continued)

ANKLE SPRAINS

In basketball, ankle sprains comprise more than 45% of all injuries, and in soccer up to 31% of all injuries are ankle sprains.[3] Uneven terrain, stepping in a hole, landing on another player's foot and sliding off the side, or muscle strength imbalance are all contributing factors to sprains in this vulnerable area.

Inversion Ankle Sprains

Acute inversion ankle sprains commonly occur when stress is applied to the ankle during plantar flexion and inversion. If the strain continues, the medial malleolus acts as a fulcrum to further invert and stretch or rupture the lateral ligaments **(Fig. 12-15)**. The peroneal tendons can absorb some strain to prevent this ligament from being injured; however, if the peroneal muscles are weak, they are unable to stabilize the joint.

around a table leg, place the foot in an elastic loop, and move the foot or leg through the range of motion. Bilateral toe raises and heel raises may be used. **Field Strategy 12-1** demonstrates several exercises used to prevent injuries to the lower leg, ankle, and foot.

SIGNS AND SYMPTOMS
The individual usually reports a cracking or tearing sound at the time of injury. Swelling and ecchymosis are rapid and diffuse. Point tenderness is localized over the lateral ligaments.

MANAGEMENT
After assessment for possible fracture, initial treatment should consist of ice therapy, compression (with or without a horseshoe pad), elevation, and restricted activity. If the individual is unable to bear weight, crutches should be used, and the individual should be referred to a physician for further assessment. **Field Strategy 12-2** summarizes the management of lateral ankle sprains.

Eversion Ankle Sprains

Eversion ankle sprains are less common than inversion ankle sprains because of the strong deltoid ligament and bony structure of the ankle joint. Most injuries to the deltoid ligament are associated with a fibula fracture, injury to the distal tibiofibular joint, or severe lateral ankle sprain. Individuals with pronated or hypermobile feet tend to be at a greater risk for eversion injuries.

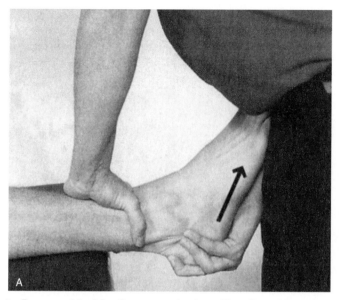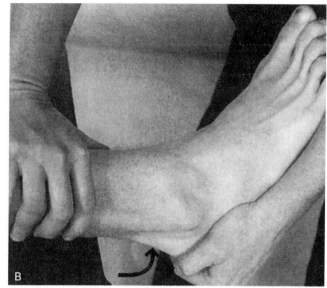

➤ FIGURE 12-21. Stress tests for the ankle collateral ligaments. **A.** Anterior drawer test. **B.** Talar tilt test.

pain should be performed last to prevent any painful symptoms from overflowing into the next movement. Perform the following motions **(Fig. 12-20)**:

- Dorsiflexion and plantar flexion of the ankle
- Pronation (eversion) and supination (inversion) of the ankle
- Toe extension and toe flexion
- Toe abduction and adduction (spread the toes; bring them back together)

STRESS TESTS

Using information gathered during the history, observation, inspection, and palpation, determine which tests most effectively assess the condition. Only those tests deemed relevant should be used.

Anterior Drawer Test

This test can assess collateral ligament integrity of the ankle. Place the individual supine and extend the foot beyond the table. Stabilize the tibia and fibula in one hand and cup the individual's heel in the other hand. To isolate the anterior talofibular ligament and anterolateral capsule, apply a straight anterior movement with slight plantar flexion and inversion **(Fig. 12-21A)**. If the talus shifts forward, the test is positive, indicating anterolateral instability.

Talar Tilt

The calcaneofibular ligament and deltoid ligaments are tested in the same position described for the anterior drawer test. Maintain the calcaneus in normal anatomic position (90° flexion). The talus is then slowly rocked between inversion and eversion **(Fig. 12-21B)**. Inversion tests the calcaneofibular ligament; eversion, the deltoid ligament.

Thompson's Test for Achilles Tendon Rupture

With the individual prone on a table, squeeze the calf muscles. A normal response elicits slight plantar flexion. Always compare bilaterally because some plantar flexion may occur if other posterior muscles are intact. A positive test, indicating a rupture of the Achilles tendon, is indicated by the absence of plantar flexion **(Fig. 12-22)**.

FUNCTIONAL TESTS

Functional tests should be performed pain-free without a limp or antalgic gait before clearing any individual for re-entry into competition. These may include any or all of the following:

- Squatting with both heels maintained on the floor
- Going up on the toes at least 20 times with no pain
- Walking on the toes for 20 to 30 feet
- Balancing on one foot at a time
- Running straight ahead, stopping, and running backwards
- Running figure-eights in large circles that slowly decrease in size

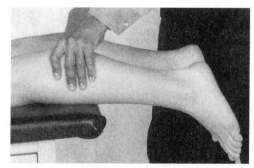

➤ FIGURE 12-22. Thompson test. Do passive compression of the calf muscles. This should produce slight plantar flexion at the ankle. If no plantar flexion occurs, suspect a possible rupture of the gastrocnemius-soleus complex or the Achilles tendon.

- Running at an angle sideways and making V-cuts
- Jumping rope for at least 1 minute
- Jumping straight up and going to a 90° squat

Summary

1. The true ankle (talocrural) joint is between the tibia, fibula, and talus. Plantar flexion and dorsiflexion occur at this joint. Motion at the subtalar joint involves inversion and eversion. The combination of calcaneal inversion, foot adduction, and plantar flexion is known as supination; calcaneal eversion is called foot abduction, and dorsiflexion is known as pronation.

2. The primary supporting structures of the plantar arches are the spring (calcaneonavicular) ligament, long plantar ligament, plantar fascia (plantar aponeurosis), and the short plantar (plantar calcaneocuboid) ligament. In addition, the tibialis posterior provides some support.

3. Lace-up ankle braces have been shown to limit all ankle motions, whereas a semirigid orthosis or an air-bladder–style brace limit only inversion and eversion. Strapping an ankle with adhesive tape to restrict inversion and eversion tends to lose its effectiveness after exercising for 20 minutes or more. Therefore, ankle braces are more effective in reducing ankle injuries.

4. Ankle sprains account for nearly 75% of all sprains in the lower leg; the majority are caused by inversion.

5. Risk factors for Achilles tendinitis include tight heel cord, foot malalignment deformities, a recent change in shoes or running surface, a sudden increase in workload (distance or intensity), and changes in the exercise environment (change in footwear or excessive hill climbing or impact-loading activities, such as jumping).

6. An acute anterior compartment syndrome is a medical emergency. Signs and symptoms include a recent history of trauma, a palpable firm mass in the anterior compartment, tight skin, and a diminished dorsalis pedis pulse.

7. Exertional compartment syndrome is characterized by exercise-induced pain and swelling that are relieved by rest. The anterior compartment is most frequently affected; if so, mild foot drop or paresthesia (or both) may be present. Fascial defects or hernias may also be present in the distal third of the leg over the anterior intramuscular septum.

8. Medial tibial stress syndrome is a periostitis along the posteromedial tibial border, usually in the distal third, not associated with a stress fracture or compartment syndrome. Signs and symptoms include point tenderness in a 3- to 6-cm area along the distal posteromedial tibial border, and pain and weakness with resisted plantar flexion or standing on tiptoe.

9. Congenital abnormalities, leg length discrepancy, muscle dysfunction (such as muscle imbalance), or a malalignment syndrome (e.g., pes cavus, pes planus, pes equinus, hammer or claw toes) can predispose an individual to several chronic foot and toe injuries.

10. Management of fractures of the lower leg, ankle, and foot should include a full assessment of sensation and circulation distal to the fracture site.

References

1. Shiba N, Kitaoka HB, Cahalan TD, and Chao EY. 1995. Shock-absorbing effect of shoe insert materials commonly used in management of lower extremity disorders. Clin Orthop, 310(1):130-136.
2. Lambson RB, Barnhill BS, and Higgins RW. 1996. Football cleat design and its effect on anterior cruciate ligament injuries: A three-year prospective study. Am J Sports Med, 24(2):155-159.
3. Renstrom P, and Johnson RJ. 1985. Overuse injuries in sports: A review. Sports Med, 2(5):316-333.
4. Brown DE. Ankle and leg injuries. In *The team physician's handbook*, edited by MB Mellion, WM Walsh, and GL Shelton. Philadelphia: Hanley & Belfus, 1997.
5. Edwards P, and Myerson MS. 1996. Exertional compartment syndrome of the leg: Steps for expedient return to activity. Phys Sportsmed, 24(4):31-46.
6. Middleton JA, and Kolodin EL. 1992. Plantar fasciitis–Heel pain in athletes. J Ath Train, 27(1):70-75.
7. Blue JM, and Matthews LS. 1997. Leg injuries. Clin Sports Med, 16(3):467-478.

Medical Emergencies and Other Conditions

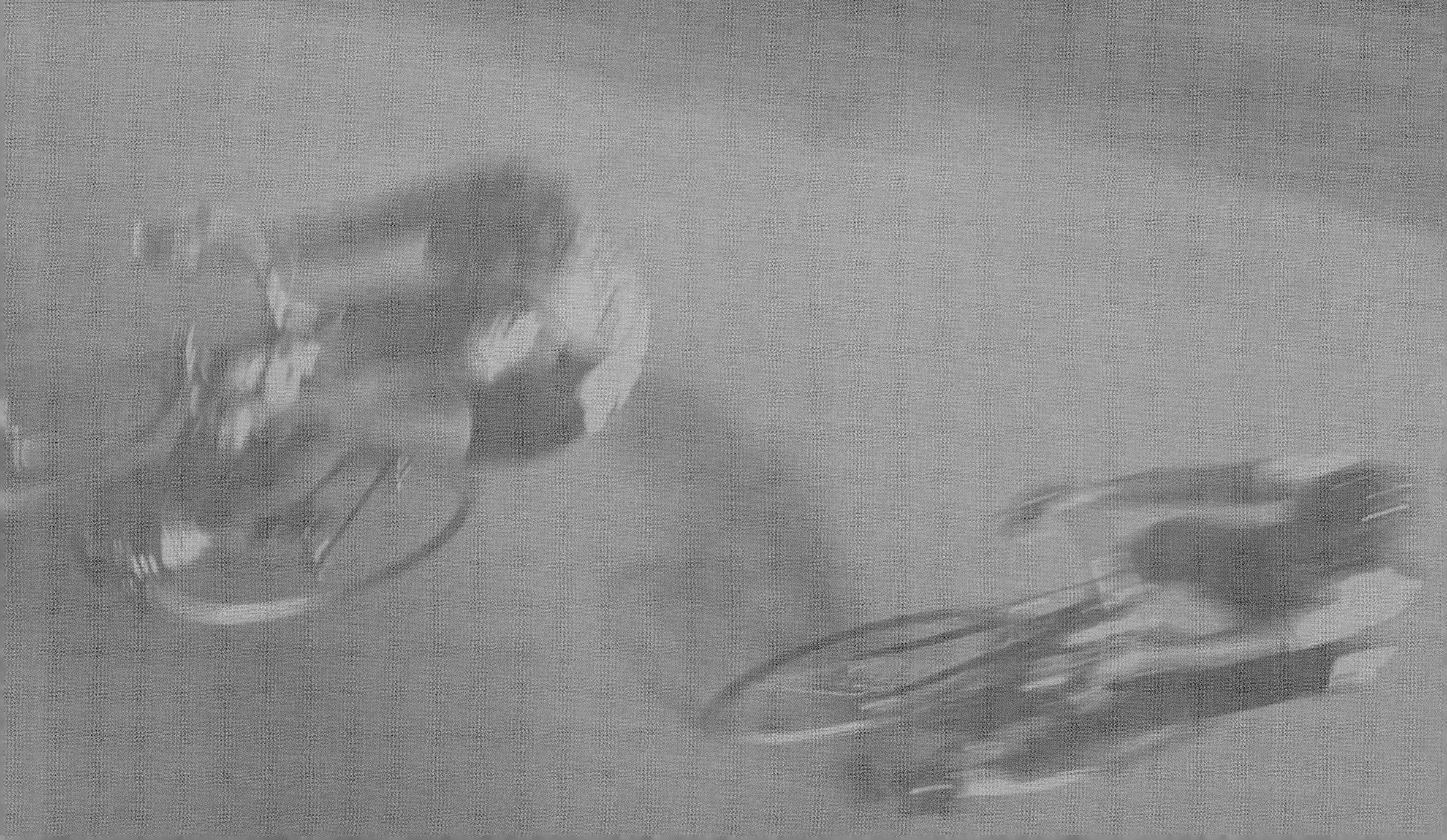

SECTION III

13

Respiratory Tract Conditions

KEY TERMS

Asthma
Bronchitis
Bronchospasm
Influenza
Pharyngitis
Purulent
Rhinorrhea
Sinusitis

OBJECTIVES

1. List the signs and symptoms of common upper respiratory tract conditions, including the common cold, sinusitis, pharyngitis, and influenza.
2. Describe strategies that can be used to prevent the common cold.
3. List the signs and symptoms of lower respiratory tract conditions, including bronchitis, bronchial asthma, and exercise-induced bronchospasm.
4. Describe the management and treatment of common respiratory tract conditions.

Conditions of the respiratory tract are common in sport participants. Many factors, such as fatigue, chronic inflammation from a localized infection, environmental factors (e.g., allergens, dust, smog), and psychological stress from difficult life events can suppress resistance to these conditions. Respiratory infections are often categorized as upper respiratory infections (URIs), which involve the nose, throat, ears, sinuses, tonsils, and associated lymph glands, or lower respiratory infections (LRIs), which involve the larynx, bronchi, and lungs. Chapter 7 has an anatomy review of the respiratory tract.

UPPER RESPIRATORY CONDITIONS

Upper respiratory infections are often caused by viruses. These conditions, although minor, can clearly affect an athlete's performance. In this section, the common cold, sinusitis, pharyngitis, and influenza are discussed.

Common Cold

The average adult has from one to six colds each year. Most of them occur in the fall and spring months. A cold can be quite contagious and can be transmitted by either person-to-person contact or airborne droplets. However, several strategies can be implemented to reduce the risk of getting a cold (**Box 13-1**).

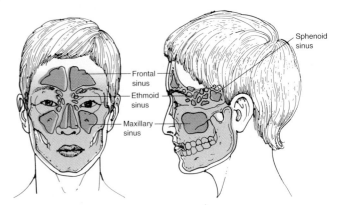

➤ FIGURE 13-1. Facial sinuses. The frontal and ethmoid sinuses are more commonly involved in sinusitis.

SIGNS AND SYMPTOMS

Symptoms usually begin 1 to 2 days after exposure and generally last 1 to 2 weeks. Symptoms include a rapid onset of clear nasal discharge, sneezing, nonproductive cough, and associated itching and puffiness of the eyes. Malaise (feeling lousy or tired), a mild sore throat, chills, and, in some cases, a low-grade fever are also present. Although most cold symptoms are benign and confined to the upper respiratory tract, colds can lead to middle ear infections and bacterial sinusitis when air flow is obstructed by swollen nasal membranes.

MANAGEMENT

Although there is no cure for the viral common cold, rest, plenty of fluids, and use of over-the-counter medications can alleviate or lessen symptoms. It is a well-known fact that vitamin C supplements can decrease the duration of cold episodes and the severity of symptoms. Likewise, zinc gluconate in the form of throat lozenges has also been shown to decrease the duration of cold episodes and the severity of symptoms if started within 24 to 48 hours of onset.[1]

Sinusitis

Sinusitis is an inflammation of the paranasal sinus caused by a bacterial or viral infection, an allergy, or environmental factors **(Fig. 13-1)**.

SIGNS AND SYMPTOMS

Nasal congestion, facial pain or pressure over the involved sinus, pain in the upper teeth, or pain and pressure behind the eyes are present. Other symptoms include **purulent** nasal discharge (nasal discharge with pus), palpable pain over the involved sinus, nighttime and daytime coughing, and, in severe cases, perinasal and eyelid swelling, fever, and chills. The individual often pinches the bridge of the nose to demonstrate the area of discomfort or reports discomfort aggravated by eyeglasses.

MANAGEMENT

This individual should see a physician for appropriate medication to control the infection, reduce mucosal edema, and allow for nasal discharge.

Pharyngitis

SIGNS AND SYMPTOMS

With **pharyngitis** (sore throat), the throat appears dark red, the tonsils appear red and swollen, and a puslike discharge may be present. Throat pain is aggravated by swallowing that may radiate along the distribution of the glossopharyngeal nerve (cranial nerve IX) to the ears. Other symptoms include **rhinorrhea** (clear nasal discharge), swollen lymph glands, hoarseness, headache, cough, a low-grade fever, and malaise. If the sore throat is caused by the bacterium *Streptococcus pyogenes* (strep throat) and is inadequately treated, peritonsillar abscess, scarlet fever, rheumatic fever, or rheumatic heart disease may result.

MANAGEMENT

Treatment for streptococcal pharyngitis includes antibiotics, such as penicillin or erythromycin.[2] In cases not involving streptococcal pharyngitis, treatment involves bed rest, plenty of fluids, warm saline gargles, throat lozenges, and mild analgesics (e.g., aspirin, ibuprofen).

Influenza

Influenza, or "flu," is a specific viral bronchitis caused by *Haemophilus influenzae* types A, B, or C. It often occurs in epidemic proportions, particularly in school-aged children.

SIGNS AND SYMPTOMS

A temperature of 39 to 39.5°C (102 to 103°F), chills, malaise, headache, general muscle aches, a hacking cough, and inflamed mucosal membranes may be present. Rapid onset of symptoms can occur within 24 to 48 hours after exposure to the virus. Sore throat, watery eyes, sensitivity to light (photophobia), and a nonproductive cough may linger for up to 5 days. The cough may progress into bronchitis.

MANAGEMENT

Initial treatment consists of rest, plenty of fluids, saltwater gargles, cough medication, and analgesics to control fever, aches, and pains. If the fever does not return to near normal within 24 hours, the individual should be seen immediately by a physician to rule out other infectious conditions.

LOWER RESPIRATORY CONDITIONS

Lower respiratory conditions result from infection or irritation from inhaled particles and substances. Bronchitis, bronchial asthma, and exercise-induced bronchospasm, formerly called exercise-induced asthma, are discussed here.

Bronchitis

Bronchitis is inflammation of the mucosal lining of the tracheobronchial tree resulting from infection or inhaled particles and substances. It is either acute or chronic.

SIGNS AND SYMPTOMS

Acute bronchitis, commonly seen in sport participants, involves bronchial swelling, mucus secretion, and increased resistance to expiration. Coughing, wheezing, and large amounts of purulent mucus are present. Chronic bronchitis is characterized by a productive daily cough for at least 3 consecutive months in 2 successive years. Irritation may result from cigarette smoke, air pollution, or infections. This condition can progress to increased airway obstruction, heart failure, and cellular changes in respiratory epithelial cells that may become malignant. Signs and symptoms include marked cyanosis, edema, large production of sputum, and abnormally high levels of carbon dioxide and low levels of oxygen in the blood. This condition is often seen simultaneously with emphysema.

MANAGEMENT

In acute bronchitis, once the stimulus is removed, the swelling decreases and airways return to normal. With chronic bronchitis, the individual should be supervised by a physician.

Bronchial Asthma

Asthma is caused by constriction of bronchial smooth muscles (**bronchospasm**), increased bronchial secretions, and mucosal swelling, all leading to an inadequate airflow during respiration (especially expiration) **(Fig. 13-2)**.

SIGNS AND SYMPTOMS

Wheezing is a common sign that results from air squeezing past the narrowed airways. Because the airways cannot fill or empty adequately, the diaphragm tends to flatten, and the accessory muscles must work harder to enlarge the chest during inspiration. This increased workload leads to a rapid onset of fatigue when the individual can no longer hyperventilate enough to meet the increased oxygen need. Acute attacks may occur spontaneously, but they are often provoked by a viral infection. A large amount of thick, yellow or green sputum is produced by the bronchial mucosa. As difficulty in breathing continues, anxiety, loud wheezing, sweating, rapid heart rate, and labored breathing are apparent. In severe cases, respiratory failure may be indicated by cyanosis, decreased wheezing, and decreased levels of consciousness.

MANAGEMENT

Individuals diagnosed with asthma typically carry medication delivered by a compressor-driven nebulizer or inhaler to alleviate the attack. Once the attack has subsided, the lungs usually return to normal.

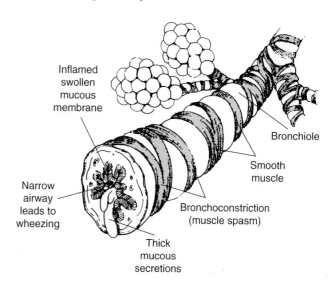

➤ **FIGURE 13-2.** Bronchospasm. An asthma attack is caused by bronchospasm that constricts the bronchiolar tubes. This spasm, combined with increased bronchial secretions and mucosal swelling, results in a characteristic loud wheezing sound heard during expiration.

Exercise-induced Bronchospasm

Exercise-induced bronchospasm (EIB), formerly known as exercise-induced asthma (EIA), affects up to 90% of asthmatics and up to 35% of those without known asthma.[3] Individuals suffering from allergies, sinus disease, or hyperventilation may be at increased risk for EIB. Bronchitis, emphysema, and other diseases affecting the bronchial tubes can exacerbate symptoms of EIB.

SIGNS AND SYMPTOMS

Common signs and symptoms include chest pain, chest tightness, or a burning sensation with or without wheezing; a regular dry cough; shortness of breath shortly after or during exercise; and stomach cramps after exercise. EIB symptoms typically appear after 8 to 10 minutes of vigorous exercise and may worsen after activity is terminated. Episodes usually remit completely within 30 to 60 minutes and do not increase airway reactivity or induce long-term deterioration in lung function.

MANAGEMENT

Management includes medications used in regular asthma treatment such as bronchodilators, cromolyn sodium, oral theophylline, and the leukotriene modifiers zafirlukast and zileitron.[3,4] However, athletes should check with the appropriate governing sport body to ensure the medication is legal for competition.

Children and young adults who have asthma and are physically fit and free of significant airway obstruction respond to exercise similar to nonasthmatic individuals. Activities such as tennis, running, and football are well tolerated if exercise includes a 5- to 10-minute stretching program followed by a 10- to 15-minute warm-up at 60% of maximum heart rate performed 30 minutes before more strenuous exercise. After warming up, athletes should pretreat themselves with two puffs of a short-acting inhaler to protect against an attack for 2 to 6 hours. After exercise, a cool-down period of several minutes of stretching or less strenuous activity allows a gradual rewarming of the airways and makes post-exercise symptoms less likely.[4] **Box 13-2** summarizes exercise strategies for individuals with EIB.

Summary

1. Viral conditions are often referred to as upper respiratory infections (URIs).
2. The common cold is quite contagious and can be transmitted by either person-to-person contact or airborne droplets. Symptoms usually begin 1 to 2 days after exposure and last for 1 to 2 weeks.
3. Sinusitis is an inflammation of the paranasal sinus

> ➤ ➤ BOX 13-2

Exercise Strategies for Exercise-Induced Bronchospasm

- Consult a physician before beginning an exercise program.
- Take medication for asthma as prescribed to achieve overall control of asthmatic symptoms, including those caused by exercise and airborne allergens.
- Use a peak flow meter as directed by a physician.
- Perform a 5- to 10-minute warm-up of moderate stretching, and work out slowly for another 10 to 15 minutes, keeping the pulse rate below 60% maximum heart rate (140 beats per minute). If symptoms occur during exercise, try to "run through" them or use the bronchodilator.
- Use a bronchodilator 15 minutes before exercise.
- Increase the time and intensity of the workout as tolerated, especially if the activity is new.
- Breathe slowly through the nose to warm and humidify the air. Exercise in a warm, humid environment, such as a heated swimming pool.
- In cold, dry environments, breathe through a mask or scarf. Alternatively, consider different locations and types of exercise during winter months, such as swimming, running, or cycling indoors.
- Avoid exposure to air pollutants and allergens whenever possible. Avoid exercise in the early morning hours, when the concentration of ragweed is the highest.
- Perform a gradual 10- to 30-minute cool-down after a vigorous workout to avoid rapid thermal changes in the airways. This can be achieved by slowing to a less intense pace while jogging, cycling, swimming, and stretching.

caused by a bacterial or viral infection, an allergy, or environmental factors.

4. If pharyngitis is caused by the bacterium *Streptococcus pyogenes* and is inadequately treated, peritonsillar abscess, scarlet fever, rheumatic fever, or rheumatic heart disease may result.
5. Bronchitis may be acute or chronic and is characterized by bronchial swelling, mucus secretion, and increased resistance to expiration.
7. Asthma is caused by a constriction of bronchial smooth muscles (bronchospasm), increased bronchial secretions, and mucosal swelling, all leading to inadequate airflow during respiration (especially expiration). Wheezing, a common sign of asthma, results from air squeezing past the narrowed airways.
8. Exercise-induced bronchospasm (EIB) affects up to 90% of asthmatics and up to 35% of those without known asthma. Key signs are a dry, regular cough within 8 to 10 minutes of the start of moderate exercise and stomach cramps after exercise.

References

1. Mossad SB, Macknin ML, Medendorp SV, and Mason P. 1996. Zinc gluconate lozenges for treating the common cold. Ann Intern Med, 125(2):81-88.
2. Mellion MB. Infections in athletes. In *The team physician's hand-book*, edited by MB Mellion, WM Walsh, and GL Shelton. Philadelphia: Hanley & Belfus, 1997.
3. Rupp NT. 1996. Diagnosis and management of exercise-induced asthma. Phys Sportsmed, 24(1):77-87.
4. Disabella V, and Sherman C. 1998. Exercise for asthma patients: Little risk, big rewards. Phys Sportsmed, 26(6):75-84.

Gastrointestinal Conditions

CHAPTER OBJECTIVES

1. List the common signs and symptoms associated with upper gastrointestinal conditions such as gastroenteritis, gastritis, dysphagia, gastroesophageal reflux, and dyspepsia (indigestion).

2. List the common signs and symptoms associated with lower gastrointestinal conditions such as diarrhea and constipation.

3. Describe the general management of upper and lower gastrointestinal conditions.

4. List other factors that may not be related to an injury or condition specific to the upper or lower gastrointestinal tract, but may adversely affect the entire gastrointestinal tract.

The gastrointestinal (GI) tract extends from the mouth to the anus, and it absorbs nutritional substances from ingested food and expels waste (see Chapter 7). In active individuals, exercise alone can induce both upper and lower GI symptoms and problems. During exercise, up to 20% of the central blood volume is shunted away from the visceral organs to the working muscles. This can result in the reduction of normal intestinal blood flow by as much as 80% to maintain an adequate central blood volume.[1] Exercised-induced shunting, as it is often called, can lead to decreased esophageal motility, erosive hemorrhagic gastritis, delayed gastric emptying, diarrhea, or intestinal bleeding. Dehydration, a high ambient temperature, and lack of acclimatization to exercise in the heat can all exacerbate this hypoperfusion of the GI tract. Nervous tension can also lead to indigestion, diarrhea, or constipation and can adversely affect sport participation. Many seemingly minor disorders, however, can be the first sign of more serious underlying conditions. If symptoms persist with any disorder, referral to a physician is warranted.

In this chapter, disorders affecting the upper GI region are discussed first, followed by disorders affecting the lower GI region. Finally, other factors that affect the entire GI tract are presented.

UPPER GASTROINTESTINAL DISORDERS

Upper GI disorders (i.e., those in the stomach and above) are caused by local irritation that results from several factors, including stress and the ingestion of caffeine, alcohol, and tomato and citric acid products. This irritation can lead to nausea, **emesis** (vomiting), bloating, abdominal cramps, and heartburn. The primary condition related to upper GI disorders is gastroenteritis, although other conditions such as gastritis and dyspepsia may also lead to GI irritation. General management includes agents with **antacids** (acid neutralizers) and diet modification.

Gastroenteritis

The incidence of **gastroenteritis**, an acute inflammation of the mucous membrane of the stomach or small intestine, is second only to upper respiratory tract infections in adolescents and young adults.[1] The condition is caused by viral or bacterial infection, allergic reaction, medication, contaminated food (food poisoning), or emotional stress.

SIGNS AND SYMPTOMS

In mild cases, increased secretion of hydrochloric acid in the stomach leads to indigestion, nausea, **flatulence** (gas), and a sour stomach. In moderate to severe cases, abdominal cramping, diarrhea, fever, and vomiting can lead to fluid and electrolyte imbalance.

MANAGEMENT

The condition is often self-limiting and usually clears in 2 to 3 days. Treatment includes eliminating irritating foods from the diet, avoiding factors that bring on anxiety and stress, and avoiding dehydration by drinking clear fluids or electrolyte-containing fluids (e.g., sport drinks). Antimotility drugs reduce movement in the small intestines and may be effective for abdominal cramps and diarrhea, but they can also prolong some infections. Return to competition is limited only by the hydration status, infective nature of the problem, complexity of the symptoms (i.e., frequent diarrhea), and reconditioning.

Gastritis

Gastritis occurs when the stomach lining becomes inflamed. It can be induced by anxiety, exercise-related hypoperfusion, nonsteroidal anti-inflammatory drugs (NSAIDs), or excessive consumption of alcohol.

SIGNS AND SYMPTOMS

Vague stomach tenderness is often accompanied by nausea, vomiting, fever, and stomach pain.

MANAGEMENT

Gastritis should be managed with an increase in clear fluids and physician referral. Drug therapy (antacids) may be contraindicated if gastric bleeding is present. If gastric bleeding does occur, exercise is contraindicated.

Gastroesophageal Reflux

When gastric juice (which is extremely acidic) regurgitates into the esophagus, it is called gastroesophageal reflux. The condition is most likely to occur when an individual eats or drinks to excess, but is also caused by conditions that force abdominal contents superiorly, such as obesity, pregnancy, and running, which causes stomach contents to splash upward with each step (runner's reflux).

SIGNS AND SYMPTOMS

Gastroesophageal reflux is associated with mild heartburn and a burning, radiating, substernal pain.

MANAGEMENT

Initial management involves use of antacids 4 hours before exercise and changes in diet, timing of meals before exercise, and activity modification.

Indigestion

Dyspepsia, or indigestion, is associated with upper GI pain. Indigestion has no identified etiology.

SIGNS AND SYMPTOMS

Irregularly occurring symptoms can range from a sense of fullness after eating to feeling as though something is lodged in the esophagus, to heartburn, nausea, vomiting, and loss of appetite. Pain and discomfort at the xiphoid region during digestion are the most common symptoms. Similar to peptic ulcers, dyspepsia can be caused by an excessive acid accumulation in the stomach and overconsumption of alcohol.

MANAGEMENT

Taking antacids 4 hours before exercise and modifying activities may help with the discomfort. If symptoms persist, immediate referral to a physician is warranted to rule out more serious abdominal conditions or diseases.

LOWER GASTROINTESTINAL DISORDERS

Lower GI disorders occur distal to the stomach. Common symptoms associated with lower GI problems include diarrhea, constipation, rectal bleeding, and hemorrhoids. Many lower GI disorders are managed by increasing dietary fiber and avoiding irritating foods.

Diarrhea

Anxiety and precompetition jitters commonly result in "nervous **diarrhea**."

SIGNS AND SYMPTOMS

Diarrhea is characterized by abnormally loose, watery stools. This is caused by food residue running through the large intestine before that organ has had sufficient time to absorb the remaining water. Prolonged diarrhea can lead to dehydration and depletion of electrolytes, particularly sodium, bicarbonate, and potassium.

MANAGEMENT

Diarrhea may respond to certain antidiarrheal medications that reduce intestinal movement, increase fluid absorption, modify intestinal bacteria, or reduce inflammation associated with diarrhea. Bismuth subsalicylate, loperamide, or diphenoxylate with atropine may help; however, these products should not be used regularly. An attempt should be made to defecate at a regular daily time, taking advantage of the morning **gastrocolic reflex** (propulsive reflex in the colon that stimulates defecation). Peristalsis and defecation can be stimulated by drinking coffee or tea, having a light meal before competition, and then jogging to stimulate the gastrocolic reflex. Exercise, specifically more than what the body is accustomed to, increases intestinal activity. Therefore, athletes may want to do the following:

- Immediately decrease the level of training and competition by 20 to 40% in both mileage and intensity until the episode passes, then build back up slowly.
- Eliminate foods that trigger bowel irritation, such as excessive juices, fresh fruits, raisin and other dried fruits, beans, lentils, and dairy products if lactose intolerance is involved.
- Limit the amount of sugar-free gum and hard candies that contain sorbitol, which can cause diarrhea.
- Improve hydration before and during exercise to increase plasma volume and decrease intestinal mucosal ischemia.

Constipation

Infrequent or incomplete bowel movements (constipation) are not a disease, but rather a description of symptoms that may indicate a more serious underlying condition. Potential causes include lack of fiber in the diet, improper bowel habits, lack of exercise, emotional distress, diabetes mellitus, pregnancy, laxative abuse, and side effects of drug (e.g., diuretics, bile acid binders, calcium supplements, aluminum antacids, antidepressants, antihistamines, antihypertensives, antispasmodics, and narcotic pain relievers).[2,3]

MANAGEMENT

Management depends on the origin. Athletes who have a low fiber diet should gradually increase the intake of high-fiber foods. Fiber absorbs water and makes feces softer and easier to eliminate. Bran cereals are the richest fiber foods, superior to salads and many vegetables and fruits. Increasing daily exercise, particularly aerobic exercise, and ensuring adequate fluid intake can alleviate symptoms. Laxatives or suppositories are useful, but they should be used sparingly and only for short-term treatment. Laxatives stimulate and promote bowel emptying. They work by holding water and swelling in the intestines, while stool softeners work by mixing fat and water into fecal matter.

In addition to medications, drinking warm clear fluids (e.g., juice, soda, or broth), particularly in the morning, can stimulate bowel activity. The body naturally wants to defecate about a half hour after consuming a warm beverage in the morning. Time should be allotted to relax and honor this urge. Drink plenty of fluids throughout the day, but do not drink more than a half-cup of prune juice. You can determine if you are drinking enough fluids by urinating every 2 to 4 hours and checking the color. The urine should be light like lemonade, not dark like apple cider. In chronic constipation, surgical intervention may be necessary.

Irritable Bowel Syndrome

Irritable bowel syndrome is one of the most common GI disorders. It is sometimes called spastic colitis, mucus colitis, or nervous colon syndrome. This condition is seen almost twice as often in women than men, particularly during menstruation and during stress. The condition is aggravated with the ingestion of fats, chocolate, caffeine, milk and dairy products, and alcohol.

SIGNS AND SYMPTOMS

The condition is usually associated with abdominal pain, bloating, gas, mucus in stools, and irregular bowel habits, including alternating diarrhea and constipation. Alternating bowel movements occur over periods of days to weeks. During episodes of constipation, stools may be hard, small, pebblelike, and difficult to eliminate. There may be a sense of incomplete evacuation; however, the passage of stool may lead to the alleviation of pain. The condition tends to be chronic and can come and go over a span of several years.

MANAGEMENT

Referral to a physician is necessary to rule out other underlying conditions. Diagnosis is made based on chronic recurrent bowel symptoms in an otherwise healthy individual. Treatment focuses on relieving stress and educating oneself on proper nutrition and eating habits, including adequate fluid and high fiber intake. Eliminating GI stimulants such as caffeinated beverages and avoiding artificial sweeteners may help. Other possible treatments include anxiety-reducing measures (e.g., regular exercise), stool softeners, fiber supplements, and prescribed antispasmodic drugs.

OTHER GASTROINTESTINAL PROBLEMS

Although certain factors may not be related to an injury or condition specific to the upper or lower GI tract, they can affect the entire GI tract. Anxiety and stress, vomiting, and food poisoning are three such conditions.

Anxiety and Stress Reaction

Performance anxiety and pregame stress are common in competing athletes. Upper GI tract function can be affected through decreased acid secretion in the stomach, slowed intestinal motility, or decreased blood flow. Continued anxiety can lead to hypersecretion of stomach acids, increased motility, or decreased transit time.

SIGNS AND SYMPTOMS

Common symptoms include a dry mouth, dyspepsia, gastroesophageal reflux, heartburn, abdominal cramping, and diarrhea.

MANAGEMENT

Treatment involves reassurance and education about the body's processes; relaxation techniques, such as deep breathing, passive and active relaxation, soothing music, smiling, and therapeutic massage; and behavior modification.

Vomiting

Vomiting is often preceded by a watering mouth and nausea. It often results from the intake of irritating foods and other intestinal irritants. Other causes are stress, excessive alcohol or other drug consumption, and food poisoning.

MANAGEMENT

Vomiting is best managed by first comforting the athlete and maintaining a clear airway. The mouth should be rinsed and monitored for repeated vomiting, followed by administering antinausea medication and clear fluids to prevent dehydration. If food poisoning is expected or if blood is found in the vomit, an immediate physician referral is necessary. Vomiting can be an early sign of pregnancy, particularly if it occurs in the morning.

Food Poisoning

The most common cause of food poisoning is contaminated food. However, food poisoning can also stem from insecticides or infectious organisms (bacteria from the salmonella group, certain staphylococci, streptococci, or dysentery bacilli) from food that is undercooked or decomposed.

SIGNS AND SYMPTOMS

Food poisoning includes varying levels of abdominal gas and pain, nausea, vomiting, low-grade fever, and diarrhea. These signs and symptoms can begin 1 to 6 hours after ingestion of contaminated foods and usually last for 1 to 3 days. Dehydration from the vomiting and diarrhea can lead to weakness, fatigue, and an increased risk of heat illness.

MANAGEMENT

Mild symptoms are treated conservatively with rapid replacement of fluids and electrolytes and administration of an antidiarrheal agent. If tolerated, light fluids, broth, bouillon with a small amount of salt, poached eggs, or bland cereals can be given. Severe cases require activation of emergency medical services. Fluids must be replaced intravenously, and pumping of the stomach contents may be necessary. If possible, samples of the vomitus should accompany the individual if he or she is transported to the nearest medical facility. This sample can help identify the food responsible for the poisoning.

Summary

1. Exercise-induced shunting can lead to decreased esophageal motility, erosive hemorrhagic gastritis, delayed gastric emptying, diarrhea, or intestinal bleeding. Dehydration, high ambient temperatures, and lack of acclimatization can all exacerbate hypoperfusion of the GI tract.

2. Many upper GI tract disorders are caused by irritation from stress or the ingestion of caffeine, alcohol, or tomato and citric acid products. These disorders result in nausea, vomiting, bloating, abdominal cramps, and heartburn.

3. Gastroenteritis is second in incidence only to upper respiratory tract infections in adolescents and adults. It is caused by viral or bacterial infection, allergic reaction, medication, contaminated food, or emotional stress. The condition is self-limiting and usually clears in 2 to 3 days. Treatment includes eliminating irritating foods from the diet, avoiding factors that bring on anxiety and stress, and avoiding dehydration.

4. Gastroesophageal reflux is associated with the regurgitation of gastric juices into the esophagus. Dyspepsia, or indigestion, is associated with upper GI pain and has no identified etiology. Both are treated with antacids taken 4 hours before exercise.

5. Diarrhea, common among runners, is caused by increased intestinal motility. Antidiarrheal medications can reduce intestinal movement, increase fluid absorption, modify intestinal bacteria, or reduce inflammation associated with diarrhea. If diarrhea is a known problem, the athlete should try to defecate before exercise and should not eat before running.

6. Anxiety and stress can lead to decreased acid secretion in the stomach, slower intestinal motility, or decreased blood flow. Continued anxiety can lead to hypersecretion of stomach acids, increased motility, or decreased transit time. Treatment involves reassurance and education about the body's processes; relaxation techniques; and behavior modification.

7. Vomiting is caused by irritating foods, intestinal irritants, stress, excessive alcohol or drug consumption, and food poisoning. Although vomiting is usually treated conservatively with antinausea medication and clear fluids to prevent dehydration, it may be an early sign of pregnancy, particularly if it occurs in the morning hours. Persistent vomiting signals a more serious condition, in which case immediate referral to a physician is warranted.

References

1. Torres JL, and Mellion MB. Gastrointestinal problems. In *The team physician's handbook*, edited by MB Mellion, WM Walsh, and GL Shelton. Philadelphia: Hanley & Belfus, 1997.
2. Martin M, and Yates WN. *Therapeutic medications in sports medicine*. Baltimore: Williams & Wilkins, 1998.
3. Consumers Union. 1998. Pillbox: Laxatives—and alternatives. Consumer Reports Health, 10(4):8-9.

15

The Diabetic Athlete

KEY TERMS:

Diabetes mellitus

Diabetic ketoacidosis

Hyperglycemia

Hypoglycemia

Ketoacidosis

Ketonuria

Nephropathy

Polyuria

Retinopathy

CHAPTER OBJECTIVES

1. Explain how insulin regulates blood glucose levels.
2. Explain the physiologic basis of diabetes.
3. Describe types 1 and 2 diabetes mellitus.
4. Contrast the signs and symptoms of insulin shock and diabetic coma.
5. Describe how to manage insulin shock and diabetic coma.
6. List physical activities that are indicated and contraindicated for a physically active individual with diabetes.

Diabetes mellitus (DM) is a chronic metabolic disorder characterized by near or absolute lack of the hormone insulin, insulin resistance, or both. The disease affects approximately 15 million Americans and ranks seventh among the leading causes of death in the United States. This disease can contribute to several other major diseases, including heart disease and stroke. Individuals with diabetes are twice as likely to develop these cardiovascular conditions as someone without diabetes.[1] Several factors increase the risk and severity of diabetes, including heredity, increasing age, minority ethnicity, obesity, being female, stress, infection, a sedentary lifestyle, and a diet high in carbohydrates and fat.

THE PHYSIOLOGIC BASIS OF DIABETES

Carbohydrates in human nutrition supply the body's cells with glucose to deliver energy to the body's systems. Upon eating, a person's blood glucose rises, stimulating the pancreas to release insulin. Under normal conditions, blood glucose ranges between 80 and 120 mg/dL. Insulin's main effect is to lower blood sugar levels, but it also stimulates amino acid uptake and fat metabolism and influences protein synthesis in muscle tissue. Insulin lowers blood sugar by enhancing membrane transport of glucose (and other simple sugars) from the blood, into body cells, especially the skeletal and cardiac muscles **(Fig. 15-1)**.

When insulin activity is absent or deficient as in diabetes, blood sugar remains high after a meal because glucose is unable to move into most tissue cells, causing blood glucose levels to increase to abnormally high levels. Increased osmotic blood

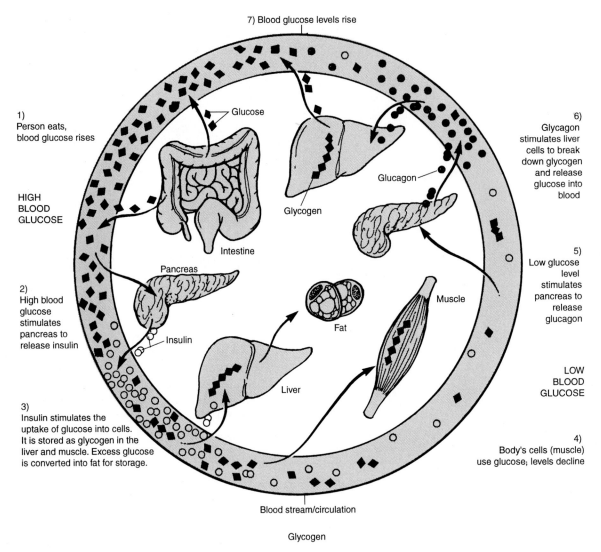

➤ **FIGURE 15-1** Maintaining a balance of blood glucose. Insulin must be available to stimulate uptake of blood glucose into the body's cells. As the cells use glucose, blood levels decline, and the liver responds by releasing glucagon into the bloodstream. Glucagon stimulates liver cells to break down stored glycogen and releases glucose into the blood, thereby raising the level of blood glucose to normal levels. (Adapted from Whitney EN, and Rolfes SR. *Understanding nutrition.* Belmont, CA: Wadsworth Publishing, 1999:1.)

pressure drives fluid from the cells into the vascular system, leading to cell dehydration. The excess glucose is passed into the kidneys, resulting in **polyuria**, a huge urine output of water and electrolytes that leads to decreased blood volume and further dehydration. Serious electrolyte losses also occur as the body rids itself of excess ketones. Because ketones are negatively charged ions, they carry positive ions out with them; as a result, sodium and potassium ions are lost. An electrolyte imbalance leads to abdominal pains, possible vomiting, and further dehydration, which stimulates excessive thirst. In response, the body shifts from carbohydrate metabolism to fat metabolism for energy. The final cardinal sign is excessive hunger and food consumption, a sign that the person is "starving." That is, although plenty of glucose is available, it cannot be used. In severe cases, blood levels of fatty acids and their metabolites rise dramatically,

producing an excess of ketoacids resulting in acidosis. Acetone, formed as a byproduct of fat metabolism, is volatile and blown off during expiration, giving the breath a sweet or fruity odor. If the condition is not rectified with insulin injection, further dehydration and **ketoacidosis** results as the ketones begin to spill into the urine (**ketonuria**). If untreated, ketoacidosis disrupts virtually all physiologic processes, including heart activity and oxygen transport. Severe depression of the nervous system leads to confusion, drowsiness, coma, and finally, death.

TYPES OF DIABETES

The National Diabetes Data Group and the World Health Organization recognize four types of DM: type 1, type 2, gestational DM, and diabetes secondary to other conditions. Each group is characterized by high blood glucose levels or **hyperglycemia**. Because athletic trainers, coaches, and sport supervisors will most likely encounter physically active individuals with type 1 or type 2 DM, these conditions will be discussed in detail, and are compared in **Box 15-1**.

Type 1 Diabetes Mellitus

In type 1, the pancreas cannot synthesize insulin. As such, the individual must obtain insulin to assist the cells in taking up the needed fuels from the blood. Formerly called insulin-dependent diabetes (IDDM) or juvenile diabetes, type I DM is considered an autoimmune disorder and is one of the most frequent chronic childhood diseases. The onset is usually acute, developing over a period of a few days to weeks. Over 95% of individuals who develop type 1 DM are under 25 years of age, with equal incidence in both sexes and an increased prevalence in the white population.[2] Individuals generally have a more severe time balancing glucose levels, the effects of exercise on the metabolic state are more pronounced, and the management of exercise-related problems are more difficult.

Type 2 Diabetes Mellitus

Formerly called non-insulin-dependent diabetes or adult-onset diabetes, type 2 DM is the most common form of diabetes (90 to 95% of all cases).[1,3] It is highly associated with a family history of diabetes, older age, obesity, and lack of exercise. It is also more common in women who have a history of gestational diabetes and in African Americans, Native Americans, and Hispanics.[2] Although the exact cause of type 2 DM is unknown, high blood glucose and insulin resistance are major contributing factors.

Onset is typically after age 40 years, but this disease is also seen in obese children. Obesity, a major factor in adults, affects nearly 90% of adults with type 2 DM. Compared with normal-weight individuals, obese people require much more insulin to maintain normal blood glucose. More insulin is produced, but as body fat increases, the number of insulin receptors and their ability to function decreases. Consequently, insulin resistance increases, and adipose and muscle tissues become less able to take up glucose. At some point, the body cannot supply enough insulin to keep up, and type 2 DM develops.

COMPLICATIONS OF DIABETES MELLITUS

In types 1 and 2 DM, glucose fails to enter into the cells; instead, it accumulates in the blood, which can lead to both acute and chronic complications. Chronically elevated blood glucose levels can damage the blood vessels and nerves, leading to circulatory and neural damage. Failure to adequately balance nutrition, exercise, insulin injections, and blood glucose levels can also cause a physically active individual to experience insulin shock or diabetic coma.

Hypoglycemia

Hypoglycemia, common in type 1 insulin-treated diabetics, can range from mild lower levels of glucose (60 to 70 mg/dL) with minimal or no symptoms to severe hypoglycemia with low levels of glucose (less than 40 mg/dL) with neurologic impairment. Although hypoglycemia can occur in any individual, it is critical when affecting type 1

➤ ➤ **BOX 15-1**

Comparison of Type 1 and Type 2 Diabetes

	TYPE 1	TYPE 2
Former names	Juvenile diabetes	Adult onset
	Insulin-dependent diabetes mellitus	Non–insulin-dependent diabetes mellitus
Age of onset	Usually before 30 years	Usually after 30 years
Type of onset	Abrupt (days to weeks)	Usually gradual (weeks to months)
Nutritional status	Almost always lean	Usually obese
Insulin production	Negligible to absent	Present, but may be in excess and ineffective because of obesity
Insulin	Needed for all patients	Necessary in only 20 to 30% of patients
Diet	Mandatory along with insulin for control of blood glucose	Proper diet alone is frequently sufficient to control blood glucose
High incidence	White population	Women with history of gestational diabetes
		African Americans
		Native Americans
		Hispanics
Family history	Minor	Common link

diabetics because their ability to recover from it is limited. In a patient with diabetes, hypoglycemia can be related to errors in dosage, delayed or skipped meals, exercise, intensity of blood glucose control, variation in adsorption of circulation insulin from subcutaneous depots, variability of insulin binding, impairment of counter-regulation, and (possibly) the use of human insulin.[3] When left untreated, this condition can lead to insulin shock.

Insulin Shock

Exercise lowers blood sugar; hence, any exercise must be counterbalanced with increased food intake or decreased amounts of insulin. If blood glucose falls below normal levels, hypoglycemia results. Contrary to the slow onset of a diabetic coma, hypoglycemia has a rapid onset. Signs and symptoms include dizziness; headache; intense hunger; aggressive behavior; pale, cold, and clammy skin; and profuse perspiration, salivation, drooling, and tingling in the face, tongue, and lips. Other observable signs include a staggering gait, clumsy movements, confusion, and a general decrease in performance.

Because glucose levels in the blood are low and insulin levels are high, treatment focuses on quickly getting 10 to 15 g of a fast-acting carbohydrate into the system. Examples include 4 oz of regular cola or 6 oz of ginger ale, 4 oz of apple or orange juice, four packets of table sugar, 2 tablespoons of raisins, or five to seven pieces of candy.[4,5] Hard candy should be given only to a conscious person who can swallow well. Chocolates, which contain a high level of fat, should not be used because the fat interferes with the absorption of sugar. If the person is unconscious or unable to swallow, roll the individual on his or her side and pay close attention to the airway: saliva should drain out of the mouth, not into the throat or airway. Place sugar or honey under the tongue so it is absorbed through the mucosal membrane. Recovery is usually rapid.

After initial recovery, the athlete should wait for 15 minutes and have blood sugar level checked. If the level is still below 70 mg/dL, if there is no meter, or if the athlete still has symptoms, give the athlete another 10 to 15 g of carbohydrates. Repeat blood testing and treatment until the blood glucose level is normalized.[4] Even when blood glucose has returned to normal, physical performance and judgment may still be impaired, or the individual may relapse if the quick sugar influx is quickly depleted. After the symptoms resolve, the individual should be instructed to have a good meal as quickly as possible to increase carbohydrates in the body. If the condition does not appear to improve, activate the emergency medical services (EMS), monitor vital signs, and treat for shock until the ambulance arrives.

Diabetic Coma

Without insulin, the body is unable to metabolize glucose, which leads to hyperglycemia in the blood. As the body shifts from carbohydrate metabolism to fat metabolism, an excess of ketoacids in the blood can lower the blood pH to 7.0 (normal pH is 7.35 to 7.45), leading to a condition called **diabetic ketoacidosis**. This condition is manifested by ketones in the breath (acetone breath), in the blood, and in the urine. Symptoms appear gradually and often occur over several days. The individual becomes increasingly restless and confused and reports a dry mouth and intense thirst. Abdominal cramping and vomiting are common. As the individual slips into coma, signs include dry, red, warm skin; eyes that appear deep and sunken; deep, exaggerated respirations; a rapid, weak pulse; and a sweet, fruity acetone breath, similar to nail polish remover.

As the name implies, diabetic coma is a serious condition and is considered a medical emergency. It is usually not possible to be certain whether an individual is in a diabetic coma or insulin shock. Therefore, give the individual glucose or orange juice if he or she is conscious. If recovery is not rapid, a medical emergency exists and EMS should be activated. The additional glucose does not worsen the condition, provided the individual is transported immediately. If the person is unconscious or semiconscious, nothing should be given orally. Instead, maintain an open airway, treat for shock, and activate EMS, who will deliver an intravenous solution of insulin to aid the athlete. **Field Strategy 15-1** summarizes the management of insulin shock and diabetic coma.

EXERCISE RECOMMENDATIONS

Controlled diabetes depends on a balance of glucose levels, insulin production, nutrition, and exercise. Before any exercise program begins, a physician should be consulted about proper diet, and normal blood glucose (BG) levels should be documented (strenuous exercise is contraindicated for some diabetics). With the advent of blood glucose self-monitoring, exercise is encouraged if certain precautions are followed. Blood glucose levels should be taken 30 minutes before and 1 hour after exercise to see how exercise affects BG. These measurements help to regulate food intake and insulin dosage.

Aerobic exercise can decrease the requirements of insulin and increase the body's sensitivity to it. Exercise can also help attain and maintain ideal body weight and decrease the risk for hypertensive diseases including cardiovascular and peripheral vascular disease, and slow the progression of diabetic **nephropathy** (kidney damage). It is recommended that all exercising diabetics should follow the guidelines listed in **Box 15-2**. Despite the benefits of exercise, type 2 diabetics who have lost protective neural sensation should not participate in treadmill walking, prolonged walking, jogging, or step exercises. Recommended exercises include low-resistance walking, swimming, bicycling, rowing, chair exercises, arm exer-

FIELD STRATEGY 15.1   MANAGEMENT OF DIABETIC EMERGENCIES

Look for a medical alert tag.

In a conscious person:

1. Administer 10 to 15 g of a fast-acting carbohydrate:
   • 4 oz of regular cola or 6 oz of ginger ale
   • 4 oz of apple or orange juice
   • 4 packets of table sugar
   • 2 tablespoons of raisins
   • 5 to 7 pieces of sugared candy

2. After initial recovery, wait 15 minutes and check the blood sugar level. If improvement is seen but the blood glucose level is still below 70 mg/dL or if symptoms still exist:
   • Ingest another 10 to 15 g of carbohydrates
   • Repeat blood testing the treatment until the blood glucose level is normalized

3. If the individual does not show improvement after the initial ingestion of carbohydrates, activate EMS.

In an unconscious person:

1. Activate EMS.

2. Roll the individual on his or her side so the saliva drains out of the mouth.

3. Maintain an open airway.

4. Place sugar or a fast-acting carbohydrate under the tongue.

5. Do not give liquids.

6. Transport to the nearest hospital.

---

cises, and other non–weight-bearing exercises. Sports that require resistance strength training are permissible as long as there are no indications of **retinopathy** (noninflammatory degenerative disease of the retina) or nephropathy. Scuba diving, rock climbing, and parachuting are strongly discouraged.

➤➤ BOX 15-2

Guidelines for Safe Exercise

• Have a routine medical examination and be cleared for activity
• Develop a balanced program of diet and exercise under a physician's supervision
• Wear an identification bracelet or necklace indicating that you are diabetic
• Eat at regular times throughout the day
• Avoid exercising at the peak of insulin action and in the evening when hypoglycemia is more apt to occur
• Adjust carbohydrate intake and insulin dosage prior to exercise
• Check blood glucose levels before, during (if possible), and after exercise
• Prevent dehydration by consuming adequate fluids before, during, and after exercise
• Have access to fast-acting carbohydrates during exercise to prevent hypoglycemia
• Avoid alcoholic beverages, or drink them in moderation
• Avoid smoking

Summary

1. Insulin is needed after carbohydrate ingestion to transfer glucose from the blood into the skeletal and cardiac muscles. It also promotes glucose storage in the muscles and liver in the form of glycogen. If little or no insulin is secreted by the pancreas, blood glucose bypasses the body cells and rises to abnormally high levels in the blood. The excess glucose is excreted in the urine, drawing large amounts of water and electrolytes with it, leading to weakness, fatigue, malaise, and increased thirst.

2. When glucose cannot enter the cells, the cells shift from carbohydrate metabolism to fat metabolism for energy. This results in dehydration and ketoacidosis, which can depress cerebral function. Acetone, a byproduct of fat metabolism, is volatile and blown off during expiration, giving the breath a sweet or fruity odor.

3. There are four types of DM. The two most common are types 1 and 2. Type 1 (insulin-dependent) DM has an onset before age 30 years in people who are not typically obese. Type 2 (non–insulin-dependent) DM has an onset after age 40 years and is the most common form of diabetes. It is highly associated with a family history of diabetes, older age, obesity, and lack of exercise.

4. Severe hypoglycemia can lead to insulin shock, which has a rapid onset. Symptoms are dizziness; headache; intense hunger; aggressive behavior; pale, cold and clammy skin; profuse perspiration, salivation, and drooling; and tingling in the face, tongue, and lips.

5. An individual will progress into a diabetic coma (hyperglycemia) over a long period. Common symptoms include a dry mouth, intense thirst, abdominal pain, confusion, and fever. Severe signs include deep respirations; rapid, weak pulse; dry, red, warm skin; and sweet, fruity, acetone breath.

6. Because it may be difficult to determine which condition is present, give a fast-acting carbohydrate to the individual. If the individual is in insulin shock, recovery is usually rapid. If recovery does not occur, activate EMS and transport the individual immediately to the nearest medical facility.

7. Aerobic, low-resistance exercise is recommended for the diabetic athlete. The program should be established under the guidance of a supervising physician.

References

1. Whitney EN, and Rolfes SR. *Understanding nutrition.* Belmont, CA: Wadsworth Publishing, 1999.
2. Mayfield M. 1998. Diagnosis and classification of diabetes mellitus: New criteria. Am Fam Phys, 58(6):1355-1363.
3. National Institutes of Health. *Diabetes in America.* Washington, DC: National Institute of Diabetes and Digestive and Kidney Diseases, 1995.
4. Jimenez CC. 1997. Diabetes and exercise: The role of the athletic trainer. J Ath Train, 32(4):339-343.
5. Seitzman A, and Anderson C. 1998. Lower your risk for lows. Diabetes Forecast, 51(6):60-65.

Acute injury Injury with rapid onset caused by traumatic episode, but with short duration.

Adhesions Tissues that bind the healing tissue to adjacent structures, such as other ligaments or bone.

Alveoli Air sacs at the terminal ends of the bronchial tree where oxygen and carbon dioxide are exchanged between the lungs and surrounding capillaries.

Amenorrhea Absence or abnormal cessation of menstruation.

Analgesic Agent that produces analgesia.

Anaphylaxis An immediate, shocklike, frequently fatal, hypersensitive reaction that occurs within minutes of administration of an allergen unless appropriate first-aid measures are taken immediately.

Anatomic position Used as a universal reference to determine anatomic direction; the body is erect, facing forward, with the arms at the side of the body, palms facing forward.

Anatomic snuffbox Site directly over the scaphoid bone in the wrist; pain here indicates a possible fracture.

Antacid Agent that neutralizes stomach acid.

Anterograde amnesia Loss of memory of events after a head injury.

Apnea Temporary cessation of breathing.

Aponeurosis A flat, expanded, tendonlike sheath that attaches a muscle to another structure.

Apophysis An outgrowth or projection on the side of a bone; usually where a tendon attaches.

Apophysitis Inflammation of an apophysis.

Appendicitis Inflammation of the appendix.

Arrhythmia Disturbance in the heart beat rhythm.

Aseptic necrosis Death or decay of tissue caused by a poor blood supply in the area.

Asthma Disease of the lungs characterized by constriction of the bronchial muscles, increased bronchial secretions, and mucosal swelling, all leading to airway narrowing and inadequate airflow during respiration.

Atherosclerosis Condition whereby irregularly distributed lipid deposits are found in the large and medium-sized arteries.

Atrophy A wasting away or deterioration of tissue because of disease, disuse, or malnutrition.

Axial force Loading directed along the long axis of a body.

Axonotmesis Damage to the axons of a nerve followed by complete degeneration of the peripheral segment, without severance of the supporting structure of the nerve.

Ballistic stretch Increasing flexibility by using repetitive bouncing motions at the end of the available range of motion.

Bankart lesion Avulsion or damage to the anterior lip of the glenoid as the humerus slides forward in an anterior dislocation.

Battery Unpermitted or intentional contact with another individual without his or her consent.

Battle's sign Delayed discoloration behind the ear caused by basilar skull fracture.

Bending Loading that produces tension on one side of an object and compression on the other side.

Bennett's fracture Fracture-dislocation to the proximal end of the first metacarpal at the carpal-metacarpal joint.

Bimalleolar fracture Fractures of both medial and lateral malleolus.

Blowout fracture Fracture of the floor of the eye orbit, without fracture to the rim; produced by a blow on the globe with the force being transmitted via the globe to the orbital floor.

Brachial plexus A complex web of spinal nerves (C5-T1) that innervate the upper extremity.

Bradykinin Normally present in blood; a potent vasodilator. Increases blood vessel wall permeability and stimulates nerve endings to cause pain.

Bronchitis Inflammation of the mucosal lining of the tracheobronchial tree characterized by bronchial swelling, mucus secretions, and dysfunction of the cilia.

Bronchospasm Contraction of the smooth muscles of the bronchial tubes causing narrowing of the airway.

Burner Burning or stinging sensation characteristic of a brachial plexus injury.

Bursa A fibrous sac membrane containing synovial fluid typically found between tendons and bones; acts to decrease friction during motion.

Bursitis Inflammation of a bursa.

Callus Localized thickening of skin epidermis caused by physical trauma, or fibrous tissue containing immature bone tissue that forms at fracture sites during repair and regeneration.

Cardiac asystole Cardiac standstill.

Carpal tunnel syndrome Compression of the median nerve as it passes through the carpal tunnel, leading to pain and tingling in the hand.

Cauda equina Lower spinal nerves that course through the lumbar spinal canal; resembles a horse's tail.

Cauliflower ear Hematoma that forms between the perichondrium and cartilage of the auricle (ear) caused by repeated blunt trauma.

Chondral fracture Fracture involving the articular cartilage at a joint.

Chondromalacia patellae Degenerative condition in the articular cartilage of the patella caused by abnormal compression or shearing forces.

Chronic injury An injury with long onset and long duration.

Circumduction Movement of a body part in a circular direction.

Clonic Movement marked by repetitive muscle contractions and relaxation in rapid succession.

Cold diuresis Excretion of urine in cold weather; caused by blood being shunted away from the skin to the core to maintain vascular volume.

Collateral ligaments Major ligaments that cross the medial and lateral aspects of a hinge joint to provide stability from valgus and varus forces.

Colles fracture Fracture involving a dorsally angulated and displaced/radially angulated and displaced fracture within 1½ inches of the wrist.

Commission Committing an act that is not legally your duty to perform.

Comparative negligence The relative degree of negligence on the part of the plaintiff and defendant, with damages awarded on a basis proportionate to each person's carelessness.

Compartment syndrome Condition in which increased intramuscular pressure brought on by activity impedes blood flow and function of tissues within that compartment.

Compression A pressure or squeezing force directed through a body that increases density.

Concussion Violent shaking or jarring action of the brain resulting in immediate or transient impairment of neurologic function.

Conjunctivitis Bacterial infection leading to itching, burning, watering, and inflamed eye; pinkeye.

Constipation Infrequent or incomplete bowel movements.

Contraindication A condition adversely affected if a particular action is taken.

Contrecoup injuries Injuries away from the actual injury site because of rotational components during acceleration.

Contusion Compression injury involving accumulation of blood and lymph within a muscle; a bruise.

Coup injuries Injuries at the site where direct impact occurs.

Cramp Painful involuntary muscle contraction, either clonic or tonic.

Crepitus Crackling sound or sensation characteristic of a fracture when the bones ends are moved.

Cruciate ligaments Major ligaments that crisscross the knee in the anteroposterior direction, providing stability in that plane.

Cryotherapy Cold application.

Curvatures A bending, as in the spine (kyphosis, scoliosis, lordosis).

Cyanosis A dark bluish or purple skin color caused by deficient oxygen in the blood.

Cyclist's palsy Paresthesia in the ulnar nerve distribution; seen when bikers lean on the handlebar for an extended period.

Dead arm syndrome Common sensation felt with a recurrent anterior shoulder subluxation and multidirectional instability.

de Quervain's tenosynovitis An inflammatory stenosing tenosynovitis of the abductor pollicis longus and extensor pollicis brevis tendons.

Detached retina Neurosensory retina separated from the retinal epithelium by swelling.

Diabetes mellitus Metabolic disorder characterized by near or absolute lack of the hormone insulin, insulin resistance, or both.

Diabetic ketoacidosis Condition in which an excess of ketoacids in the blood can lower the blood pH to 7.0; manifested by ketones in the breath, blood, and urine.

Diarrhea Loose or watery stools.

Diffuse injuries Injury over a large body area, usually caused by low velocity–high mass forces.

Diplopia Double vision.

Diuretics Chemicals that promote the excretion of urine.

Dural sinuses Formed by tubular separations in the inner and outer layers of the dura mater, these sinuses function as small veins for the brain.

Duty of care Standard of care measured by what is learned, or should have been learned, in the professional preparation of an individual charged with providing health care.

Dyspepsia Gastric indigestion.

Dyspnea Labored or difficult breathing.

Ecchymosis Superficial tissue discoloration.

Edema Swelling resulting from a collection of exuded lymph fluid in interstitial tissues.

Elasticity The ability of a muscle to return to normal length after either lengthening or shortening.

Emesis Vomiting.

Epicondylitis Inflammation and microrupturing of the soft tissues on the epicondyles of the distal humerus.

Epidermis The outer epithelial portion of the skin.

Epiphyseal fracture Injury to the growth plate of a long bone in children and adolescents; may lead to arrested bone growth.

Epistaxis Profuse bleeding from the nose; nosebleed.

Erb's point Located 2 to 3 cm above the clavicle at the level of the transverse process of the C6 vertebra; compression over the site may injure the brachial plexus.

Excitability A muscle's ability to respond to a stimulus; irritability.

Expressed warranty Written guarantee that states the product is safe for consumer use.

Extensibility The ability of a muscle to be stretched or to increase in length.

Extensor mechanism Complex interaction of muscles, ligaments, and tendons that stabilize and provide motion at the patellofemoral joint.

Extrinsic Origination outside of the part where something is found or upon which it acts; denoting especially a muscle.

Extruded tooth Tooth driven in an outwardly direction.

Extruded disc Condition in which the nuclear material bulges into the spinal canal and runs the risk of impinging adjacent nerve roots.

Exudate Material composed of fluid, pus, or cells that has escaped from blood vessels into surrounding tissues after injury or inflammation.

Facet joint Joint formed when the superior and inferior articular processes mate with the articular process of adjacent vertebrae.

Fasciitis Inflammation of the fascia surrounding portions of a muscle.

Fibroblast A cell present in connective tissue capable of forming collagen fibers.

Flatulence Presence of an excessive amount of gas in the stomach and intestines.

Flexibility Total range of motion at a joint dependent on normal joint mechanics, mobility of soft tissues, and muscle extensibility.

Focal injuries Injury in a small concentrated area, usually caused by high velocity–low mass forces.

Foreseeability of harm Condition whereby danger is apparent, or should have been apparent, resulting in an unreasonably unsafe condition.

Fracture Disruption in the continuity of a bone.

Frontal plane A longitudinal (vertical) line that divides the body or any of its parts into anterior and posterior portions.

Gamekeeper's thumb Sprain of the metacarpophalangeal (MCP) joint of the thumb; the thumb is in near extension and is forcefully abducted away from the hand, tearing the ulnar collateral ligament at the MCP joint.

Ganglion cyst Benign tumor mass commonly seen on the dorsal aspect of the wrist.

Gastritis Inflammation, especially mucosal, of the stomach.

Gastrocolic reflex Propulsive reflex in the colon that stimulates defecation.

Gastroenteritis Inflammation of the mucous membrane of the stomach or small intestine.

Glenoid labrum Soft tissue lip around the periphery of the glenoid fossa that widens and deepens the socket to add stability to the joint.

Hallux The first, or great, toe.

Heat cramps Painful involuntary muscle spasms caused by excessive water and electrolyte loss.

Hemarthrosis Collection of blood within a joint or cavity.

Hematoma A localized mass of blood and lymph confined within a space or tissue.

Hematuria Blood or red blood cells in the urine.

Hemothorax Condition involving the loss of blood into the pleural cavity but outside the lung.

Heparin An anticoagulant that is a component of various tissues and mast cells.

Hernia Protrusion of abdominal viscera through a weakened portion of the abdominal wall.

Hip pointer Contusions caused by direct compression to an unprotected iliac crest that crushes soft tissue and sometimes the bone itself.

Histamine A powerful stimulant of gastric secretion, a constrictor of bronchial smooth muscle, and a vasodilator (capillaries and arterioles) that causes a fall in blood pressure.

Homeostasis The state of a balanced equilibrium in the body's various tissues and systems.

Hyperglycemia Abnormally high levels of glucose in the circulating blood that can lead to diabetic coma.

Hyperhydration Overhydration; excess water consumption of the body.

Hyperthermia Elevated body temperature.

Hypertrophic cardiomyopathy Excessive hypertrophy of the heart, often of obscure or unknown origin.

Hypertrophy General increase in bulk or size of an individual tissue not caused by tumor formation.

Hyphema Hemorrhage into the anterior chamber of the eye.

Hypoglycemia Abnormally low levels of glucose in the circulating blood that can lead to insulin shock.

Hypothalamus A region of the diencephalon that forms the floor of the third ventricle of the brain; responsible for thermoregulation and other autonomic nervous mechanisms underlying moods and motivational states.

Hypothenar The fleshy mass of muscle and tissue on the medial side of the palm.

Hypothermia Decreased body temperature.

Hypovolemic shock Shock caused by a reduction in volume of blood, as from hemorrhage or dehydration.

Hypoxia A reduced concentration of oxygen in air, blood, or tissue, short of anoxia.

Idiopathic Of unknown origin or cause.

Impingement syndrome Chronic condition caused by repetitive overhead activity that damages the supraspinatus tendon, glenoid labrum, long head of the biceps brachii, and subacromial bursa.

Implied warranty Unwritten guarantee that the product is reasonably safe when used for its intended purpose.

Indication A condition that could benefit from a specific action.

Infectious mononucleosis An acute illness associated with the Epstein-Barr herpetovirus; characterized by fever, sore throat, enlargement of lymph nodes and spleen, and leukopenia that changes to lymphocytosis.

Inflammation Pain, swelling, redness, heat, and loss of function that accompany musculoskeletal injuries.

Influenza Acute infectious respiratory tract condition characterized by malaise, headache, dry cough, and general muscle aches.

Informed consent Consent given by a person of legal age who understands the nature and extent of any treatment and available alternative treatments before agreeing to receiving treatment.

Innominate Without a name; used to describe anatomic structures.

Intrinsic In anatomy, denoting those muscles of the limbs whose origin and insertion are both in the same limb.

Intruded tooth Tooth driven deep into the socket in an inwardly direction.

Ischemia Local anemia caused by decreased blood supply.

Ischemic necrosis Death of a tissue caused by decreased blood supply.

Jersey finger Rupture of the flexor digitorum profundus tendon from the distal phalanx caused by rapid extension of the finger while actively flexed.

Jones fracture A transverse stress fracture of the proximal shaft of the fifth metatarsal.

Kehr's sign Referred pain down the left shoulder indicative of a ruptured spleen.

Ketoacidosis Condition caused by excess accumulation of acid or loss of base in the body; characteristic of diabetes mellitus.

Ketonuria Enhanced urinary excretion of ketone bodies.

Kyphosis Excessive curve in the thoracic region of the spine.

Legg-Calvé-Perthes disease Avascular necrosis of the proximal femoral epiphysis seen especially in young males ages 3 to 8 years.

Little leaguer elbow Tension stress injury of the medial epicondyle commonly seen in adolescents.

Little league shoulder Fracture of the proximal humeral growth plate in adolescents caused by repetitive rotational stresses during pitching.

Lordosis Excessive convex curve in the lumbar region of the spine.

Lumbar plexus Interconnected roots of the first four lumbar spinal nerves.

Malaise Lethargic feeling of general discomfort; out-of-sorts feeling.

Mallet finger Rupture of the extensor tendon from the distal phalanx caused by forceful flexion of the phalanx.

Malocclusion Inability to bring the teeth together in a normal bite.

Marfan syndrome Inherited connective tissue disorder affecting many organs, but commonly resulting in the dilation and weakening of the thoracic aorta.

Mast cells Connective tissue cells that carry heparin, which prolongs clotting, and histamine.

McBurney's point A site one-third the distance between the anterior superior iliac spine and umbilicus that, with deep palpation, produces rebound tenderness indicating appendicitis.

Meninges Three protective membranes that surround the brain and spinal cord.

Meningitis Inflammation of the meninges of the brain and spinal column.

Menisci Fibrocartilaginous discs found within a joint that reduce joint stress.

Mitral valve prolapse A condition in which redundant tissue is found on one or both leaflets of the mitral valve. During a ventricular contraction, a portion of the redundant tissue on the mitral valve pushes back beyond the normal limit and, as a result, produces an abnormal sound followed by a systolic murmur as blood is regurgitated back through the mitral valve into the left atrium; often called a click-murmur syndrome.

Muscle cramp A painful, involuntary contraction that is either clonic (alternating contraction and relaxation) or tonic (continued contraction over time).

Muscle spasm A short, involuntary contraction caused by reflex action biochemically derived or initiated by a mechanical blow to a nerve or muscle.

Myocardial infarction Heart attack.

Myositis Inflammation of connective tissue within a muscle.

Myositis ossificans Accumulation of mineral deposits within muscle tissue.

Nephropathy Any disease of the kidney.

Neurapraxia Injury to a nerve that results in temporary neurologic deficits followed by complete recovery of function.

Neurotmesis Complete severance of a nerve.

Nonunion fracture Failure of normal healing of a fractured bone.

Nystagmus Abnormal jerking or involuntary eye movement.

Oligomenorrhea Infrequent menstrual cycles or menstruation that involves scant blood flow.

Omission Failing to perform a legal duty of care.

Osgood-Schlatter disease Inflammation or partial avulsion of the tibial apophysis due to traction forces.

Osteitis pubis Stress fracture to the pubic symphysis caused by repeated overload of the adductor muscles or repetitive stress activities.

Osteochondral fracture Fracture involving the articular cartilage and underlying bone.

Osteochondritis dissecans Localized area of avascular necrosis that results in complete or incomplete separation of joint cartilage and subchondral bone.

Osteochondrosis Any condition characterized by degeneration or aseptic necrosis of the articular cartilage because of limited blood supply.

Osteopenia Condition of reduced bone mineral density that predisposes the individual to fractures.

Otitis externa Bacterial infection involving the lining of the auditory canal; swimmer's ear.

Otitis media Localized infection in the middle ear secondary to upper respiratory infections.

Paresthesia Abnormal sensations, such as tingling, burning, itching, or prickling.

Paronychia A fungal or bacterial infection in the folds of skin surrounding a fingernail or toenail.

Patellofemoral joint Gliding joint between the patella and patellar groove of the femur.

Patellofemoral stress syndrome Condition whereby the lateral retinaculum is tight, or the vastus medialis oblique is weak, leading to lateral excursion and pressure on the lateral facet of the patella; causes a painful condition.

Pericardial tamponade Compression of venous return to the heart caused by increased volume of fluid in the pericardium; usually caused by direct trauma to the chest.

Periorbital ecchymosis Swelling and hemorrhage into the surrounding eyelids; black eye.

Periostitis Inflammation of the periosteum (outer membrane covering the bone).

Peritonitis Irritation of the peritoneum that lines the abdominal cavity.

Pes cavus High arch.

Pes planus Flat feet.

Phagocytosis Process by which white blood cells surround and digest foreign particles, such as bacteria and necrotic tissue.

Pharyngitis Viral, bacterial, or fungal infection of the pharynx that causes a sore throat.

Phonophoresis The introduction of anti-inflammatory drugs through the skin with the use of ultrasound.

Photophobia Abnormal sensitivity to light.

Plantar fascia Specialized band of fascia that covers the plantar surface of the foot and helps support the longitudinal arch.

Pneumothorax Condition whereby air is trapped in the pleural space, causing a portion of a lung to collapse.

Polyuria Excessive excretion of urine that causes a huge urine output of water and electrolytes and leads to decreased blood volume and further dehydration.

Postconcussion syndrome Delayed condition characterized by persistent headaches, blurred vision, irritability, and inability to concentrate.

Prolapsed disc Condition in which the eccentric nucleus produces a definite deformity as it works its way through the fibers of the annulus fibrosus.

Pronation Inward rotation of the forearm; palms face posteriorly. At the foot, combined motions of calcaneal eversion, foot abduction, and dorsiflexion.

Prostaglandins Active substances found in many tissues, with effects such as vasodilation, vasoconstriction, and stimulation of intestinal or bronchial smooth muscle.

Purulent Containing, consisting of, or forming pus.

Q-angle Angle between the line of quadriceps force and the patellar tendon.

Raccoon eyes Delayed discoloration around the eyes from anterior cranial fossa fracture.

Reflex Action involving stimulation of a motor neuron by a sensory neuron in the spinal cord without involvement of the brain.

Retinopathy Noninflammatory degenerative disease of the retina.

Retrograde amnesia Forgetting events before an injury.

Rhinitis Inflammation of the nasal membranes with excessive mucus production resulting in nasal congestion and postnasal drip.

Rhinorrhea Clear nasal discharge.

Rotator cuff The SITS muscles (supraspinatus, infraspinatus, teres minor, and subscapularis) hold the head of the humerus in the glenoid fossa and produce humeral rotation.

Sacral plexus Interconnected roots of the L4-S4 spinal nerves that innervate the lower extremities.

Saddle joint A biaxial-like condyloid joint with both concave and convex areas, but with freer movement, like the carpometacarpal joints of the thumbs.

Sagittal plane A longitudinal (vertical) line that divides the body or any of it parts into right and left portions.

Sciatica Compression of a spinal nerve caused by a herniated disc, annular tear, myogenic or muscle-related disease, spinal stenosis, facet joint arthropathy, or compression from the piriformis muscle.

Scoliosis Lateral rotational spinal curvature.

Screwing-home mechanism Rotation of the tibia on the femur at the end of extension to produce a "locking" of the knee in a closed packed position.

Shear force A force directed parallel to a surface.

Shock Collapse of the cardiovascular system when insufficient blood cannot provide circulation for the entire body.

Sign Objective measurable physical findings that you can hear, feel, see, or smell during the assessment.

Sinusitis Inflammation of the paranasal sinuses.

Smith's fracture Volar displacement of the distal fragment of the radius; sometimes called a reversed Colles fracture.

Snapping hip syndrome A snapping sensation either heard or felt during motion at the hip.

Solar plexus punch A blow to the abdomen with the muscles relaxed resulting in an immediate inability to catch one's breath.

Spondylolisthesis Anterior slippage of a vertebra resulting from complete bilateral fracture of the pars interarticularis.

Spondylolysis A stress fracture of the pars interarticularis.

Sports medicine Area of health and special services that applies medical and scientific knowledge to prevent, recognize, manage, and rehabilitate injuries related to sport, exercise, or recreational activity.

Sprain Injury to ligamentous tissue.

Standard of care What another minimally competent professional educated and practicing in the same profession would have done in the same or similar circumstance to protect an individual from harm.

Stenosing Narrowing of an opening or stricture of a canal; stenosis.

Stitch in the side A sharp pain or spasm in the chest wall, usually on the lower right side, during exertion.

Strain Amount of deformation with respect to the original dimensions of the structure; injury to the musculotendinous unit.

Stress The distribution of force within a body; quantified as force divided by the area over which the force acts.

Stress fracture Fracture resulting from repeated loading with relatively low magnitude forces.

Subconjunctival hemorrhage Minor capillary ruptures in the eye globe.

Subungual hematoma Hematoma beneath a fingernail or toenail.

Sudden death A nontraumatic, unexpected death that occurs instantaneously or within a few minutes of an abrupt change in an individual's previous clinical state.

Supination Outward rotation of the forearm; palms facing forward. At the foot, combined motions of calcaneal inversion, foot adduction, and plantar flexion.

Symptom Subjective information provided by an individual regarding his or her perception of the problem.

Syncope Fainting or lightheadedness.

Tachycardia Rapid beating of the heart, usually applied to rates over 100 beats per minute.

Tendinitis Inflammation of a tendon.

Tenosynovitis Inflammation of a tendon sheath.

Tensile force A pulling or stretching force directed axially through a body or body part.

Tension pneumothorax Condition in which air continuously leaks into the pleural space, causing the mediastinum to displace to the opposite side and compressing the uninjured lung and thoracic aorta.

Thenar The fleshy mass of muscle and tissue on the lateral palm; the ball of the thumb.

Thermoregulation The process by which the body maintains body temperature; primarily controlled by the hypothalamus.

Thermotherapy Heat application.

Thoracic outlet syndrome Condition whereby nerves or vessels become compressed in the root of the neck or axilla, leading to numbness in the arm.

Tibiofemoral joint Dual condyloid joints between the tibial and femoral condyles that function primarily as a modified hinge joint.

Tinnitus Ringing or other noises in the ear caused by trauma or disease.

Torsion force Twisting around an object's longitudinal axis in response to an applied torque.

Tort A wrong done to an individual whereby the injured party seeks a remedy for damages suffered.

Transverse plane A horizontal line that divides the body into superior and inferior portions.

Triage Assessing all injured individuals to determine priority of care.

Unconsciousness Impairment of brain function wherein the individual lacks conscious awareness and is unable to respond to superficial .sensory stimuli.

Valgus An opening on the medial side of a joint caused by the distal segment moving laterally.

Valsalva maneuver Holding one's breath against a closed glottis, resulting in sharp increases in blood pressure.

Varus An opening on the lateral side of a joint caused by the distal segment moving medially.

Vasoconstriction Narrowing of the blood vessels; opposite of vasodilation.

Vasodilation Enlarging of the blood vessels; opposite of vasoconstriction.

Volkmann's contracture Ischemic necrosis of the forearm muscles and tissues caused by damage to the blood flow.

Wedge fracture A crushing compression fracture that leaves a vertebra narrowed anteriorly.

Yield point (elastic limit) The maximum load that a material can sustain without permanent deformation.

Zone of primary injury Region of injured tissue before vasodilation.

Zone of secondary injury Region of damaged tissue after vasodilation.

In this index, page numbers in *italics* designate figures; page numbers followed by the letter "t" designate boxes or tables; *see also* cross-references designate related topics or more detailed topic breakdowns.